LEG ULCERS
DIAGNOSIS AND MANAGEMENT

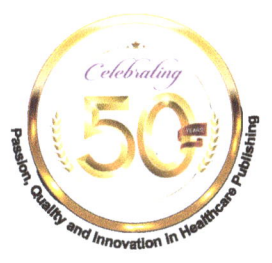

LEG ULCERS
DIAGNOSIS AND MANAGEMENT

Editors

S Sacchidanand
MBBS MD DVD DHA FRCP(GI)

Vice Chancellor
Rajiv Gandhi University of Health Sciences
Bengaluru, Karnataka, India

Eswari L
MBBS MD DVL FRGUHS (Dermatosurgery) FAADV (Dermatopathology)

Associate Professor
Department of Dermatology
Bangalore Medical College and Research Institute
Bengaluru, Karnataka, India

Shilpa K
MBBS MD DVL FRGUHS (Dermatosurgery)

Associate Professor
Department of Dermatology
Bangalore Medical College and Research Institute
Bengaluru, Karnataka, India

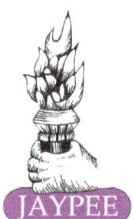

JAYPEE BROTHERS MEDICAL PUBLISHERS
The Health Sciences Publisher
New Delhi | London | Panama

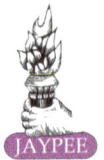

Jaypee Brothers Medical Publishers (P) Ltd

Headquarters
Jaypee Brothers Medical Publishers (P) Ltd
4838/24, Ansari Road, Daryaganj
New Delhi 110 002, India
Phone: +91-11-43574357
Fax: +91-11-43574314
Email: jaypee@jaypeebrothers.com

Overseas Offices
J.P. Medical Ltd
83 Victoria Street, London
SW1H 0HW (UK)
Phone: +44 20 3170 8910
Fax: +44 (0)20 3008 6180
Email: info@jpmedpub.com

Jaypee-Highlights Medical Publishers Inc
City of Knowledge, Bld. 235, 2nd Floor
Clayton, Panama City, Panama
Phone: +1 507-301-0496
Fax: +1 507-301-0499
Email: cservice@jphmedical.com

Jaypee Brothers Medical Publishers (P) Ltd
Bhotahity, Kathmandu, Nepal
Phone: +977-9741283608
Email: kathmandu@jaypeebrothers.com

Website: www.jaypeebrothers.com
Website: www.jaypeedigital.com

© 2019, Jaypee Brothers Medical Publishers

The views and opinions expressed in this book are solely those of the original contributor(s)/author(s) and do not necessarily represent those of editor(s) of the book.

All rights reserved. No part of this publication may be reproduced, stored or transmitted in any form or by any means, electronic, mechanical, photocopying, recording or otherwise, without the prior permission in writing of the publishers.

All brand names and product names used in this book are trade names, service marks, trademarks or registered trademarks of their respective owners. The publisher is not associated with any product or vendor mentioned in this book.

Medical knowledge and practice change constantly. This book is designed to provide accurate, authoritative information about the subject matter in question. However, readers are advised to check the most current information available on procedures included and check information from the manufacturer of each product to be administered, to verify the recommended dose, formula, method and duration of administration, adverse effects and contraindications. It is the responsibility of the practitioner to take all appropriate safety precautions. Neither the publisher nor the author(s)/editor(s) assume any liability for any injury and/or damage to persons or property arising from or related to use of material in this book.

This book is sold on the understanding that the publisher is not engaged in providing professional medical services. If such advice or services are required, the services of a competent medical professional should be sought.

Every effort has been made where necessary to contact holders of copyright to obtain permission to reproduce copyright material. If any have been inadvertently overlooked, the publisher will be pleased to make the necessary arrangements at the first opportunity. The **CD/DVD-ROM** (if any) provided in the sealed envelope with this book is complimentary and free of cost. **Not meant for sale.**

Inquiries for bulk sales may be solicited at: jaypee@jaypeebrothers.com

Leg Ulcers: Diagnosis and Management

First Edition: **2019**

ISBN 978-93-5270-939-7

Contributors

Amina Asfiya MI MD
Senior Resident
Department of Dermatology
Yenepoya Medical College
Mangaluru, Karnataka, India

Amrita Hongal MBBS MD DNB
Senior Resident
Department of Dermatology
Bangalore Medical College and Research Institute
Bengaluru, Karnataka, India

Aniketh Venkataram MBBS MS MCH
Consultant Plastic Surgeon
The Venkat Center for Skin and Plastic Surgery
Bengaluru, Karnataka, India

Anju George MD DNB FRGUHS
Senior Resident
Department of Dermatology
Christian Medical College
Vellore, Tamil Nadu, India

Aseem Sharma MD DNB MBA
Assistant Professor (Dermatology)
Lokmanya Tilak Municipal Medical College and General Hospital
Mumbai, Maharashtra, India

Biju Vasudevan MD DVL FRGUHS (Dermatosurgery)
Professor
Department of Dermatology
Base Hospital Lucknow
Lucknow, Uttar Pradesh, India

Brijesh Nair MD
Consultant Dermatologist
Military Hospital
Jaipur, Rajasthan, India

Deepak HS MBBS DDVl FRGUHS
Consultant Dermatologist
SD Dermatz Skin Clinic
Bengaluru, Karnataka, India

Divya Gorur MBBS MD DVL FRGUHS
Consultant Dermatologist
Oliva Skin and Hair Clinic
Chennai, Tamil Nadu, India

Eswari L MBBS MD DVL FRGUHS (Dermatosurgery) FAADV (Dermatopathology)
Associate Professor
Department of Dermatology
Bangalore Medical College and Research Institute
Bengaluru, Karnataka, India

Gayatri Gupta MD (Dermatology)
Assistant Professor
Department of Dermatology
Base Hospital Lucknow
Lucknow, Uttar Pradesh, India

Heera Ramesh MBBS
Junior Resident Dermatology
Bangalore Medical College and Research Institute
Bengaluru, Karnataka, India

Kavya Thimmaiah MBBS
Junior Resident
Department of Dermatology
Bangalore Medical College and Research Institute
Bengaluru, Karnataka, India

Madhulika Mhatre MD FRGUHS (Aesthetic Dermatology) FIADVL (Trichology)
Consultant Dermatologist
Wockhardt Hospitals
Mulekar Clinic
Mumbai, Maharashtra, India

Manjunath Shenoy MD DNB
Professor and Head
Department of Dermatology
Yenepoya Medical College
Mangaluru, Karnataka, India

Nagesh TS MD DNB
Professor
Department of Dermatology
Sapthagiri Institute of Medical Sciences and Research Center
Bengaluru, Karnataka, India

Reena Rai MD
Professor
Department of Dermatology
PSG Institute of Medical Science and Research
Coimbatore, Tamil Nadu, India

S Sacchidanand MBBS MD DVD DHA FRCP(GI)
Vice Chancellor
Rajiv Gandhi University of Health Sciences
Bengaluru, Karnataka, India

Sachin S MBBS
Junior Resident
Department of Dermatology
Bangalore Medical College and Research Institute
Bengaluru, Karnataka, India

Savitha AS MD DNB FRGUHS (Dermstosurgery)
Associate Professor
Department of Dermatology
Sapthagiri Institute of Medical Sciences and Research Center
Bengaluru, Karnataka, India

Shashi Kumar BM MD (DVL) FIADVL (Dermatopathology)
Associate Professor
Department of Dermatology
Mandya Institute of Medical Sciences
Mandya, Karnataka, India
Honorary Treasurer
Indian Association of Dermatologists, Venereologists and Leprologists (IADVL)
Vice President, IADVL Karnataka Branch

Shilpa K MBBS MD DVL FIADVL (Trichology)
Associate Professor
Department of Dermatology
Bangalore Medical College and Research Institute
Bengaluru, Karnataka, India

Shivakumar Patil MBBS MD DVL
Associate Professor
Department of Dermatology
Jawaharlal Nehru Medical College
Belgaum, Karnataka, India

Shwetha S MBBS MD DVL
Assistant Professor
Department of Dermatology
Sambhram Institute of Medical Science and Research
Bengaluru, Karnataka, India

Smitha Segu MCH (Plastic Surgery)
Professor
Department of Plastic Surgery
Bangalore Medical College and Research Institute
Bengaluru, Karnataka, India

Sneha M MD
Senior Resident
Department of Dermatology
Sapthagiri Institute of Medical Sciences and Research Center
Bengaluru, Karnataka, India

Sravan CPS DNB (Peripheral Vascular Surgery)
Resident
Jain Institute of Vascular Sciences (JIVAS)
A Unit of Bhagwan Mahaveer Jain Hospital (BMJH)
Bengaluru, Karnataka, India

Suhas S MCh (Plastic Surgery)
Assistant Professor
Department of Plastic Surgery
Bangalore Medical College and Research Institute
Bengaluru, Karnataka, India

Ujwal M MBBS
Junior Resident
Department of Dermatology
Bangalore Medical College and Research Institute
Bengaluru, Karnataka, India

Vaibhav Lende DNB (Peripheral Vascular Surgery)
Resident
Jain Institute of Vascular Sciences (JIVAS)
A Unit of Bhagwan Mahaveer Jain Hospital (BMJH)
Bengaluru, Karnataka, India

Vivekanand MBBS MS (General Surgery) FVES (Dusseldorf University)
Head of Department and Consultant Vascular Surgeon
Jain Institute of Vascular Sciences (JIVAS)
A Unit of Bhagwan Mahaveer Jain Hospital (BMJH)
Bengaluru, Karnataka, India

Yuvasri Gunasekaran MBBS
Junior Resident
Department of Dermatology
PSG Institute of Medical Science and Research
Coimbatore, Tamil Nadu, India

Preface

The management of leg ulcers was initially the domain of surgeons which later extended to vascular surgeons, plastic surgeons and of course the dermatologists. Many a times dermatologists are the first to encounter patients with venous ulcers, vasculitic ulcers, pyoderma gangrenosum and very importantly neuropathic ulcers due to diabetes and leprosy. Hence, leg ulcers are challenging which requires a liaison of multispecialty to efficiently manage and relieve the ailing patients who are burdened by the chronicity of the condition.

We felt that managing leg ulcers was the need of the hour and so undertook this task of writing a comprehensive book on Leg ulcers, involving expert dermatologists from across the country who are experienced in the field, and also experts from the fraternity of vascular surgery and plastic surgery. The chapters encompass the basic anatomy, physiology of leg ulcers, to pathology and investigations dedicated chapters to individual type of ulcers based on etiology and also the therapeutics and recent advances up-to-date.

This book has been designed to be of benefit to residents and consultants across specialties of dermatology, surgery, vascular surgery and plastic surgery. Hope we succeed in our endeavor which is aimed at relieving and helping the patients suffering from the ever burdening leg ulcers.

We thank all the authors who have taken immense interest and have devoted time contributing their knowledge and expertise to bring about this book.

S Sacchidanand
Eswari L
Shilpa K

Acknowledgments

We are immensely grateful to all the patients who have consented to use their photographs in our book, knowing that it serves the greater purpose of helping patients suffering from leg ulcers at large. We learn from them to become more efficient in managing their conditions.

We would like to thank Shri Jitendar P Vij (Group Chairman), Mr Ankit Vij (Managing Director), Ms Chetna Malhotra Vohra (Associate Director-Content Strategy), Ms Prerna Bajaj (Development Editor), and all the staff of M/s Jaypee Brothers Medical Publishers (P) Ltd, New Delhi, India, for their efforts and input enabling timely publication of the book.

Contents

1. Epidemiology and Socioeconomic Impact 1
Shashi Kumar BM, Savitha AS
- Epidemiology   1
- Etiology   1
- Social and Economic Impact   2
- Psychological Problems   3

2. Venous Anatomy of the Lower Extremity 5
Madhulika Mhatre, Aseem Sharma, Aniketh Venkataram
- Superficial Venous System   5
- Deep Venous System   9
- Perforating Veins   9
- Accompanying Nerves   10
- Applied Anatomy   10

3. Pathology of Leg Ulcers 13
Divya Gorur, Heera Ramesh
- Pathophysiology of Venous Leg Ulcer   13
- Pathophysiology of Arterial Ulcers   14
- Vasculitic Ulcers   15
- Neuropathic and Diabetic Foot Ulcer   15
- Ulcerating Skin Diseases   16
- Infectious Diseases   17
- Drugs   17
- Malignancy (Ulcerating Tumors)   17
- Hematological Disorders   17
- Clotting Disorders   17

4. Microbiology of Leg Ulcers 19
Amrita Hongal, Ujwal M
- Sample Collection and Analysis Methods   19
- Pathogenesis and the Flora   19

5. Wound Healing 23
Shivakumar Patil, Kavya Thimmaiah
- Hemostasis   23
- Inflammation   24
- Proliferation   24
- Remodeling of Connective Tissue   25
- Scarless Healing   26
- Chronic Wound   26

Factors Influencing Wound Healing 26
Healing of Skin Wounds 27
Wound Strength 27

6. History Taking and Examination in Chronic Leg Ulcers — 28
Shilpa K, S Sacchidanand
History Taking 28
Physical Examination 29

7. Venous Leg Ulcers — 37
Amina Asfiya, Manjunath Shenoy
Etiopathogenesis 37
Classification of Chronic Venous Insufficiency 38
Clinical Features 38
Venous Ulcer 39
Arterial Disease 39
Diagnostic Evaluation 40
Management 41
Venous Ulcer Recurrence 45
Criteria for Specialist Referral for Appropriate Management 45

8. Diabetic Foot Ulcers — 47
Vivekanand, Vaibhav Lende, Sravan CPS
Epidemiology 47
Pathophysiology 47
Biomechanics and Foot Pressures 50
Presentation and Diagnosis 50
Management 52
The Charcot Foot 56

9. Neuropathic Ulcers — 61
Savitha AS, S Sacchidanand
Causes of Neuropathic Ulcers 61
Etiopathogenesis 61
Stages of Ulcer Formation 62
Clinical Features 62
Approach to Patient with Neuropathic Ulcer 63
Management of Ulcer 63

10. Ischemic Ulcers, Pyoderma Gangrenosum and Vasculitic Ulcers — 68
Biju Vasudevan, Gayatri Gupta
Ischemic (Arterial) Ulcers 68
Risk Factors 68
Pathogenesis 69
Clinical Features 69
Management 73
Pyoderma Gangrenosum 80
Definition 80
Epidemiology 80
Etiology 80

Pathogenesis 80
Associations 80
Clinical Features 81
Differential Diagnosis 82
Diagnosis 82
Treatment 82
Prognosis 83
Vasculitic Ulcer 83
Introduction 83
Clinical Features and Management 84

11. Principles of Leg Ulcer Management — 87
Anju George

12. Investigations and Radiological Diagnosis of Leg Ulcers — 94
Shwetha S, Deepak HS
Investigations for Leg Ulcers due to Venous Insufficiency and Dependency 94
Investigations for Arterial Cause of Leg Ulcers 99
Investigations for Ulcer Secondary to Vasculitis 103
Neuropathic Ulcers 104
Hereditary Sensory Neuropathy Type 1C: Charcot–Marie–Tooth Disease 107
Laboratory Screening Tests for Clotting Disorders 108
Metabolic Causes of Leg Ulcers 108
Infectious Causes of Leg Ulcer 108
Hematological Causes of Leg Ulcers 108
Investigating Atypical Leg Ulcers 108

13. Topical Therapy for Leg Ulcers — 114
Nagesh TS, Sneha M
History and Physical Examination 114
Management of Leg Ulcer 114

14. Systemic Therapy of Leg Ulcers — 120
Brijesh Nair
Pentoxifylline 120
Aspirin 121
Zinc 121
Antibiotics/Antimicrobials 121
Systemic Steroids 122
Phlebotonics/Flavonoids 122
Fibrinolytic Enhancers 123
Prostaglandin and Prostacycline Analogues 123

15. Compression Therapy and Dressings — 126
Shilpa K, S Sacchidanand, Sachin S
Mechanism of Compression Stockings 126
Types of Compression Stockings 126
Grading the Strength of Compression Stockings 126
Assessment to be done Before Prescribing Compression Therapy 128
Dressings 129

16. Role of Skin Grafting in Managing Leg Ulcers — 136
Smitha Segu, Suhas S
Applied Anatomy of Skin   136
Stem Cells in Skin and Skin Regeneration   137
Common Ulcers and Role of Skin Grafts   138
Optimization of the Wound Bed   138
Negative Pressure Wound Therapy (Vacuum-Assisted Closure Therapy)   139
Hyperbaric Oxygen Therapy   139
Pre-Requisites of Wound Bed for Split Thickness Skin Graft   140
Contraindications for Skin Grafting   140
Skin Graft   140
Skin Graft Storage   145
Complications   145
Recent Advances in Skin Replacement   146

17. Role of Platelet Rich Plasma and Platelet Rich Fibrin in Managing Leg Ulcers — 148
Reena Rai, Yuvasri Gunasekaran
Role of Platelet-Derived Products   148
Platelet Rich Plasma   149
Platelet Rich Fibrin   151

18. Novel Research and Recent Advances in Managing Leg Ulcers — 155
Eswari L, S Sacchidanand
The Role of Stem Cells   155
Biopharmaceutical Agents   156
Endothelial Progenitor Cell Therapy   156
Novel Drug Delivery Systems   156
Biologically Active Skin Graft Substitutes/Tissue Engineered Skin Equivalents   159
Acellular Regenerative Tissue Scaffold   160
Human Amniotic Cellular/Tissue Based Products   161
Topical Therapy   161
Dressings   162
Balneotherapy   162
Oral Nutritional Supplements   162
Photodynamic Therapy   162
Negative Pressure Wound Therapy   163
Hyperbaric Oxygen Therapy   163
Electrical Stimulation   164
Pulsed Radiofrequency Electromagnetic Field   164
Surgical Therapy   164

Index — 169

CHAPTER 1

Epidemiology and Socioeconomic Impact

Shashi Kumar BM, Savitha AS

INTRODUCTION

Leg ulcers are a common problem causing great physical and mental distress to patients. Ulcers are defined as wounds with full thickness defect and slow healing tendency. Ulcers of skin can result in complete loss of the epidermis, often portions of the dermis and even subcutaneous fat.[1] A chronic wound, which is below the knee and does not show any tendency to heal even with appropriate therapy for 3 months or is still not fully healed at 12 months is chronic lower limb ulcer.[2] Chronic nonhealing leg ulcers occupy considerable space in surgical wards. Often these ghastly looking ulcers emit offensive smell posing difficulty in daily dressing for the surgeon. These ulcers involve a wide variety of spectrum of severity, etiology, and pathology with significant morbidity and mortality. Leg ulcers also significantly interfere with the lifestyle of the patient causing considerable loss of work hours and enormous healthcare costs.[3]

EPIDEMIOLOGY

The prevalence of chronic leg ulcers (CLUs) in the community ranges from 1.9% to 13.1% causing significant morbidity.[4] Almost, 10% of the population have the risk of developing a chronic wound in the course of a lifetime, with a wound-related mortality rate of 2.5%.[5] Wide geographical variations exist in both the etiology and prevalence of chronic wounds. Studies from India are limited. In a study by Shukla VK et al., the estimated the prevalence of chronic wounds was 4.5 per 1,000 population and incidence of acute wounds was more than double at 10.5 per 1,000 population.[6] In the UK and Switzerland, the estimated annual incidence of leg ulcers are 3.5 and 0.2 per 1,000 individuals, respectively. In the US, about 15% of the elderly population suffer from chronic wounds. The main causes of chronic ulcers in them are pressure ulcers (bedsores), venous stasis ulcers, and diabetic (neuropathic) foot ulcers. Every year, 2-3 million more Americans are diagnosed with various types of chronic wounds.[7,8]

Age

With the increase in the elderly population due to good healthcare, the incidence of ulceration is also rising. Atherosclerotic risk factors like obesity, diabetes, and smoking are high in the elderly. CLUs affect 0.6-3% of those aged over 60 years, increasing to over 5% of those aged over 80 years.[9] Strandness et al. observed the average age of patient with nondiabetic ulcer to be 63 years and Tassiopoulos et al. in their study of 1,249 limbs recorded the mean age of patients to be 59 years.[10,11] According to the study in Ireland, the overall prevalence was 0.12% but it was 1.03% in the patients aged 70 years and over.[12] Mukherjee et al. in their study of nondiabetic leg ulcers found predominantly patients in age group of 30-50 years.[3]

Sex

Sex incidence varies. The overall difference in incidence of leg ulcers between women and men probably reflects the greater number of women with longer lifespan, thereby increasing the overall rate for women.[13]

ETIOLOGY

The most common type of leg ulcer is venous ulcer, the others being neuropathic ulcer and arterial ulcers according to most of the Western and European studies.[9] Venous diseases accounted for majority of cases (81%) of ulcers followed by arterial disease (16.3%), while ulceration due to diabetic neuropathy and rheumatoid vasculitis was unusual in a study from Ireland.[12] Another study reported a 35.5% prevalence of varicose veins and 1.5% prevalence of severe chronic venous insufficiency with an ulcer or ulcer scar.[14] A study from Germany made the observation that venous insufficiency was the predominant causative factor in 47.6% and arterial insufficiency in 14.5% and 17.6% of ulcers were due to combined arterial and venous insufficiency.[15] A study from one center in India reported leprosy (40%), diabetes (23%), venous disease (11%), and trauma (13%) as causes of lower-extremity wounds. Other causes included atherosclerosis and tuberculosis. Inappropriate treatment of acute traumatic wounds was the foremost cause for wounds becoming chronic.[6] The etiology of chronic wounds in the hospital setting is different from that seen in the community. While hospital-based studies are easier to carry out, they do not reflect the true population-based statistics. In a community-based study from Northern India, the prevalence of chronic wounds was 4.48 per 1,000 population with lower-extremity involvement being much more common than the involvement of the upper extremity.[16] The most common etiology for chronic ulcers in the above study was untreated or improperly treated acute traumatic wound followed by diabetes. In contrast, most studies indicate that diabetic ulcers are the most common cause of lower-extremity ulceration in the hospital setting.[17] Table 1 lists the causes of leg ulcers.

Table 1: Causes of leg ulcers.

Acute	Trauma	Injury
		Burns
	Vascular	Vasculitis
		Arterial
	Infections	Bacterial
	Hematological	Sickle cell anemia
Chronic	Vascular	Venous
		Arterial
	Infections	Fungal
		Protozoal
		Leprosy
	Neuropathic	Diabetes
		Leprosy
		Syringomyelia
		Tabes dorsalis
	Tumors	Basal cell carcinoma
		Squamous cell carcinoma
	Others	Pyoderma gangrenosum
		Necrobiosis lipoidica

SOCIAL AND ECONOMIC IMPACT

Chronic leg ulcers impact virtually every aspect of daily life:
- Pain is common
- Sleep is often impaired
- Mobility and work capacity tend to be restricted
- Personal finances are often adversely affected
- Chronic leg ulcer is usually associated with significant morbidity, high cost of healthcare, loss of productivity, and reduced quality of life.[9]

Cost of Healthcare

Venous Ulcer

Venous diseases are consuming 1–2% of the healthcare budgets of European countries. In France too, the costs of venous disease represented 2.6% of the total healthcare budget in 1995, thus confirming other data from European studies and an early health survey in the United States.[18] Similarly in the United States, treatment costs for venous ulcers in more than 6 million patients approached $2.5 billion (£1.6 billion; €1.8 billion), and 2 million workdays were lost annually because of venous ulcer disease.[19] A recent prospective study performed in 23 specialized wound centers throughout Germany calculated the mean total cost of a venous ulcer per patient per year to be €9,569 [€8,658 (92%) direct costs and €911 (8%) indirect costs].[20]

Diabetic Ulcer

According to the Center for Disease Control and Prevention, in 2007, diabetes and its complications cost the exchequer $174 billion of which $116 billion were in direct costs and the rest $58 billion were indirect costs such as loss of productivity, disability, and early mortality. In a study in which patients with diabetic foot ulcers (DFUs) were prospectively followed up, it was shown that 54% patients healed in 2 months, 19% healed in 3–4 months, and 27% healed in more than 5 months. Healing without amputation costs an average of $6,664 against healing by amputation, which averaged $44,790.[19] Presence of vascular disease and neuropathy adds to the costs of treating DFUs. In India, the expenditure incurred in treating DFUs varied from ₹10,000 in patients in urban areas to ₹6,260 in patients in rural areas. Patients in urban areas spent a significantly higher amount on medications as well as for laboratory tests and consultations than patients in rural areas. The median costs of surgical treatment were also considerably higher in urban patients (₹21,000 vs ₹6,500). Expenditure increased with increased duration of diabetes as well as with the number of complications in both groups. In a recently published study, the cost of treating DFU in five different countries was estimated based on a hypothetical model. While the cost of treatment varied from the lowest in Tanzania to the highest in the United States for two different types of DFUs, the burden for the patient cannot be determined by the adjusted absolute cost but by the patients' responsibility for bearing the cost. The cost to the patient is a function of both insurance cover and annual per capita purchasing power parity (PPP) adjusted gross domestic product (GDP). The authors concluded that India is the most expensive country for treatment of DFU, where approximately 5.7 years of income are required to pay for treatment compared to only 3 months of income in Chile and in China.[21]

Risk of Amputation and Economic Loss

In the United States, nearly 71,000 lower-limb amputations were performed in people with diabetes in 2004 costing approximately 3 billion dollars per year. 67% of all lower-extremity amputations have diabetes. Every year, 5% of diabetics develop foot ulcers and 1% require amputation. Recurrence rate of DFUs is 66%, and the amputation rate rises to 12% with subsequent ulcerations. Amputation rates also rise with increasing age varying from 3.9 per 1,000 in diabetics who are less than 65 years of age to 7.9 per 1,000 in diabetics more than 75 years of age. The 5-year survival rate after a major lower-extremity amputation is about 50%. Once amputation occurs, 50% will develop an ulcer in the contralateral limb within 5 years. According to estimates, a staggering $9 billion were spent on the treatment of DFUs in 2001.[22]

Loss of Work

Loss of work may be either due to inability to carry out the work because of disability or forced abstainism from work for medical management. The loss of income results in huge economic burden on patient and family. Venous ulcers are responsible for a staggering $2 billion in lost wages. Accurate assessment, prompt treatment, and suitable follow-up are essential for minimizing the long-term disability caused by chronic wounds.[23]

PSYCHOLOGICAL PROBLEMS

Severe pain in ulcers can lead to irritation, depression, and reduced social activity. Bad odor can have adverse psychological effects like self-loathing and feelings of disgust. Limitations of routine activities due to pain and immobility increase the dependence on others, which hampers social life. Guarnera et al. reported that women with venous ulcers had more pain and worse quality of life than men. Visual analog scale showed a higher value during dressing change. There was direct correlation between pain and quality of life, being worse for ulcers with longer duration and larger area.[24] It has been documented that elderly had worse health-related quality-of-life issues as did those with pain and nonhealing ulcers. Pain, itching, altered appearance, loss of sleep, functional limitation, and disappointment with treatment were identified as the psychological effects of chronic ulceration.[25]

Health-related quality of life (HRQOL) is worse in diabetics with complications than in diabetics without complications. The reduced mobility and restriction of daily activities caused by foot ulcers adversely affect HRQOL. DFU patients suffer from huge negative psychological and social effect including reduction in social activities, increased family tensions for patients and their caregivers, limited employment, and financial hardship.[26]

Due to the above reasons, wound management should also include recommendations to improve quality of life in these patients.

CONCLUSION

Leg ulcers tend to be chronic and debilitating causing a huge impact on the personal, social, and economic life of patient. Venous leg ulcers are the most commonly reported ulcers to date, but with the increase in the incidence of diabetes, diabetic ulcers will be more prevalent in future.

REFERENCES

1. Van Gent WB, Wilschut ED, Wittens C. Management of venous ulcer disease. Br Med J. 2010;341(7782):1092-6.
2. Kahle B, Hermanns HJ, Gallenkemper G. Evidence based treatment of chronic leg ulcers. Dtsch Arztebl Int. 2011;108(14):231-7.
3. Mukherjee S, Raza MA, Bansal P, et al. A prospective, open label, clinical study for evaluation of management of chronic non-healing, non-diabetic leg ulcers in a tertiary care hospital. Int Surg J. 2015;2(4):560-5.
4. Rayner R, Carville K, Keaton J, et al. Leg ulcers: atypical presentations and associated comorbidities. Wound Pract Res. 2009;17(4):168-85.
5. Sasanka CS. Venous ulcers of the lower limb: where do we stand? Indian J Plast Surg. 2012;45(2):266-74.
6. Shukla VK, Ansari MA, Gupta SK. Wound healing research: a perspective from India. Int J Low Extrem Wounds. 2005;4(1):7-8.
7. Cheng CF, Sahu D, Tsen F, et al. A fragment of secreted Hsp90α carries properties that enable it to accelerate effectively both acute and diabetic wound healing in mice. J Clin Invest. 2011;121(11):4348-61.

8. Mekkes J, Loots MA, Van Der Wal AC, et al. Causes, investigation and treatment of leg ulceration. Br J Dermatol. 2003;148(3):388-401.
9. Agale SV. Chronic Leg Ulcers: Epidemiology, Aetiopathogenesis, and Management. Ulcers. 2013;2013:9.
10. Strandness DE, Priest RE, Gibbons GE. Combined clinical and pathologic study of diabetic and non-diabetic peripheral arterial disease. Diabetes. 1964;13:366-72.
11. Tassiopoulos AK, Golts E, Oh DS, et al. Current concepts in chronic venous ulceration. Eur J Vasc Endovasc Surg. 2000;20(3):227-32.
12. O'Brien JF, Grace PA, Perry IJ, et al. Prevalence and aetiology of leg ulcers in Ireland. Irish J Med Sci. 2000;169(2):110-2.
13. Margolis DJ, Bilker W, Santanna J, et al. Venous leg ulcer: incidence and prevalence in the elderly. J Am Acad Dermatol. 2002;46:381-6.
14. Faria E, Blanes L, Hochman B, et al. Health-related quality of life, self-esteem, and functional status of patients with leg ulcers. Wounds. 2011;23(1):4-10.
15. Korber A, Klode J, Al-Benna S, et al. Etiology of chronic leg ulcers in 31,619 patients in Germany analyzed by an expert survey University Clinic. J Dtsch Dermatol Ges. 2011;9(2):116-21.
16. Gupta N, Gupta SK, Shukla VK, et al. An Indian community based epidemiological study of wounds. J Wound Care. 2004;13:323-5.
17. Sen CK, Gordillo GM, Roy S, et al. Human skin wounds: a major and snowballing threat to public health and the economy. Wound Repair Regen. 2009;17(6):763-71.
18. Gupta SK. Impact of ulceration. In: Khanna AK, Tiwary S (Eds). Ulcers of lower extremity. New Delhi: Springer; 2016: p. 10.
19. Phillips T, Stanton B, Provan A, et al. A study of the impact of leg ulcers on quality of life: financial, social, and psychological implications. J Am Acad Dermatol. 1994;31:49-53.
20. Purwins S, Herberger K, Debus ES, et al. Cost-of-illness of chronic leg ulcers in Germany. Int Wound J. 2010;7:97-102.
21. Cavanagh P, Attinger C, Abbas Z, et al. Cost of treating diabetic foot ulcers in five different countries. Diabetes Metab Res Rev. 2012;28 (Suppl 1):107-11.
22. Driver VR, Fabbi M, Lavery LA, et al. The costs of diabetic foot: The economic case for the limb salvage team. J Vasc Surg. 2010;52:17S-22S.
23. Alexander SJ. Time to get serious about assessing and managing psychosocial issues associated with chronic wounds. Curr Opin Support Palliat Care. 2013;7:95-100.
24. Guarnera G, Tinelli G, Abeni D, et al. Pain and quality of life in patients with vascular leg ulcers: an Italian multicentre study. J Wound Care. 2007;16(8):347-51.
25. Goodridge D, Trepman E, Embil JM. Health-related quality of life in diabetic patients with foot ulcers: literature review. J Wound Ostomy Continence Nurs. 2005;32(6):368-77.
26. Fejfarova V, Jirkovska A, Dragomirecka E, et al. Does the diabetic foot have a significant impact on selected psychological or social characteristics of patients with Diabetes mellitus? J Diab Res. 2014;2014:371938.

CHAPTER 2

Venous Anatomy of the Lower Extremity

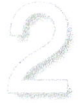

Madhulika Mhatre, Aseem Sharma, Aniketh Venkataram

INTRODUCTION

Historically, microcirculation of the lower limb has not been given its due importance or diligence, with a description of a functional, three-pronged system comprising the superficial plexus, the deep plexus and the interconnecting communicators, as described in older literature. These were based primarily on cadaveric studies, and basic radiological assessment. In recent times, however, with the advent of the Doppler ultrasound, and emerging radiographic modalities like endoscopic ultrasonography, invasive intravascular ultrasound, and digital subtraction venography, the microvasculature of the venous system has been delineated in great detail.

The papillary dermal plexus drains into the reticular venous plexus, which further terminates into the superficial veins through vertical channels. The fascia of the deep muscle is a fulcrum for the deep and superficial compartments, the former comprising vasculature from the skin above, and the latter till the bone below. The venous vasculature is, thus, subdivided into the superficial venous plexus, deep venous plexus, communicators (intracompartmental), perforators communicating veins connect veins within a compartment, perforators connect veins between the superficial and deep compartments; hence, the nosology, and the plantar reservoir vein complex.

The complex interplay between these deep compartments, the perforators and the communicators, and the three muscular pumps, viz., the foot, the calf, and the thigh pumps, help to maintain circulation in the lower limb and prevent acute and venous insufficiency of the venous system.

The learning objective of this chapter includes knowledge of normal anatomical make-up of the lower extremity veins, its anatomical variants, and aberrations. It shall be covered under the subheadings of (Fig. 1):
- Superficial veins
- Deep venous plexus
- Perforators
- Accompanying structures.

SUPERFICIAL VENOUS SYSTEM

Synonyms: Superficial compartment, subcutaneous plexus group

This compartment shows the most anatomic variability in terms of venous structure and distribution. The small plantar (Lejar's plexus) and dorsal subcutaneous veins mark its origin, forming the venous plexus of the foot. They lie in the superficial fascia over the surface of deep fascia. Most of their blood flows to the deep veins through perforating veins. The dorsal arch is formed at the level of proximal metatarsals by small superficial veins and give off the great (medially) and small (laterally) saphenous veins (Fig. 2). Other tributaries include the medial and dorsal digital veins, and the marginal veins.

Great Saphenous Vein

Synonyms: Long saphenous vein

Course

This is the longest vein, the human body has. Originating from the medial marginal vein and the medial dorsal venous arch, the great saphenous vein (GSV) crosses the distal third of the medial surface of the tibia obliquely. It then ascends slightly behind the medial border and crosses

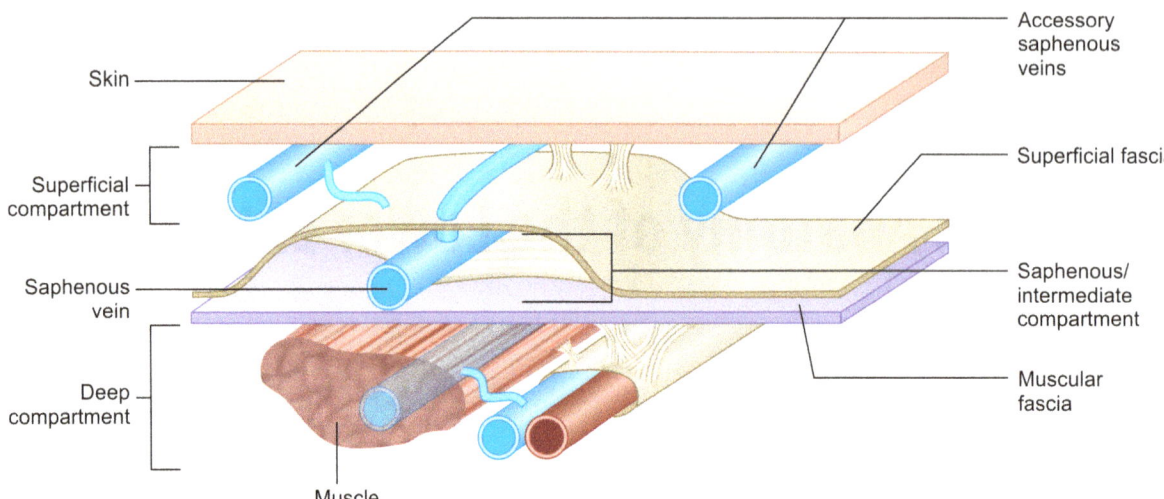

Fig. 1: The compartments. The saphenous fascia forms the superior border of saphenous compartment and the inferior border is formed by the muscle fascia. It contains the saphenous veins and the saphenous nerve. The accessory saphenous vein overlies this compartment, below the dermis.

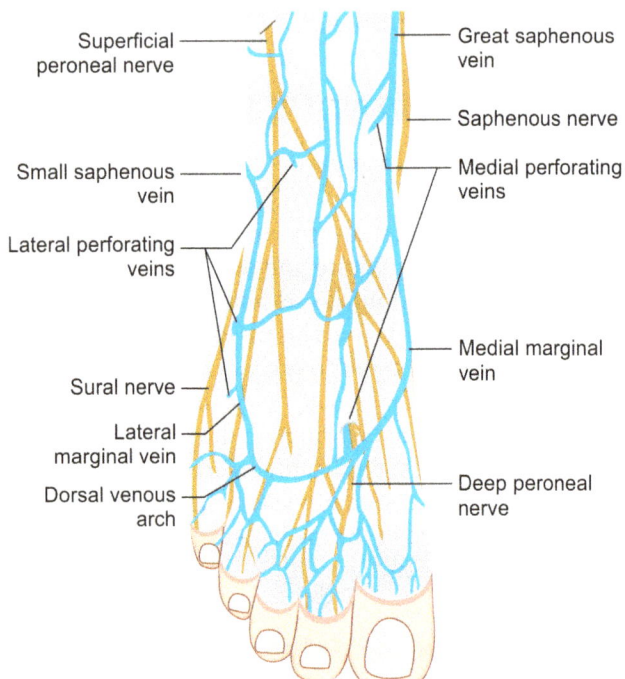

Fig. 2: Superficial and perforating veins of the foot and ankle.

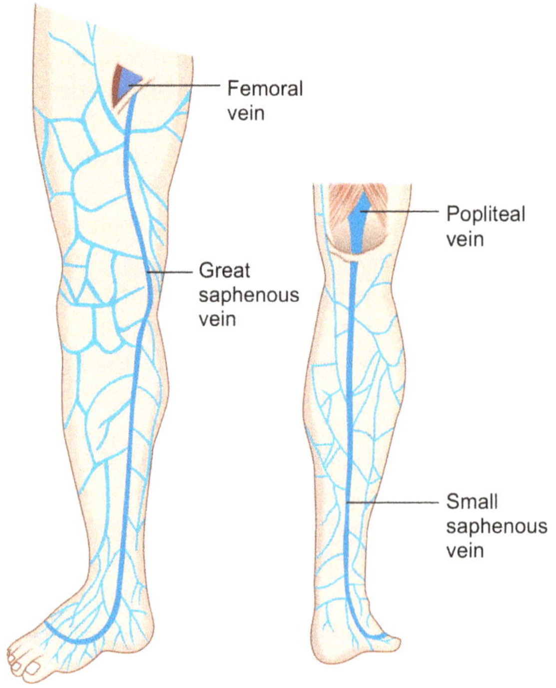

Fig. 3: Anatomical course of the greater and smaller saphenous veins.

the knee, posteromedially, to the medial tibiofemoral condyles. It further runs up and connects with femoral vein at saphenofemoral junction (SFJ), through fossa ovalis—saphenous, in the femoral triangle. As discussed, the anatomic variability of the GSV renders it unreliable for surface markings (Figs. 3 and 4).

Tributaries

- *Calf tributaries—arch veins*: GSV gives off two main tributaries, the anterior and posterior arch veins and many other unnamed communications with small saphenous vein (SSV). The "da Vinci vein" or posterior arch vein drains the medial side, and joins the GSV, distal

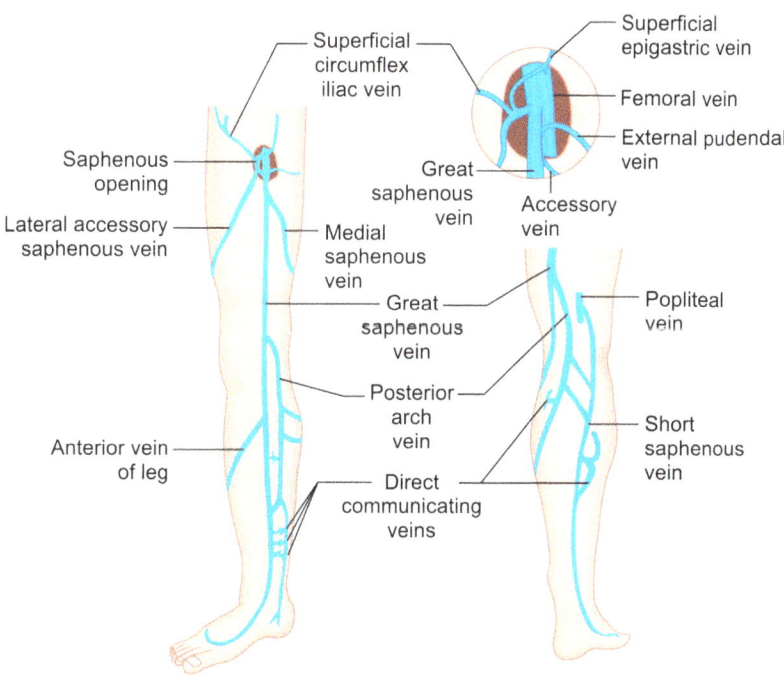

Fig. 4: Tributaries of the saphenous veins along their respective courses.

to knee. Cockett perforators, invariably connect the posterior tibial vein to the posterior arch vein.
- *Thigh tributaries—accessory saphenous veins*: GSV receives the lateral and medial accessory saphenous veins. The lateral vein drains the anterolateral thigh, while the medial vein drains the posteromedial aspect of the thigh.
- Before piercing the cribriform fascia, the GSV gives off the following branches:
  - Superficial circumflex iliac
  - Superficial epigastric
  - Superficial external pudendal
  - Deep external pudendal (immediately before termination after piercing the femoral sheath).

The Eye of Horus: Horus was the Egyptian God of the sky. A sonographic peculiarity can be found in the anatomical association of the various fascias involving the inferior extremity veins. The saphenous fascia, lies in front of the saphenous canal, and the fascia lata, behind it. Together with the saphenous vein in the center, they form the "Eye of the Egyptian", or the "Horus Eye" (Figs. 5A and B).

Small Saphenous Vein

Synonyms: Lesser saphenous, short saphenous

Course

It begins on dorsal venous arch (lateral aspect), opposite to the GSV origin, runs posterior to the lateral malleolus, and emerges lateral to the calcaneal tendon. At the upper leg, the SSV empties at the saphenopopliteal junction (SPJ) into the popliteal vein, between the gastrocnemius muscle heads. Anatomic aberrations include the SSV terminating into the GSV, or even rarely, the femoral vein (Figs. 3 and 4).

Tributaries

Named: Giacomini, an eponym for an Italian anatomist, is a large communicant vein between the GSV and SSV.

Junctions

Saphenofemoral Junction

It is best described as a venous star with five main tributaries. Due to high variability and anatomical aberrations, the branches at this confluence have never been delineated.

Saphenopopliteal Junction

The termination of the SPJ is highly variable. A universal classification divided Types A, B, and C. Type A is the classical SPJ. Type B is when the SSV empties into the SPJ with another cranial extension into the GSV or SFJ. Type C is when there is no SPJ, but the vein empties higher up.

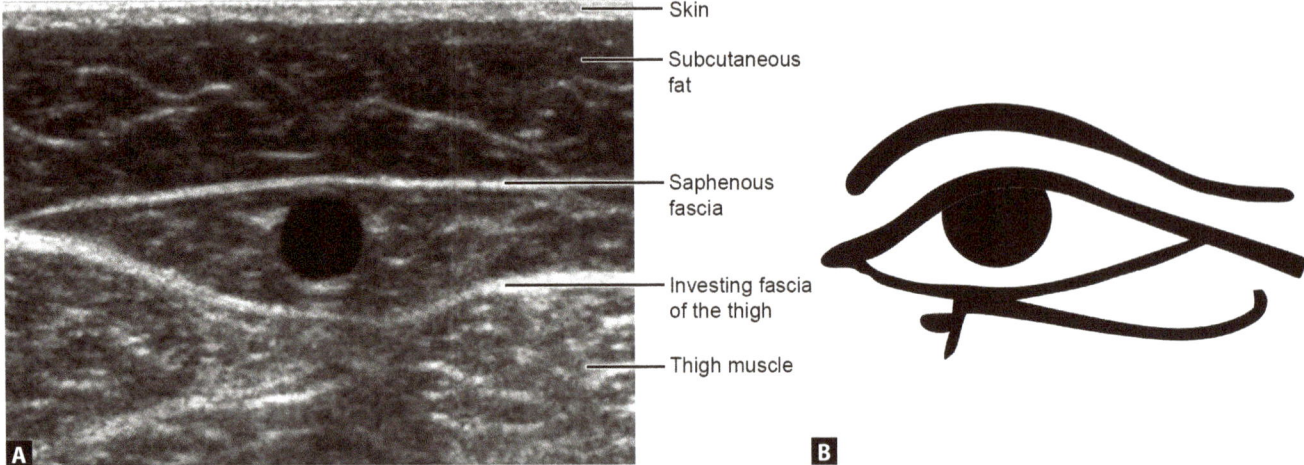

Figs. 5A and B: (A) The Eye of Horus; (B) Schematic representation of the Egyptian eye.
Source: Dr Sandhya Dey, Consultant Radiologist, Mumbai.

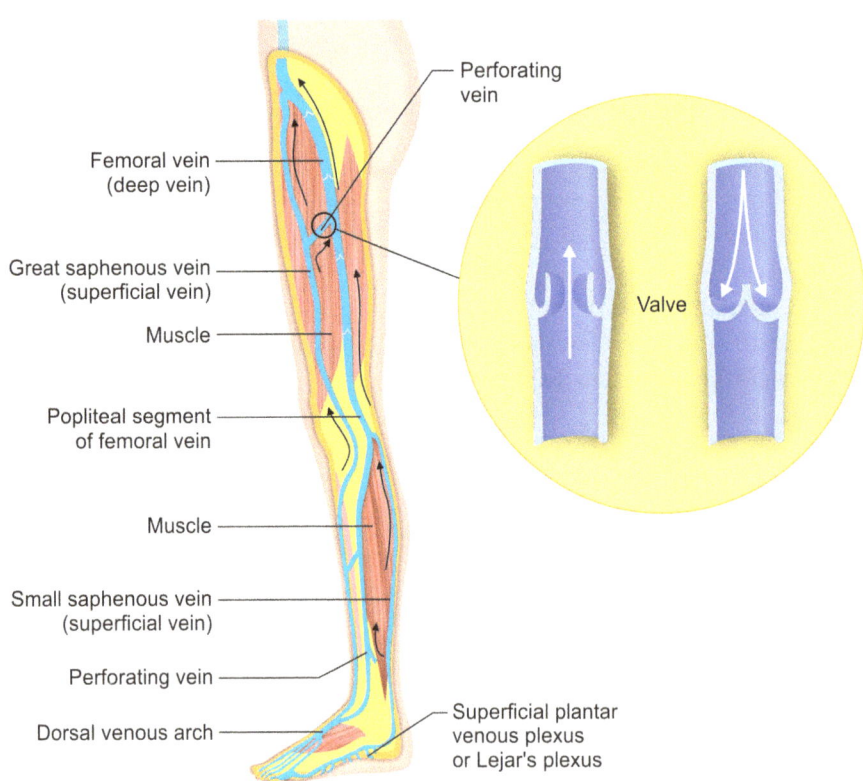

Fig. 6: The valvular system of the superficial veins of the inferior extremity.

Valves

Bicuspid valves exist direct flow to the heart. These are larger valves at termination of venous trunks. The GSV usually has 6–14 valves, up to 20, more in number in the leg, compared to the thigh. One valve called the preterminal valve is present as GSV pierces through the cribriform fascia and the terminal valve at the SFJ (Fig. 6).

The SSV has 4–13 valves, which are more closely spaced, with the highest valve at the termination of the SSV.

DEEP VENOUS SYSTEM

Synonyms: Deep fascial plexus group, venae comitantes, submuscular plexus

Often paired, the deep veins are known as "venae comitantes" or (artery) accompanying veins, by virtue of flanking major vessels.

Course

The deep plantar arch accumulates blood from metatarsum and phalanges. At the ankle, the medial and lateral plantar veins form the posterior tibial vein. The major dorsal deep veins (dorsalis pedis) form the anterior tibial veins.

The posterior tibial veins drain the GSV and posterior arch veins via perforators. They then pierce the soleus muscle and continue as the popliteal vein.

The anterior tibial veins drain the muscles of the anterior compartment. They branch to form the peroneal veins forms. The anterior tibial and peroneal veins form the tibioperoneal trunk, which drains into the popliteal vein.

The profunda femoris vein drains the lateral thigh and receives perforators form the lateral accessory saphenous vein, which joins the femoral vein to form the common femoral vein, which receives the GSV at the SFJ. It also receives the medial and lateral circumflex femoral veins, and continues as the external iliac vein (Fig. 7).

The deep veins of the foot and distal calf have many valves at 2 cm intervals. The thigh deep veins have very few valves.

Venous Sinuses—The Gastrocnemius–Soleus Muscle Pump

These large, thin-walled blood-filled spaces located mostly in the soleus (<20 sinuses in number) and to a lesser extent in gastrocnemius, formed by superficial, deep, and the perforator complex. They can house a significant volume of blood, thereby functioning as peripheral heart chambers. Their primary function is to aid circulation by enforcing venous return against the gravitational pull. The draining veins have valves, which are vital for the efficiency of the peripheral muscle pump.

PERFORATING VEINS

They form connections between the superficial and deep venous plexi. They are classified as: indirect and direct.
- *Indirect*—connects superficial and deep veins through muscular veins.
- *Direct*—GSV and SSV are large direct perforators (Figs. 8 to 10).

Small direct perforators have been grouped and enumerated on the basis of anatomic levels in the lower limb (Fig. 11).

Thigh:
- *Dodds*—to popliteal vein
- *Hunterian*—to superficial femoral vein.

Calf:
- *Lateral*: Peroneal perforators; SSV to the peroneal vein. Named ones include the *Bassi* perforator (lateral malleolus)
- *Anterior*: Premalleolar, mid-crural; drain GSV into anterior tibial vein.

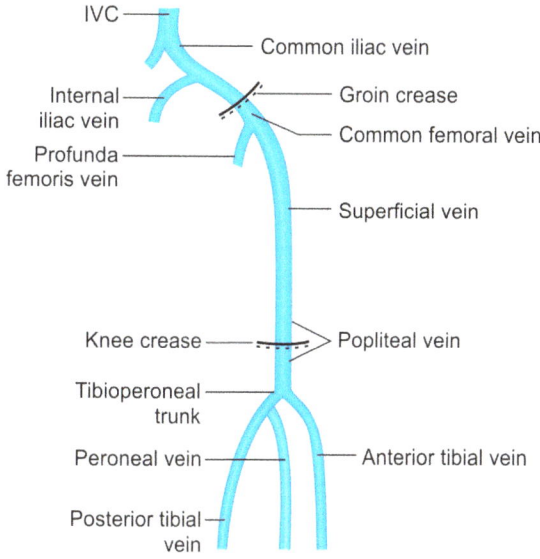

Fig. 7: The deep venous plexus of the lower limb.

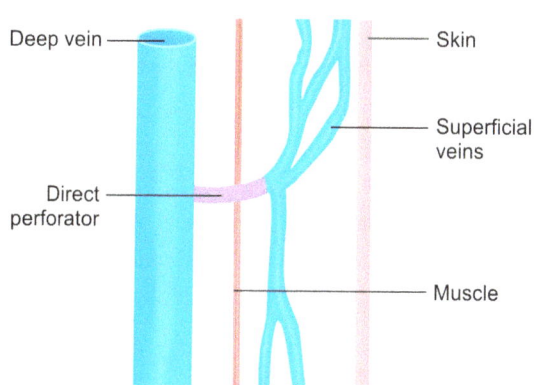

Fig. 8: Direct perforating veins.

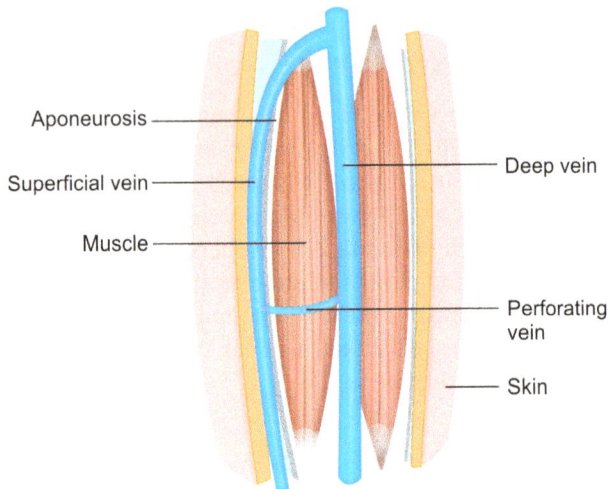

Fig. 9: Representative diagram of the anatomical location of the perforators.

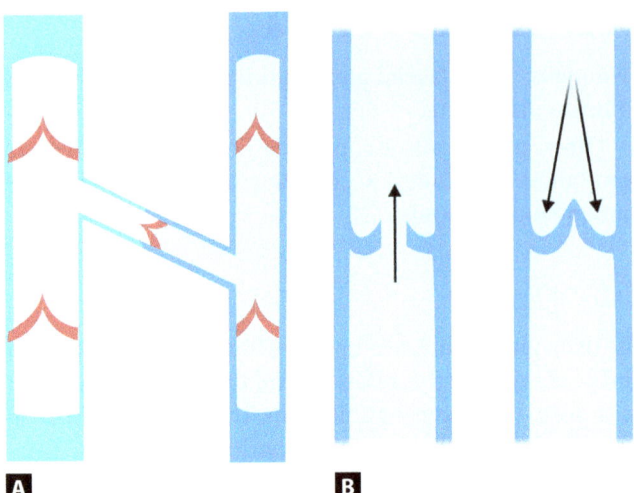

Figs. 10A and B: The perforators and valves allowing unidirectional flow.

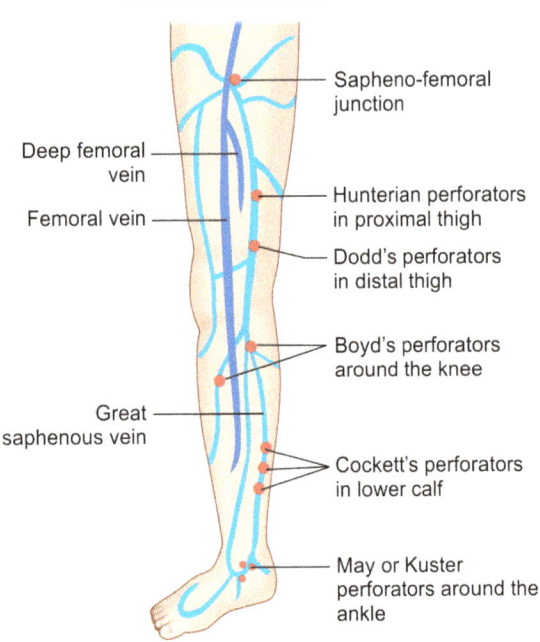

Fig. 11: Eponymous perforators of the lower limb.

- *Medial*:
  - *Cockett I (behind malleolus)*—connects GSV to posterior tibial veins
  - *Cockett II (7–10 cm from medial malleolus)*
  - *Cockett III (10–12 cm from malleolus)*.

Paratibial Perforators

- *Boyd's* perforators—connect the GSV to the popliteal veins.
- Ankle perforator—*May and Kuster*
- *Foot*—connects the superficial venous arch to the dorsalis pedis vein; less than 10 in number.

In 2001, the International Union of Angiology (IUA) retracted this named nosology and aimed to rename the perforators as per draining veins (Table 1).

ACCOMPANYING NERVES

Saphenous Nerve

The cutaneous branch of femoral nerve originates in the thigh. It accompanies the superficial femoral artery, deep to the Sartorius. The nerve then travels close to the GSV, which makes venesection, phlebotomy, or venous ablation almost impossible without nerve injury. Eventually, it terminates by supplying skin over the medial leg and foot.

Sural Nerve

This is the cutaneous branch of tibial nerve. It originates between the gastrocnemius muscle heads, and terminated by supplying posterolateral skin over the leg and lateral foot.

APPLIED ANATOMY

Venous diseases can be divided into:
- *Diseases due to thrombosis*:
  - Superficial thrombophlebitis
  - Deep vein thrombosis.
- *Diseases due to insufficiency*:
  - Varicose veins
  - Lipodermatosclerosis

Table 1: The revised International Union of Angiology (IUA) nosology (2002).

Current and historical nomenclature of perforating veins of the lower extremity

Location	Current nomenclature	Eponym
Foot perforators	Dorsal foot PV	
	Medial foot PV	
	Lateral foot PV	
	Plantar foot PV	
Ankle perforators	Medial ankle PV	May's or Kuster's
	Anterior ankle PV	
	Lateral ankle PV	
Leg perforators	Medial leg PV Paratibial PV • Posterior tibial PV Anterior leg PV Lateral leg PV Posterior leg PV • Medial gastrocnemius PV • Lateral gastrocnemius PV • Intergemellar PV • Para-Achilean PV	Boyd's, Sherman's, 24 cm Cockett's I, II, and III
Knee perforators	Medial knee PV	
	Suprapatellar PV	
	Lateral knee PV	
	Infrapatellar PV	
	Popliteal fossa PV	

(PV: perforator vein)

- Chronic venous insufficiency—venous ulceration
- Stasis dermatitis.

CONCLUSION

To conclude, the venous anatomy of the lower limb is both unreliable and unpredictable. Common patterns with specific anatomic variability, when studied and understood, help comprehend venous pathology better, and additionally, help in identifying disease patterns venous diseases, albeit not fatal primarily, do impact quality of life severely, if left untreated. For this very reason, a thorough knowledge of this chapter is quintessential.

BIBLIOGRAPHY

1. Ballard J, Bergan J. Chronic Venous Insufficiency. London: Springer London; 2000.
2. Caggiati A, Bergan J, Gloviczki P, et al. Nomenclature of the veins of the lower limbs: An international interdisciplinary consensus statement. J Vasc Surg. 2002;36(2):416-22.
3. Caggiati A, Bergan JJ, Gloviczki P, et al. International Interdisciplinary Consensus Committee on Venous Anatomical Terminology. Nomenclature of the veins of the lower limb: extensions, refinements, and clinical application. J Vasc Surg. 2005;41(4):719-24.
4. Caggiati A, Bergan JJ. The Saphenous vein: derivation of its name and its relevant anatomy. J Vasc Surg. 2002;35(1):172-5.
5. Caggiati A, Phillips M, Lametschwandtner A, et al. Valves in small veins and venules. Eur J Vasc Endovasc Surg. 2006;32(4):447-52.
6. Carradice D, Chetter I. Minimally invasive treatment of venous insufficiency using endovenous laser ablation. Kingston: University of Hull; 2011.
7. Cavezzi A, Labropoulos N, Partsch H, et al. Duplex ultrasound investigation of the veins in chronic venous disease of the lower limbs—UIP Consensus Document. Part II: Anatomy. Phlebology. Journal Venous Dis. 2006;21(4):168-79.
8. Cavezzi A, Labropous, Partsch H, et al. Duplex Ultrasound Investigation of the Veins in Chronic Venous Disease of the Lower Limbs—UIP Consensus Document. Part II. Eur J Vasc Endovasc Surg. 2006;31(3):288-99.
9. Currie S, Kennish S, Flood K. Essential radiological anatomy for the MRCS. Cambridge: Cambridge University Press; 2009.
10. Delis KT, Knaggs AL, Khodabakhsh P. Prevalence, anatomic patterns, valvular competence, and clinical significance of the Giacomini vein. J Vasc Surg. 2004;40(6):1174-83.
11. Dodd H, Cockett FB. Surgical anatomy of the veins of the lower limb. In: Dodd H, Cockett FB (Eds). The pathology and surgery of the veins of the lower limb. London: E&S Livingstone; 1996. pp. 28-64.
12. Earthslab.com. (2018). Nerves of Foot. [online] Available from https://www.earthslab.com/anatomy/nerves-of-the-foot/. [Accessed December, 2018].
13. Englund R. Duplex Scanning For Recurrent Varicose Veins. ANZ J Surg. 1996;66(9):618-20.
14. Fan CM. How I Decide to Ablate a Refluxing Perforator. Endovascular Today. 2015;2:68-73.
15. Flandershealth.us. (2018). Anatomy of the Lower Extremity Veins—Varicose Veins. [online] Available from https://www.flandershealth.us/varicose-veins/anatomy-of-the-lower-extremity-veins.html. [Accessed December, 2018].
16. Gezamo Z, Gloviczki P. Venous Embryology and Anatomy. In: Bergan JL (Ed). The Vein Book, 1st edition. United Kingdom: Taylor & Francis; 2007. pp. 15-25.
17. Green D. Sclerotherapy for the permanent eradication of varicose veins: Theoretical and practical considerations. J Am Acad Dermatol. 1998;38(3):461-75.
18. Kalra M, Gloviczki P. Surgical treatment of venous ulcers: role of subfascial endoscopic perforator vein ligation. Surg Clin North Am. 2003;83(3):671-705.
19. Kuster G, Lofgren EP, Hollinshead WH. Anatomy of the veins of the foot. Surg Gynecol Obstet. 1968;127(4):817-23.
20. Lanzer P. Panvascular medicine. 2nd edition, UK: Springer; 2009.

21. Ludbrook J. Musculovenous pumps of the human lower limb. Am Heart J. 1966;71(5):635-41.
22. May R. Nomenclature of the surgically most important connecting veins. In: May R, Partsch H, Staubesand J (Eds). Perforating veins. Baltimore: Urban & Schwartzenberg; 1981. pp. 13-18.
23. Monahan T, Chander R. Ultrasound assessment of great saphenous vein insufficiency. J Vascr Diag. 2015;2015:15-21.
24. Mózes G, Carmichael S, Gloviczki P. Surgical Anatomy of the Veins of the Lower Limb. Persp Vasc Surg. 2000;13(2):0107-16.
25. Mozes G, Carmichael SW, Gloviczi P. Development and anatomy of the venous system. In: Gloviczki P (Ed). Handbook of venous disorders, 2nd edition. London (UK): Arnold publishers; 2001. pp. 14-22.
26. Mozes G, Gloviczki P, Menawat SS, et al. Surgical anatomy for endoscopic subfascial division of perforating veins. J Vasc Surg. 1996;24(5):800-8.
27. Mozes G, Gloviczki P. New Discoveries in Anatomy and New Terminology of Leg Veins: Clinical Implications. Vasc Endovasc Surg. 2004;38(4):367-74.
28. Mühlberger D, Morandini L, Brenner E. Venous valves and major superficial tributary veins near the saphenofemoral junction. J Vasc Surg. 2009;49(6):1562-9.
29. Pascarella L, Mekenas L. Ultrasound Examination of the patient with primary venous insufficiency. In: Bergan JL (Ed). The Vein Book, 1st edition. United Kingdom: Taylor & Francis; 2007. pp. 177-83.
30. Reich-Schupke S, Stücker M. Nomenclature of the veins of the lower limbs—current standards. JDDG. 2010;9(3):189-94.
31. Sam RC, Silverman SH, Bradbury AW. Nerve injuries and varicose vein surgery. Eur J Vasc Endovasc Surg. 2004;27(2):113-20.
32. Schweighofer G, Mühlberger D, Brenner E. The anatomy of the small saphenous vein: fascial and neural relations, saphenofemoral junction, and valves. J Vasc Surg. 2010;51(4):982-9.
33. Shah DM, Chang BB, Leopold PW, et al. The anatomy of the greater saphenous venous system. J Vasc Surg. 1986;3(2):273-83.
34. Sherman RS. Varicose veins: Anatomic findings and an operative procedure based upon them. Ann Surg. 1944;120:222-32.
35. Thomson H. The surgical anatomy of the superficial and perforating veins of the lower limb. Ann R Coll Surg Engl. 1979;61:198-205.
36. Travell J, Simons D. Myofascial pain and dysfunction. Philadelphia: Lippincott Williams and Wilkin; 1992.
37. Uhl J, Gillot C. Anatomy of the veno-muscular pumps of the lower limb. Phlebology: The Journal of Venous Disease. 2014;30(3):180-193.
38. Vaidyanathan S, Ajay K. Chronic venous disorders of the lower limbs. India: Springer India Private; 2016.
39. Vaidyanathan S. Chronic venous disorders of the lower limbs. India: Springer India Private;2016.
40. Zamboni P, Mendoza E, Gianesini S. Saphenous vein-sparing strategies in chronic venous disease. united kingdom: Springer; 2018.
41. Zygmunt J, Pichot O, Dauplaise T. Venous anatomy. Practical Phlebology: Venous Ultrasound. USA: CRC Press; 2013.

CHAPTER 3

Pathology of Leg Ulcers

Divya Gorur, Heera Ramesh

INTRODUCTION

Leg ulcer is a relatively common condition affecting middle and elderly population, causing significant morbidity in terms of chronicity, mobility, pain, and sleep deprivation. Leg ulcers are defined as break in continuity of skin, extending to dermis. Chronic leg ulcer is a chronic wound of the leg that shows no tendency to heal after 3 months of appropriate treatment or incompletely healed at 12 months.[1]

The etiology of leg ulcers are many, in order to provide correct diagnosis and management, the clinician should have a sound knowledge regarding the causes and also brief pathogenesis of leg ulcers in order to investigate and treat the patient (Table 1).

PATHOPHYSIOLOGY OF VENOUS LEG ULCER (FLOWCHART 1)

The most common cause of leg ulcers are venous leg ulcers (VLUs), accounting for 60–80% of all leg ulcers. They are defined as open lesions between the knee and ankle joint that occur in the presence of venous disease.[2] The prevalence of VLUs is between 0.18% and 1%[3] which increases to 4% after the age of 65. The advanced stage of chronic venous disease and lipodermatosclerosis results in venous leg ulcers.[4]

Venous Hypertension and Stasis

Valvular incompetence and calf muscle pump insufficiencies lead to increased pressure in the distal veins of the leg resulting in venous hypertension. Valvular incompetence may be due to primary (no underlying cause) or secondary causes like deep vein thrombosis, perforator insufficiency, or arteriovenous fistulas. Venous hypertension changes the

Table 1: Causes of leg ulcers.

Vascular	Venous, arterial, mixed, Martorell hypertensive ischemic leg ulcer
Neuropathic	Diabetes, tabes, leprosy trophic ulcers, syringomyelia
Traumatic	Injury, pressure, burns
Infections	Bacterial, fungal, protozoa
Tumors	Squamous cell carcinoma, basal cell carcinoma, malignant melanoma
Hematological	Sickle cell disease, cryoglobulinemia
Vasculitis and panniculitis	Pyoderma gangrenosum, necrobiosis lipoidica, systemic lupus erythematosus (SLE), polyarteritis nodosa (PAN), etc.

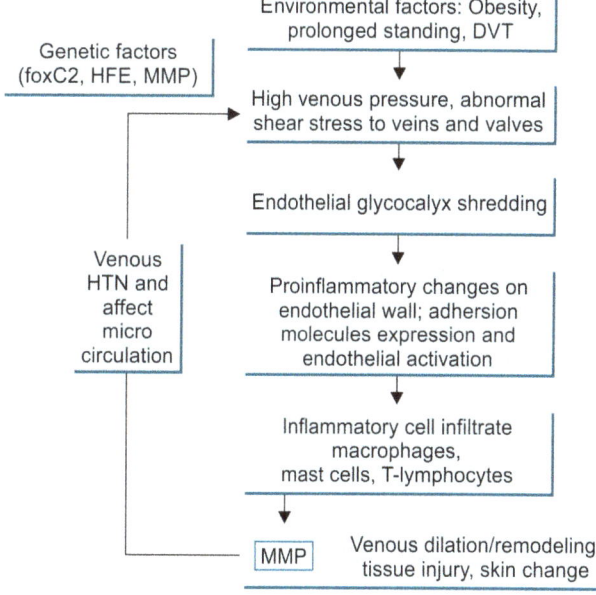

Flowchart 1: Pathophysiology of venous leg ulcers.

DVT: deep vein thrombosis; HTN: hypertension; MMP: matrix metalloproteinases.

pressure gradient between the arteriolar and venular end of the capillaries which results in sluggish movement of the blood within the capillaries and increases adherence of white blood cells (WBCs) and platelets to the endothelium.[5,6]

Fibrin Cuff Theory

Fibrin gets deposited around distended capillary beds leading to raised intravascular pressure. This causes enlargement of endothelial pores resulting in further increased fibrinogen deposition in the interstitium. The "fibrin cuff" which surrounds the capillaries (Fig. 1) forms a permeability barrier reducing nutrient supply and oxygen permeability by 20-fold, resulting in tissue hypoxia, impaired wound healing, fibrosis and ulceration.[7]

Inflammation and Release of Cytokines

The damaged endothelium along with sluggish blood flow initiates leukocyte activation leading to release of proteolytic enzymes and free radicals, which escapes through the leaky vessel walls and damages the capillary wall further and the surrounding tissue resulting in ulceration (Fig. 2). The inflammatory cells, growth factors and cytokines get trapped in the fibrin cuff promote severe uncontrolled inflammation in surrounding tissue preventing proper wound healing.

These damaged capillary wall become increasingly permeable to various macromolecules, accentuating fibrin deposition. Occlusion by leukocytes also causes local ischemia, tissue hypoxia along with reperfusion damage.

Inflammation

Dysregulation of various pro-inflammatory cytokines and growth factors like tumor necrosis factor-α (TNF-α),

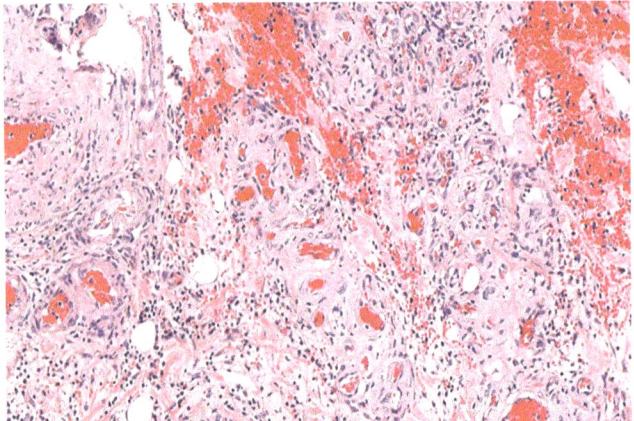

Fig. 1: Fibrin cuff around capillaries.

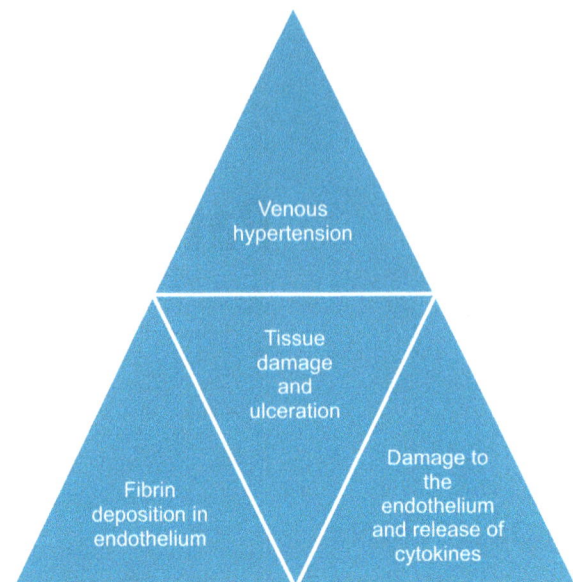

Fig. 2: Pathophysiology of venous leg ulcers.

transforming growth factor (TGF-β) and matrix metalloproteinases lead to chronicity of the ulcers.[8]

Other factors include prothrombin and factor V mutations; deficiency of antithrombin, protein C and S; presence of antiphospholipid antibodies, deficiencies and hyperhomocysteinemia.

PATHOPHYSIOLOGY OF ARTERIAL ULCERS (FLOWCHART 2)

A reduction in blood supply causes death of tissue in the area being fed by the affected artery. Ulcer development due to arterial occlusion is often rapid with deep destruction of subcutaneous tissue extending to bone. Earliest changes are: the affected limb looks pale, and there is a noticeable lack of hair. Ischemic leg ulcer could be due to extramural strangulation, mural thickening or intramural restriction of blood flow. There is often considerable overlap with ill-defined pathogenesis. Arterial leg ulcers occur as a result of reduced arterial blood flow leading to tissue hypoxia.[9]

Arterial or arteriolar occlusion can result from atherosclerosis or emboli.

Atherosclerosis is the most common cause and the risk factors are hypercholesterolemia, hypertension, cigarette smoking, and diabetes mellitus.

The initial mechanical or toxic injury may be due to hypoxia, hemodynamic stress, toxic metabolites (e.g. tobacco, homocysteine), or infectious agents (herpes virus, cytomegalovirus, Chlamydia etc.). The final

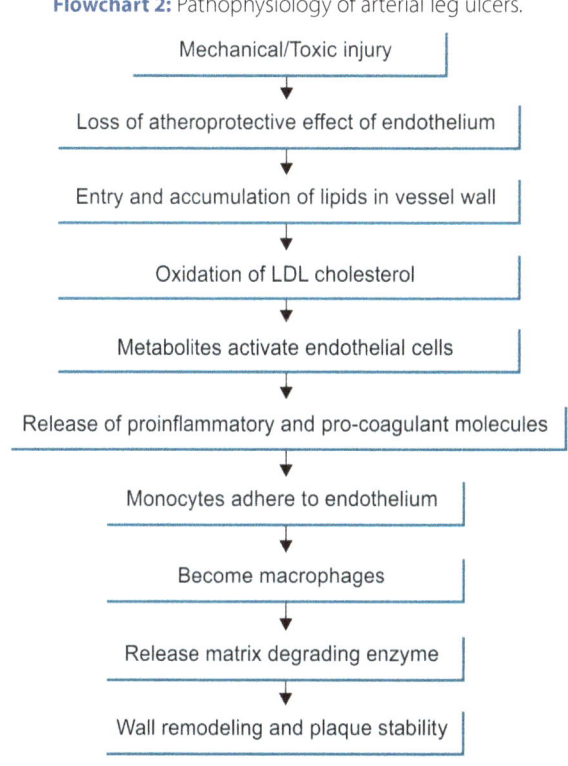

Flowchart 2: Pathophysiology of arterial leg ulcers.

(LDL: Low-density lipoprotein)

outcome is a loss of the various atheroprotective effects of normal endothelium, which include its anti-adhesive properties, barrier function and anti-proliferative effect on the underlying smooth muscle cells. One of the early events is entry and accumulation of lipids in the vessel wall. Oxidation of these low-density lipoprotein (LDL) cholesterol produces metabolites that activate endothelial cells with expression of proinflammatory (e.g., leukocyte adhesion molecules) and procoagulant molecules as well as decrease in protective substances (e.g., nitric oxide). Circulating monocytes adhere to activated endothelium and exposed matrix, become macrophages, and scavenge lipid. These macrophages release matrix degrading enzymes, which may be involved in wall remodeling and plaque stability.

T-lymphocytes are also recruited, and both of these inflammatory cells elaborate an array of cytokines [interleukin-1 (IL-1), TNF-α, and TGF-β)], which potentiate the inflammation. Platelets adhere to dysfunctional endothelium, exposed matrix and monocytes-macrophages adding to the inflammatory cascade.

Amplification occurs by means of numerous potential positive feedback loops between cytokines and growth factors (both autocrine and paracrine) in which persistent inflammatory activation is the central feature.[10]

VASCULITIC ULCERS

Vasculitis is immunologically mediated angiocentric inflammation, the histological hallmark of which is predominant neutrophilic infiltration, extravasation of red blood cells (RBCs), fibrinoid necrosis of the vessel wall. All these events lead to narrowing of lumen, formation of thrombus, focal ischemia and ulceration. Extravasation of RBCs manifests as palpable purpura (Fig. 3).

This sequence of events is associated with collagen vascular disease, infection, drug reaction or malignancy. Small vessel vasculitis where dermal vessels are affected manifests as palpable purpura, vesicobullous lesions and superficial ulcers with regular borders. Vasculitis of larger vessels like muscular arteries presents as erythematous, tender nodules; punched-out ulcers with irregular borders or gangrene along with systemic symptoms.

Due to the anatomic features of the postcapillary venules and the hydrostatic pressure which governs the microcirculation physiology, skin is one of the first and most commonly involved structures. The raised hydrostatic pressure in the lower limbs makes it the most common and first site of appearance of vasculitic lesions.[11]

The pathogenesis of hypoxia and ulceration in vasculitis is: occlusion by macromolecular or cold-predictable complexes (cryoproteins, paraproteins), intimal hyperplasia, platelet thrombosis, fibrin deposition, postinflammatory fibrosis.

NEUROPATHIC AND DIABETIC FOOT ULCER

In diabetic ulcers apart from neuropathy, infection and microvascular occlusion interplay in the formation of ulcer.

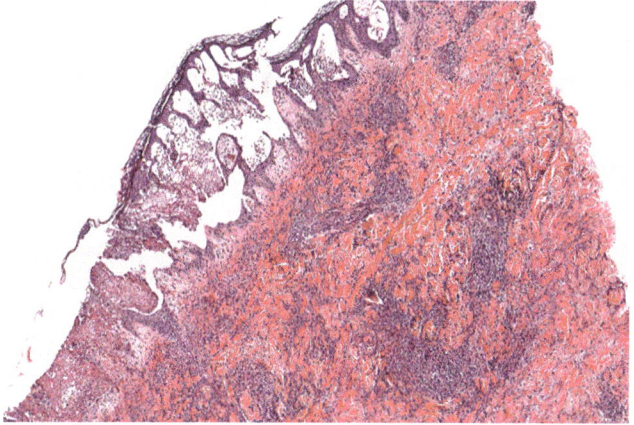

Fig. 3: Subepidermal bulla, neutrophilic infiltration, extravasation of red blood cells, fibrinoid necrosis of the vessel wall in bullous vasculitis.

Neuropathies in diabetics have the sensory, motor and autonomic components.

Sensory neuropathy leads to inability in detecting trauma to the lower extremities. The affected area is subjected to repeated trauma, excessive pressure from weight-bearing and mobility, which goes unnoticed.[12,13]

Motor neuropathy leads to imbalance in the movement of foot due to damage in innervations of the affected intrinsic foot muscles. This produces anatomic foot deformities that create abnormal bony prominences gradually contributing to skin breakdown and ulceration.

Damage to autonomic nerve fibers leads to diminished sweating. The overlying skin becomes xerotic; with impaired barrier function develops fissures and a subsequent development of ulceration and infection. Autonomic denervation reduces the tone of vascular smooth muscle, causes bone demineralization and osteolysis.[14]

Hyperglycemia results in inhibition of the synthesis of nerve cell myoinositol, antioxidant deficiency leading to the abnormal glycation of nerve cell protein, abnormal activation of protein kinase C, ultimately leading to ischemia and nerve dysfunction.

Role of Hyperglycemia in Peripheral Vascular Disease

Persistent hyperglycemic state leads to endothelial cell dysfunction, smooth cell abnormalities, decreases in endothelium-derived vasodilators, increase in thromboxane A2, all of which contribute to vasoconstriction and plasma hypercoagulability. This along with pre-existing risk factors like smoking, hypertension, and hyperlipidemia potentiates vascular occlusion. The internal milieu of procoagulant state results in ischemia and ulceration of affected foot in diabetic patients.[14]

Diabetes is the most common cause of neuropathic ulcer; others are Hansen's disease, neurological disorders.

ULCERATING SKIN DISEASES

Several skin disorders present with ulceration as the first symptom [pyoderma gangrenosum (PG), pemphigoid and other bullous diseases, panniculitis, periarteritis nodosa, erythema induratum (Bazin), malignant atrophic papulosis (Degos), erythema exudativum multiforme, sarcoidosis, erythema elevatum diutinum, Behçet disease (BD), cutaneous discoid and systemic lupus erythematosus, scleroderma, lichen planus, keratosis actinica, contact dermatitis, fat necrosis/pancreatic fat necrosis, trench foot, insect bites, lymphedema, lipedema, myxedema, erythermalgia/erythromelalgia, perniosis (chilblains), hemangioma, Stewart–Bluefarb syndrome].[15]

The most impressive ulcerating dermatosis is PG. PG causes deep necrotic ulcers, usually with an elevated violaceous border, and the ulceration is progressive if left untreated.[15]

Pyoderma gangrenosum is considered part of the spectrum of the neutrophilic disease. Impaired phagocytosis by neutrophils has been suggested in the pathogenesis of PG. Neutrophil analysis in PG showed evidence of abnormal neutrophil trafficking and aberrant integrin oscillations. IL-8, a potent leukocyte chemotactic agent, has been shown to be over expressed in PG ulcers (Fig. 4).

In the recently described "PAPA syndrome" (pyogenic sterile arthritis, PG and acne) there is an over expression of the *IL-16* gene and the IL-16 protein is chemotactic to neutrophils. It can be concluded that the factors triggering/maintaining the various immunological/neutrophil abnormalities are multiple and include genetic predisposition, parainflammatory, paraneoplastic or para-immune phenomena. The predisposed patient experiences an inciting event such as minor trauma, and instead of normal response that recognizes and removes the damaged tissue, the patient's abnormal response results in lesions of PG.[16]

Pyoderma gangrenosum can also arise as a consequence of drug therapy like propylthiouracil, pegfilgastrim (granulocyte stimulating factor), gefinib (epidermal growth factor receptor inhibitor), and isotretinoin.[16]

Behçet's disease is another dermatological cause of leg ulcers. Association with human leukocyte antigen-B51 (HLA-B51) is known as the strongest genetic susceptibility

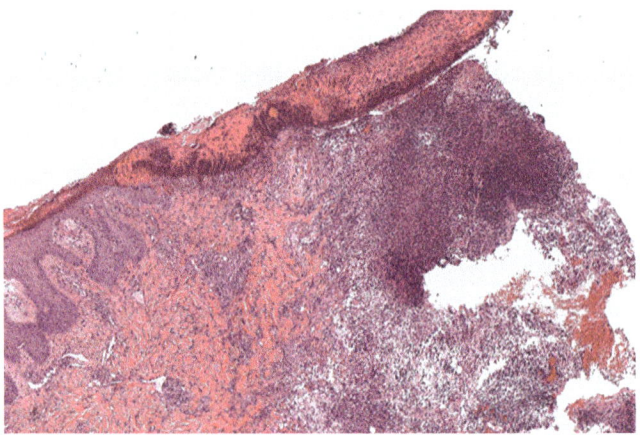

Fig. 4: Epidermal necrosis with dermal neutrophilia with vasculitis seen in Pyoderma Gangrenosum.

factor for BD. Recent genome-wide association studies have confirmed this relationship, and reported new susceptibility genes (IL-10, IL-23R, IL-12RB2) for the disease. A triggering infectious agent could operate through molecular mimicry, and the disease could subsequently be perpetuated by an abnormal immune response to an auto-antigen in the absence of ongoing infection. Several potential bacteria have been investigated but the most commonly implicated microorganism is *Streptococcus sanguis*. Recent data have showed that the T cell homeostasis perturbation consisted mainly of Th1 and Th17 expansions, while regulatory T-cell response was suppressed. Cytokine such as IL-17, IL-23 and IL-21 play a significant role in the pathogenesis of BD. Inflammatory cells within BD inflammatory lesions include mostly neutrophils, CD4 (+) T cells, and cytotoxic cells. Lastly, endothelium dysfunction has been clearly established.[17]

INFECTIOUS DISEASES

Some microorganisms can cause tissue necrosis, such as the notorious β-hemolytic *Streptococcus pyogenes*. Acquired immune deficiency due to human immunodeficiency virus (HIV)-infection reintroduced ulcerative conditions that were thought to be eradicated, such as tertiary lues and ulcerating tuberculosis, and may be associated with atypical, large ulcers caused by herpes simplex or cytomegalovirus. In addition, bacillary angiomatosis, caused by *Rochalimae* species and histoplasmosis must be included in the differential diagnosis of ulcerations occurring in HIV disease. Leishmaniasis, atypical mycobacteria, ulcus tropicum and deep mycotic infections should also be considered.[15]

DRUGS

Steroid (intralesional injection), vaccination ulcer (BCG), halogens, ergotamin, methotrexate, hydroxyureum, paravasal injection of cytostatic and other drugs, granulocyte-colony stimulating factor can also cause ulceration.[15]

MALIGNANCY (ULCERATING TUMORS)

Basal cell carcinoma, squamous cell carcinoma, malignant melanoma, metastasis, pseudoepitheliomatous hyperplasia, epithelioma (Marjolin ulcer), lymphoma, leukemia, cutaneous T-cell and B-cell lymphoma, Hodgkin disease, sarcoma, lymphosarcoma, rhabdomyosarcoma, hemangiosarcoma, lymphangiosarcoma, Kaposi and pseudo-Kaposi sarcoma, including metastases, may present with skin ulceration as the first symptom. The two most frequent ulcerating tumors of the skin are basal cell carcinoma (ulcus rodens) and squamous cell carcinoma, which may occur anywhere on the body, with a preference for sun-exposed skin. Malignancies (predominantly squamous cell carcinoma, sometimes fibro sarcoma) can also develop secondarily in chronic leg ulcers, especially in ulcers of longer duration, probably as a consequence of the continuously increased cell division in and around the ulcer.[15]

HEMATOLOGICAL DISORDERS

Several forms of anemia (sickle cell anemia, thalassemia, hereditary spherocytosis, glucose-6-phosphate dehydrogenase deficiency) have been associated with lower leg ulceration.[15]

In sickle cell anemia, an increased number of activated endothelial cells has been found in the circulation, and it is hypothesized that an interaction between sickle cells and endothelial cells causes increased expression of endothelial cell adhesion molecules, which promotes thrombotic vaso-occlusion. In addition, in the other hematological conditions (e.g. essential thrombocythemia, thrombotic thrombocytopenic purpura, cryoglobulinemia, (Fig. 5) polycythemia, leukemia, dysproteinemia), micro vascular thrombosis is the most likely pathogenetic factor.[15]

CLOTTING DISORDERS

Hypercoagulable disorders may cause ulceration, either indirectly as a consequence of venous thrombosis, or directly by thrombus formation in small arteries, arterioles, capillaries or venules. A growing number of hereditary

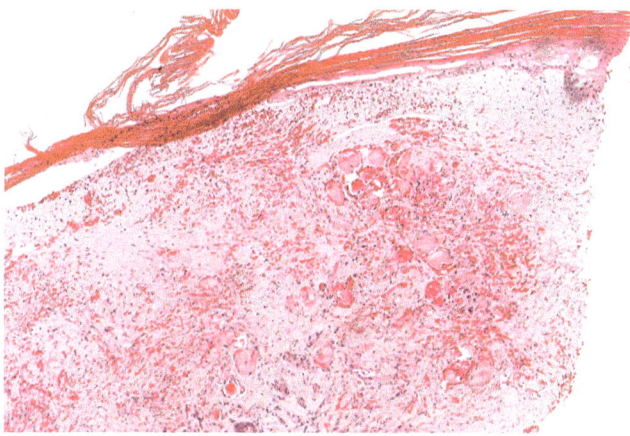

Fig. 5: Vasculopathy, thrombin in the capillaries seen in cryoglobulinemia.

or acquired conditions predisposing to thrombosis have been identified, such as the antiphospholipid syndrome, deficiency of antithrombin III, protein C or protein S or abnormal clotting factors (factor V Leiden, factor II mutant).[15]

CONCLUSION

Leg ulcers are known for their chronicity and morbidity. A comprehensive clinical examination of the affected limb, ulcer and the patient along with detailed history is essential to establish the etiology without which appropriate management is difficult. Many a times there are multiple causes and risk factors which have to be addressed. A good clinician should have sound knowledge of the etiology and pathogenesis for overall management of patients with leg ulcers.

REFERENCES

1. Agale SV. Chronic Leg Ulcers: Epidemiology, Aetiopathogenesis, and Management. Ulcers. 2013.
2. Scottish Intercollegiate Guideline Network (19988). The Care of Patients with Chronic Leg Ulcer (Guideline 26). [online] Available from https://gneaupp.info/wp-content/uploads/2014/12/The-care-of-patients-with-chronic-leg-ulcer.pdf [Accessed December 2018].
3. Cornwall JV, Doré CJ, Lewis JD. Leg ulcers: Epidemiology and aetiology. Br J Surg. 1986;73:693-6.
4. Vasudevan B. Venous leg ulcers: Pathophysiology and Classification. Indian Dermatol Online J 2014;5:366-70.
5. Irving G, Hargreaves S. Venous and arterial leg ulceration. InnovAiT. 2009;2:415-22.
6. Meissner MH, Moneta G, Burnand K, et al. The haemodynamics and diagnosis of venous disease. J Vasc Surg. 2007; 46 (Suppl S):4S-24S.
7. Burnand KG, Whimster I, Naidoo A, et al. Pericapillary fibrin in the ulcer-bearing skin of the leg: The cause of lipodermatosclerosis and venous ulceration. Br Med J (Clin Res Ed). 1982;285:1071-2.
8. Higley HR, Ksander GA, Gerhardt CO, et al. Extravasation of macromolecules and possible trapping of transforming growth factor-beta in venous ulceration. Br J Dermatol. 1995;132:79-85.
9. C Moffatt. Leg ulcers. In: Murray S (Ed). Vascular Disease. London: Whurr Publishers; 2001. pp. 200-37.
10. Townsend CM, Beauchamp RD, Evers BM, et al. Peripheral Arterial Occlusive Disease. Sabiston Textbook of Surgery: The Biological Basis of Modern Surgical Practice, 18th edition. Philadelphia: Elsevier; 2007. pp. 1945-6.
11. Papi M, Papi C. Vasculitic Ulcers. Int J Low Extrem Wounds. 2016;15:6-16.
12. Pendsey SP. Understanding diabetic foot. Int J Diabetes Dev Ctries. 2010;30:75-9.
13. Bowering CK. Diabetic foot ulcers: Pathophysiology, assessment, and therapy. Can Fam Physician. 2001;47:1007-16.
14. Clayton W Jr, Elasy T. A Review of the Pathophysiology, Classification, and Treatment of Foot Ulcers in Diabetic Patients. Clin Diabetes. 2009;27:52-8.
15. Mekkes JR, Loots MA, Van Der Wal AC, et al. Causes, investigation and treatment of leg ulceration. Br J Dermatol. 2003;148: 388-401.
16. Bhat RM. Pyoderma gangrenosum: An update. Indian Dermatol Online J. 2012;3:7-13.
17. Houman MH, Bel Feki N. Physiopathologie de la maladie de Behçet. La Revue de Médecine Interne. 2014;35: 90-6.

CHAPTER 4

Microbiology of Leg Ulcers

Amrita Hongal, Ujwal M

INTRODUCTION

Infections are among those complications of leg ulcers that have a pronounced effect on wound healing as well as on the patient's quality of life and the cost of wound management. Infections of the leg ulcers result in major source of morbidity in an individual's life and important cause of amputation. The impact of microorganisms on leg ulcers is studied extensively to assess their role in wound healing. Few experts consider quantity of microbes as the critical factor in determining wound healing, while others consider presence of specific organisms (qualitative) in delayed wound healing.

The function of intact skin is to prevent pathogenic invasion of the underlying tissue. An ulcer is a discontinuity of the skin and provides a portal for microbes. Leg ulcers occur due to break in the physiology of skin from varied etiology like arterial, venous, lymphatic, neuropathic, infective, trauma, and malignancy, resulting in circumscribed necrosis of skin, and extending deeper sometimes to the fascia, muscles, or up to deeper bone; with stagnant granulation and slower coverage by epidermis migrating from the ulcer margins.[1] Not all ulcers are infected.

SAMPLE COLLECTION AND ANALYSIS METHODS

Infected leg ulcers frequently have multidrug-resistant pathogens, particularly after performance of procedures and use of several antibiotics. Evaluation of infection includes a thorough clinical examination supplemented with necessary laboratory tests and imaging studies. The presence of a leg ulcer should indicate an associated infection.[2]

The microbiota of leg ulcers is polymicrobial and several studies have shown that most of the ulcers with no clinical signs of infection contained more than one bacterial species.[3] It is difficult to compare the microbial flora due to use of dissimilar methods of specimen collection and analysis as well as difference in patient demographics, in the etiological factors and infection status of ulcers.[4]

The most simple and common qualitative sampling method is cotton-tipped swabs (Fig. 1). Needle aspiration of deep tissue, culture of biopsy material, and irrigation followed by aspiration are suitable methods to assess quantitative and semiquantitative microbiology. Use of a selective culture media grows specific bacterial strains. Culture-based techniques are biased toward growth of organisms under standard laboratory conditions. Molecular genomic methods can assess the quantity and quality of microbes in a less biased way. Sequencing and analysis of 16S ribosomal RNA genes have demonstrated an under-representation of true diversity of microbes and their burden by culture-based methods.[5]

PATHOGENESIS AND THE FLORA

Following skin injury, the colonization of eroded surface by local bacterial flora takes place. The organisms that are commonly isolated are *Staphylococcus aureus* and Group B streptococci (Fig. 2), though bacteria need not be the primary etiological factor.

Staphylococcus aureus has been isolated in varying frequencies from infected and noninfected leg ulcers.[3] In addition, a number of aerobic species (Fig. 3) have been implicated including many species of *Escherichia coli, Klebsiella, Proteus, Enterobacter*, and *Enterococcus*.[6] In addition to the aerobes, the anaerobes (obligate

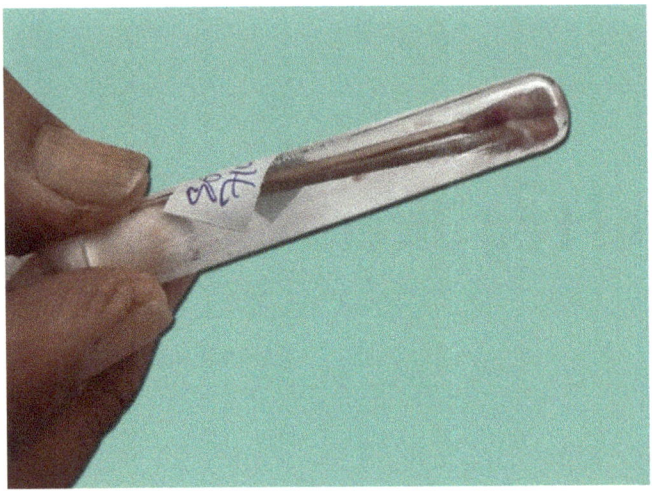
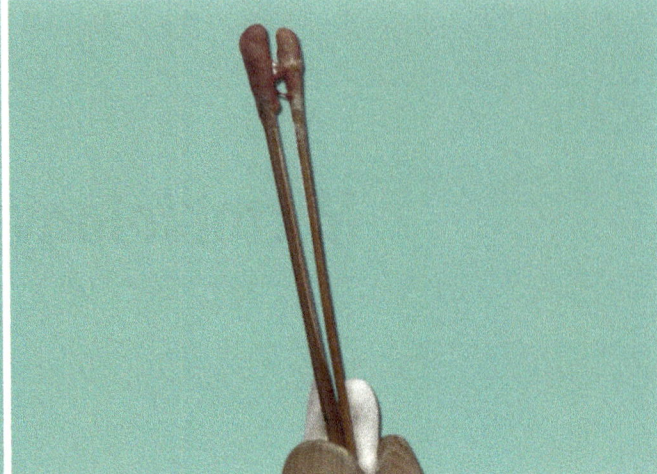

Fig. 1: Cotton tipped swabs used for sample collection.

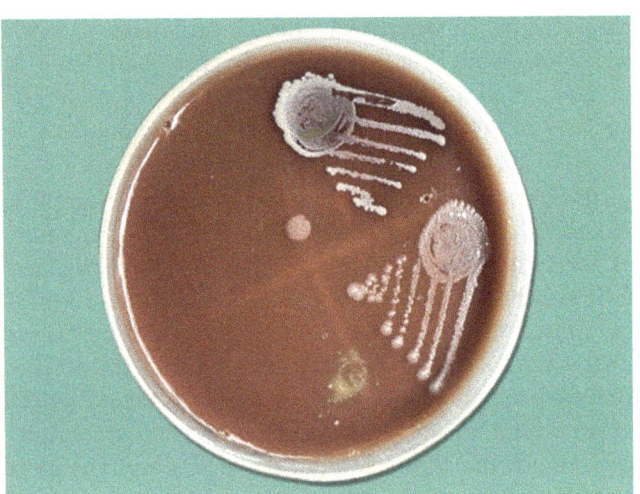

Fig. 2: Culture of swabbed material.

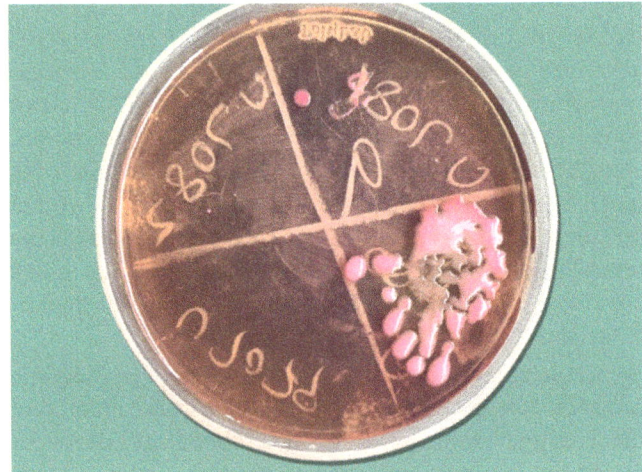

Fig. 3: Culture on McConkey Agar.

and facultative) have been isolated from leg ulcers, most commonly being the *Peptostreptococcus* species and *Prevotella* species. In the study by Bowler PG,[6] a coexistence of aerobic-anaerobic microbiota in leg ulcers was demonstrated, but the correlation between a specific pathogen and wound infection was lacking. The interplay between ulcer and bacteria can be arranged into four levels: (1) contamination, (2) colonization, (3) critical colonization, and (4) infection (Fig. 4).

Contamination and colonization by microbes do not inhibit healing, but critical colonization is a stage at which bacteria begin to interfere with wound healing.[7] In presence of one of the following infection of the ulcer is suspected: pyrexia, increased pain, increase in ulcer size, increasing erythema of surrounding skin, or lymphangitis (Box 1).[8]

Box 1: Signs of infection.
- Pyrexia or fever
- Increased pain
- Increased ulcer size
- Increased erythema of the surrounding skin
- Lymphangitis

Leg ulcers by their chronicity in nature do not exhibit the above classical signs and symptoms of infections and an extended list has been suggested to identify infection, which includes serous exudate plus existing inflammation, discoloration of granulation tissue, friable granulation tissue, foul odor, delayed healing, and wound breakdown.[9]

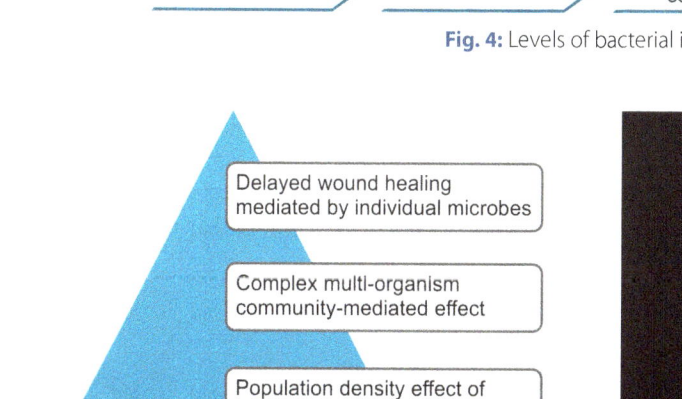

Fig. 4: Levels of bacterial infection.

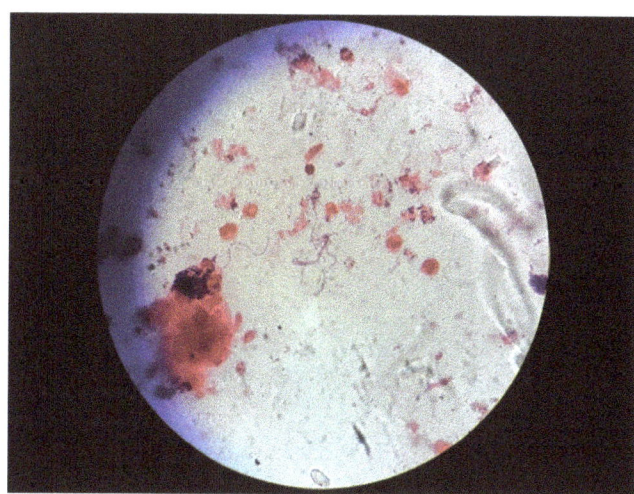

Fig. 5: Mechanism of delayed wound healing.

Fig. 6: Gram's stain of swab material with complex microbiota.

S. aureus, beta hemolytic streptococci, and *Pseudomonas* species are more likely to impair the wound healing.[10] Study by Schmidtchen et al.,[11] supports the role of *Pseudomonas* species in delayed wound healing as they express a major metalloproteinase called elastase, induce degradation of complement C3, antiproteinases, kininogens, fibroblast proteins, and proteoglycans in vitro. As important is the number of different species of colonizing bacteria, the total number of organisms per gram of tissue is another important cause in delayed wound healing. A mechanism has been suggested by which microorganisms delay wound healing (Fig. 5):

- Delayed wound healing mediated by individual microbes
- Complex multiorganism community-mediated effect
- Population density effect of microorganisms
- Secondary subclinical host-mediated inflammatory response.[12]

Infected leg ulcers can be from bacterial, fungal, or protozoan infection. The common clinical presentations are erysipelas, ulcerating pyoderma, ecthyma gangrenosum, necrotizing fasciitis, gas gangrene, and Maduramycosis (Fig. 6). Delayed diagnosis and treatment of these infections increase the risk of mortality. Early and vigorous surgical debridement improves the survival. Targeted antibiotic therapy in addition to repeated surgical debridement is the mainstay of therapy of infected leg ulcers.[13,14]

More research is needed to know the interactions between microorganisms, antibiotics, and antibiotic resistance in chronic wounds patients and the general population.[5]

REFERENCES

1. Olszewski WL. Role of bacteria in pathogenesis of lower leg ulcers. In: Khanna A, Tiwary S (Eds). Ulcers of the Lower Extremity. New Delhi: Springer; 2016.
2. Nath G, Kumar G. Microbiology of ulcers. In: Khanna A, Tiwary S (Eds). Ulcers of the Lower Extremity. New Delhi: Springer; 2016.
3. Hansson C, Hoborn J, Möller A, et al. The microbial flora in venous leg ulcers without clinical signs of infection. Acta Derm Venereol. 1995;75:24-30.
4. Davies CE, Wilson MJ, Hill KE, et al. Use of molecular techniques to study microbial diversity in the skin: chronic wounds reevaluated. Wound Repair Regen. 2001;9:332-40.
5. Misic AM, Gardner SE, Grice EA. The Wound Microbe: Modern approaches to examining the role of microorganisms in impaired chronic wound healing. Adv Wound Care. 2014;3(7):502-10.
6. Bowler PG, Davies BJ. The microbiology of infected and noninfected leg ulcers. Int J Dermatol. 1999;38(8):573-8.
7. Schultz GS, Sibbald RG, Falanga V, et al. Wound bed preparation: a systematic approach to wound management. Wound Repair Regen. 2003;11:1-28.
8. Douglas WS, Simpson NB. Guidelines for the management of chronic venous leg ulceration. Report of a multidisciplinary workshop. Br J Dermatol. 1995;132:446-52.

9. Gardner SE, Frantz RA, Doebbeling BN. The validity of the clinical signs and symptoms used to identify localized chronic wound infection. Wound Repair and Regeneration. 2001;9:178-86.
10. Trengove NJ, Stacey MC, McGechie DF, et al. Qualitative bacteriology and leg ulcer healing. J Wound Care. 1996;5(6):277-80.
11. Schmidtchen A, Holst E, Tapper H, et al. Elastase-producing *Pseudomonas aeruginosa* degrade plasma proteins and extracellular products of human skin and fibroblasts, and inhibit fibroblast growth. Microb Pathog. 2003;34(1):47-55.
12. Ebrighr JR. Microbiology of Chronic Leg and Pressure Ulcers: Clinical Significance and Implications for Treatment. Nurs Clin N Am. 2005;40:207-16.
13. Khanna R, Meena RN, Mukunda MV, et al. Infective Leg Ulcers. In: Khanna A, Tiwary S (Eds). Ulcers of the Lower Extremity. New Delhi: Springer: 2016.
14. Howell-Jones RS, Wilson MJ, Hill KE, et al. A review of the microbiology, antibiotic usage and resistance in chronic skin wounds. J Antimicrob Chemother. 2005;55:143-9.

CHAPTER 5

Wound Healing

Shivakumar Patil, Kavya Thimmaiah

INTRODUCTION

Healing, a critical step in the evolution and survival of humankind is the process of restoration of tissue architecture and function.

The earliest documented reference to the process of healing dates back to early 2,200 BC. Since ancient times, a wide variety of substances such as mud, clay, plants and herbs were fashioned to be used as plasters. Honey, grease, lint and even wine were used as antibacterial agents and also as a physical barrier. The Hippocratic collection about wound healing has an interesting anecdote: "For an obstinate ulcer, sweet wine and a lot of patience should be enough".[1] If only it were enough!

In keeping with the rapid progress in the field of medicine, the art of wound healing has also undergone extensive research which has translated into the need for introducing fellowship programs dedicated to wound healing.

Wound healing is the response of the body to any kind of external or internal stimuli to injury. The stimuli can be varied; physical, chemical, infectious, immunological, electric or thermal.[2,3] The process of wound healing is accomplished by varying degrees of:
- Regeneration
- Scar formation.

Regeneration is seen when the injury is mild, the injury being restricted to the epithelium. Regeneration can occur either by proliferation of uninjured cells at the site or by proliferation of tissue stem cells provided the underlying basement membrane is intact.

Scar formation is seen when the injury is severe or if the underlying connective tissue framework has been damaged. The repair process in these cases is achieved by a combination of varying degrees of residual tissue regeneration and deposition of connective tissue. The resultant scar is tough, firm and provides structural stability.

Wound healing involves the following overlapping and precise processes:[4]
- Hemostasis
- Inflammation
- Proliferation of keratinocytes (re-epithelization), blood vessels (angiogenesis) and fibroblasts (fibroplasia)
- Remodeling of connective tissue.

HEMOSTASIS

It occurs immediately following injury.
- The primary response is vasoconstriction which restricts the loss of blood
- A clot (Fig. 1) is formed followed by platelet degranulation and the deposition of a fibrin meshwork

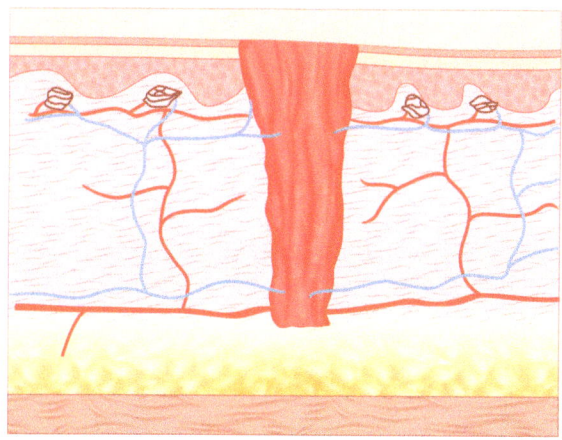

Fig. 1: Section of skin with wound covered by hemostatic plug.

- A host of pro-inflammatory cytokines and growth factors are released
- The blood vessels at the site, under the influence of vascular endothelial growth factor (VEGF) show increased vascular permeability leading to edema.

INFLAMMATION

It occurs by transmigration of inflammatory cells (Fig. 2) through the vessel walls and generally lasts from the initiation of injury up to 2 days.

- *Neutrophils*: These are the early response cells. They are present in the greatest numbers 24 hr after the injury. They are responsible for a diverse range of functions; including the production of more pro-inflammatory cytokines (further recruitment of inflammatory cells), release of proteases (breakdown), clearance of wound debris and formation of reactive oxygen species (antimicrobial).
- *Macrophages*: Monocytes transmigrate through the vessel wall and differentiate into macrophages. The role of macrophages in wound healing is complex. Macrophages can be activated via two pathways; classical pathway and the alternative pathway. Classically activated macrophages (M1) are microbicidal (production of reactive oxygen species) and pro-inflammatory. Alternatively, activated macrophages (M2) are anti-inflammatory and produce growth factors which help in tissue repair and fibrosis. Wound healing entails a switch from M1 to M2 phenotype. This is a critical step, the failure of which results in a chronic wound.[5,3]
- *Lymphocytes*: The role of lymphocytes in wound healing is not very well-defined. The dendritic epidermal T cells are thought to help in the keratinocyte proliferation after activation following inflammation.[4] It is also postulated that CD4+ T cells play an active role whereas CD8+ cells play an inhibitory role. An impaired healing is observed when there is delayed T cell infiltration into the site of injury.[4]

PROLIFERATION

Concurrent with the process of inflammation, the process of epithelial regeneration begins around 48 hr and can last for up to 14 days.

Re-epithelialization

In the first 24–48 hr, epithelial cells from both ends of the wound begin to migrate towards the center where they meet in the midline.[6] Fibroblastic growth factor-2 (FGF-2) and epidermal growth factor (EGF) play a pivotal role in this migration.[7,2] Epidermal stem cells which normally reside in the hair follicle niche also differentiate to form keratinocytes and contribute to re-epithelialization. The migrated keratinocytes then synthesize the underlying basement membrane (Fig. 3). A continuous layer is thus reestablished which acts as a barrier to microbial infection.

Angiogenesis

The formation of new blood vessels is a critical step of the healing process as new blood vessels are required for the transportation of nutrients and oxygen to the regenerative tissue.[4]

Angiogenesis (Fig. 4) can occur by sprouting of existing capillaries or by recruitment of bone marrow derived

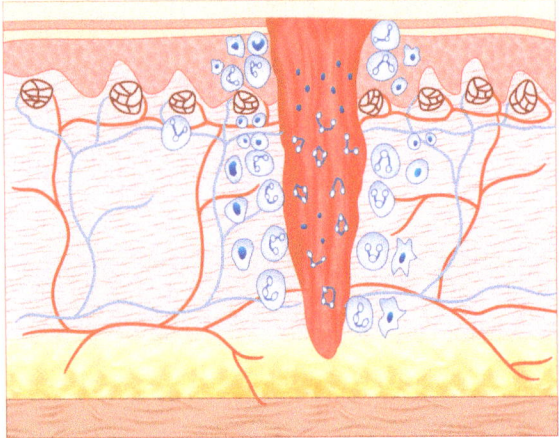

Fig. 2: Section of skin showing stage of inflammation with neutrophils and macrophages aggregated at the wound site.

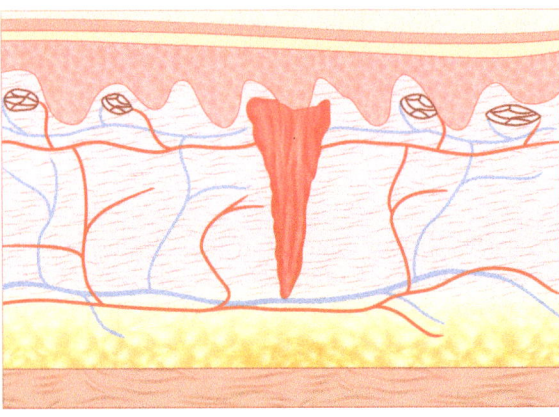

Fig. 3: Stage of re-epithelialization.

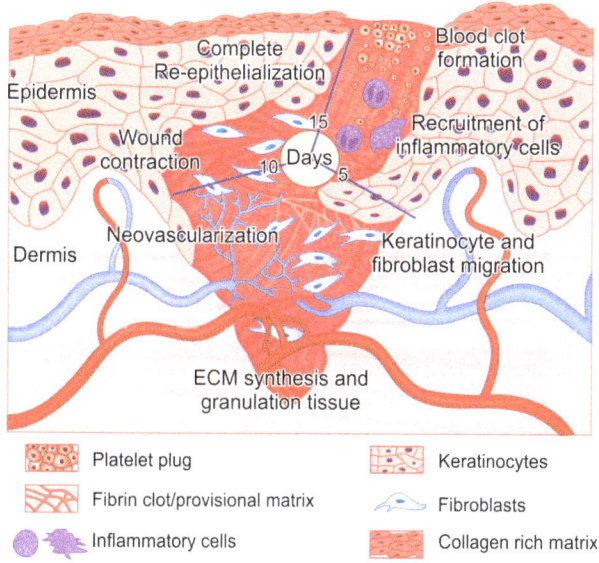

Fig. 4: Stage of angiogenesis.

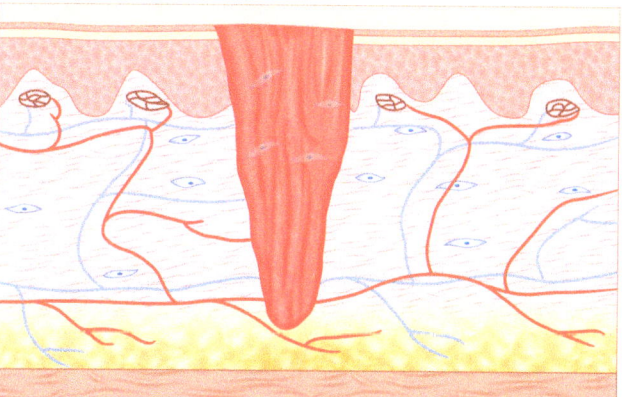

Fig. 5: Showing formation of granulation tissue with fibroblasts involved in wound retraction process.

stem cells under the effect of growth factors like vascular endothelial growth factor-A (VEGF-A).

The sprouting of capillaries begins with the dilation of the vessel wall at the site of injury followed by the vessel sprouting over an extracellular matrix scaffold. The endothelial cells begin to migrate towards the site and proliferate to form rudimentary tube like structures. These newly formed blood vessels are initially leaky but later become structurally sound with the recruitment of pericytes and smooth muscle cells under the influence of Angiopoietin 1 and 2.[2]

Angiogenesis depends on:
- *VEGF*: The production of VEGF at the site of injury is stimulated by platelet derived growth factor (PDGF) and transforming growth factor-α (TGF-α). VEGF have a variety of effects on angiogenesis including stimulation of endothelial cell migration, proliferation and formation of vascular lumina.
- *FGF*: It promotes proliferation of endothelial cells and epithelial cells.
- *Notch signaling*: Regulates sprouting and branching of vessels.

Formation of Granulation Tissue

Begins by day 4 of injury. At the site of injury, alternatively activated macrophages secrete transforming growth factor-β (TGF-β). The deposition of connective tissue is brought about by the fibroblasts which migrate from the periphery towards the site of injury and proliferate under the influence of TGF-β. These fibroblasts start depositing extracellular matrix, particularly collagen type III.[3] They also produce glycosaminoglycans and proteoglycans.[4] Newly formed blood vessels which are maximally seen by day 5, are leaky and give an edematous, reddish and granular appearance and hence the name granulation tissue/proud flesh (Fig. 5). Myofibroblasts which are rich in smooth muscle actin accumulate at the borders and begin the process of wound contraction.[3] Excessive activity of myofibroblasts can lead to skin contractures later.[8] Over a period of time, the cellular elements like the fibroblasts decrease and the amount of connective tissue increases.

REMODELING OF CONNECTIVE TISSUE

The collagen formed is subjected to a remodeling process (Fig. 6) which begins 2–3 weeks after the injury and can last for up to a year. Here the Type III collagen is gradually replaced by Type I collagen so that the maximum tensile strength is achieved.[9,3] The collagen bundles are generally thicker and slightly haphazardly arranged.[3]

The amount of collagen deposited is dependent not only on the production of collagen, but also on the degradation of collagen by matrix metalloproteinases (MMP) whose action is terminated by the inhibitors of matrix metalloproteinases.[2]

There are 4 families of metalloproteinases:
- *Interstitial collagenases*: Degrade Type I, II and III collagen
- *Gelatinases*: Type IV collagen and gelatin
- *Stromeolysins*: Type IV collagen and proteoglycans
- *Cysteine Proteinase (Cathepsin B)*: Lyse laminin of basement membrane (BM) and collagen IV, I and III.

Matrix metalloproteinases are produced in an inactive precursor form by a variety of cells and are activated at

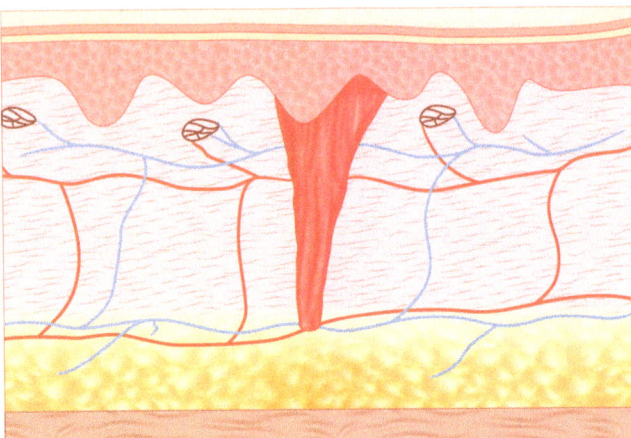

Fig. 6: Stage of connective tissue remodeling.

the site of injury by proteases. The tissue inhibitors of matrix metalloproteinases (TIMP's) are produced by the mesenchymal cells and they serve to terminate the function of MMP's. The delicate balance between these determines the type of scar formed.

Thus, the resultant scar comprises of dense and structurally strong connective tissue covered by the epidermis. But the dermal appendages which are damaged are permanently lost.

SCARLESS HEALING[8-11]

Several animal studies threw light on a highly interesting and potentially therapeutic finding; the presence of scarless healing in the fetus. The fetal wound healing process culminates in normal appearing epidermis containing epidermal appendages and normal collagen patterning. Studies have shown that the shift from scarless to scarring healing occurs around 24 weeks of gestation in humans.

This scarless healing in the fetus is postulated to be due to several reasons:
- Lack of inflammatory cells like neutrophils and macrophages in the fetus
- Interleukins 6 and 8 are seen in high levels in adult healing, fetal healing shows interleukin 10
- TGF β1 and β2 levels are higher in adult healing but TGF β3 levels are found to be higher in fetal healing
- Myofibroblasts are absent in the fetus.

CHRONIC WOUND[12]

The wound becomes chronic when:
- Inflammatory phase persists for prolonged periods of time
- Impaired M1 to M2 switch of macrophages
- High rate/early degradation of growth factors
- Lower amount of granulation tissue production
- High levels of matrix metalloproteinases/low levels of TIMP's

FACTORS INFLUENCING WOUND HEALING[2,4,6]

The following factors affect the wound healing process:
- *Advancing age*:
  - Altered inflammatory response
  - Delay in every stage of the healing process
  - Aged males have delayed wound healing as compared to aged females.
- Presence of infection
- *Diabetes*:
  - Hyperglycemia results in increased generation of reactive oxygen species resulting in oxidative stress
  - Advanced glycation end products retard healing
  - Diabetics have dysregulated inflammatory cell functions
  - Decreased VEGF and increased MMP activity is present.
- *Nutritional status*:
  - Glucose deficiency: Reduced adenosine triphosphate (ATP) synthesis
  - Protein deficiency: Affects proliferative and remodeling stage
  - Vitamin C deficiency: Vitamin C is required for hydroxylation of procollagen, and has antioxidant effect
  - Vitamin A deficiency: Altered modulation of cellular differentiation
  - Vitamin E deficiency: Vitamin E is an antiscarring and antioxidant agent.
- *Medication glucocorticoids*: Cause weak scar formation due to anti-inflammatory effects and reduced collagen synthesis
- *Mechanical factors*: Increased local pressure, increased wound tension
- *Poor perfusion*: Old age and diabetics
- *Obesity*: Adipokines secreted by adipocytes alter the immune response, improved by weight loss
- Foreign bodies at site of injury
- Type and extent of injury.

HEALING OF SKIN WOUNDS

Depending on the extent of injury and repair process needed, the healing of skin wounds is divided into the following two types:
1. Healing by first intention
2. Healing by second intention.

Healing by first intention takes place when the damage is restricted to the epithelium and the repair takes place by epithelial regeneration.

Healing by second intention takes place when the area of injury is large and irregular. The repair process also involves a combination of regeneration and scar formation.

Healing by second intention as compared to healing by primary intention involves a more intense inflammatory reaction with abundant formation of granulation tissue to fill the large defect. Healing process takes a longer time, also wound contraction by myofibroblasts is more pronounced in healing by second intention.

WOUND STRENGTH[2]

- 1 week: 10%
- 3 months: 70–80% of normal.

CONCLUSION

Wound healing is a complex interaction of cascade of cellular events leading to re-epithelialization, reconstitution and restoration of the tensile strength of the ulcerated skin.

REFERENCES

1. Shah JB. The history of wound care. J Am Col Certif Wound Spec. 2011;3(3):65-66.
2. Kumar V, Abbas AK, Fausto N, et al. Tissue renewal, repair and regeneration. Pathologic basis of Disease. 8th Edition. Philadelphia: Elsevier Saunders; 2010: pp. 79-110.
3. Gonzalez AC, Costa TG, Andrade ZA, et al. Wound healing - A literature review. An Bras Dermatol. 2016;91(5):614-20.
4. Guo S, Dipietro LA. Factors affecting wound healing. J Dent Res. 2010;89(3):219-29.
5. Herter EK, Landén NX. Non-Coding RNAs: New players in skin wound healing. Adv Wound Care. 2017;6(3):93-107.
6. Harsh Mohan. Inflammation & Repair. Textbook of Pathology. 7th Edition. New Delhi: Jaypee Brothers Medical Publishers; 2015: pp. 116-4.
7. Li Y, Zhang J, Yue J, et al. Epidermal stem cells in skin wound healing. Adv Wound Care. 2017;6(9):297-307.
8. Marshall CD, Hu MS, Leavitt T, et al. Cutaneous scarring: Basic science, current treatments, and future directions. Adv Wound Care. 2018;7(2):29-45.
9. Barnes LA, Marshall CD, Leavitt T, et al. Mechanical forces in cutaneous wound healing: Emerging therapies to minimize scar formation. Adv Wound Care. 2018;7(2):47-56.
10. Erickson JR, Echeverri K. Learning from regeneration research organisms: The circuitous road to scar free wound healing. Dev Biol. 2018;433(2):144-54.
11. Leavitt T, Hu MS, Marshall CD, et al. Scarless wound healing: Finding the right cells and signals. Cell Tissue Res. 2016;365(3): 483-93.
12. Larouche J, Sheoran S, Maruyama K, et al. Immune regulation of skin wound healing: Mechanisms and novel therapeutic targets. Adv Wound Care. 2018;7(7):209-31.

CHAPTER 6

History Taking and Examination in Chronic Leg Ulcers

Shilpa K, S Sacchidanand

INTRODUCTION

The evaluation and management of lower extremity ulcers are an essential yet difficult task for a dermatologist. Because many a times the differential diagnosis and treatment of chronic and nonhealing leg ulcers include conditions and therapeutic modalities, which are beyond the domain of dermatologist and often intrude on almost every major medical and surgical subspecialty. However in majority of the patients, the ulcers are caused by venous insufficiency, peripheral arterial occlusive disease, or neuropathies with very few cases due to other uncommon conditions. Evaluation in chronic leg ulcers should include proper history, clinical examination and relevant investigations depending on history and clinical findings.

HISTORY TAKING

A stepwise workup with thorough history taking, physical examination, and bedside diagnostic tests are essential to assess the nature of a patient's underlying disease. Later, these findings may be supplemented with confirmatory diagnostic tests. Initial evaluation should begin in the office setting with a thorough history. The history should include the following things.

History Pertaining to Venous Insufficiency

- Occupation of the patient—certain occupations requiring standing for long duration like teachers, conductors can predispose to development of venous insufficiency.
- Symptoms suggestive of venous insufficiency as listed in Box 1.

Box 1: Symptoms suggestive of venous insufficiency.
- Swelling of lower limbs
- Dragging pain on standing for long duration
- Tightness/heaviness of legs
- Skin irritation/pruritus
- Tingling
- Muscle cramps
- Cosmetically unacceptable linear swellings
- Skin pigmentation
- Ulceration

- Worsening of symptoms during the course of the day and with prolonged standing.
- Specific features about the pain must include the degree to which the pain interferes with the patient's day-to-day life and work.
- The duration for which the patient can stand before the pain or swelling appears.
- The history regarding age of onset of varicose veins is important to rule out congenital abnormality such as Klippel-Trenaunay syndrome, which begins very early in life.
- Relevant medical and surgical history of the past should include previous deep vein thrombosis, pulmonary embolism, cellulitis, limb or pelvic surgery, trauma.
- History regarding previous treatments for varicose veins, like operative and percutaneous procedures.
- History pertaining to ulcer like the number, location, duration, prior treatments, the course and treatment of all current ulcers.

History in relation to arterial disease includes history of/history suggestive of:
- Pre-existing disorders that predispose to the development of arterial occlusion like diabetes, thyroid disease, coronary artery disease, hyperlipidemia, renal disease, hypertension, strokes.
- Alcohol and tobacco use
- Collagen vascular disorders, vasculitis
- Hypercoagulable status with embolization
- Any tumors pressing on arteries
- Claudication pain, cold, and clammy extremities
- Bluish discoloration in relation to cold
- Discoloration of digits or autoamputation

History in relation to neuropathic disorders includes history of/history suggestive of:
- Diabetes mellitus
- Hansen's disease
- Familial neuropathies
- Spontaneous painless blistering of hands and soles
- Difficulty in wearing footwear, dryness of skin
- Pricking and burning sensation on foot and hands.

History in Relation to Miscellaneous Conditions

- Preexisting skin conditions (malignant and premalignant ulcerating conditions)
- History of trauma as a source of infections
- History of any metabolic disorders
- Gross swelling of limbs suggestive of lymphatic obstruction
- Endocrine disorders—thyroid disorders, diabetes
- Gastrointestinal diseases due to association with pyoderma gangrenosum, bowel bypass syndrome.
- Renal disorders presenting as Kyrle's disease, reactive perforating collagenosis, calciphylaxis.
- Hematological disorders, autoimmune blistering disorders of skin, nutritional deficiencies, genetic, and mechanical blistering disorders.

History in Relation to Ulcers

- Number, size, location of ulcers
- Onset, progression, and duration of ulcers
- History of discharge—quantity, color, odor
- Associated symptoms—painless, painful, itching, burning sensation, pricking sensation
- Surrounding skin changes.

PHYSICAL EXAMINATION

A proper history should be followed by thorough physical examination, which includes general physical examination along with careful examination of lower extremities.

Prerequisites
- Examination should be done in a well lit and warm room
- It is suitable to undress the patient allowing complete exposure of lower limbs from groin to toes.

Ulcer Examination

Ulcer examination is very important as its morphology gives clue to the underlying cause. Ulcer-specific examination should include recording the location and size, shape, edge, base, border of each ulcer, percentage of necrotic tissue, granulation tissue, and fibrinous tissue on the ulcer bed and the magnitude and odor of the exudate. Findings in ulcers of various etiologies have been tabulated in Table 1 (Figs. 1 to 6).

Examination of Skin around the Ulcers

The perilesional skin should be examined to know its hair distribution, induration, intactness, maceration, dryness, scaling, weeping, cellulitis, hyperkeratosis and signs of inflammation like erythema, tenderness, edema, increased temperature, and so forth. Scarring from previous ulceration, atrophie blanche, gangrenous digits, clubbing, cyanosis, obvious varicose veins, livedo reticularis, and perilesional

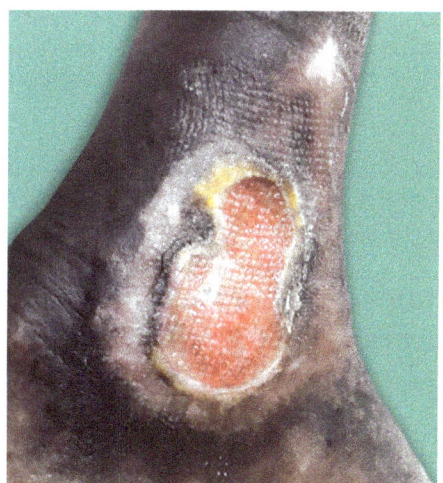

Fig. 1: Irregular shallow ulcer in gaiter area due to venous insufficiency also note the pigmentation and sclerosis in surrounding skin.

Table 1: Findings in ulcers of various etiologies.

Etiology	Site of ulcer	Size and shape Floor	Edge/border	Surrounding skin	Pain/other symptoms
Venous insufficiency	Gaiter area	Irregular shallow ulcers of varied size Typically "wet" with moderate to heavy exudate (Figs. 1 and 2)	Sloping edges	Indurated, inflamed, weeping, edema, varicose veins, hair loss, hyperpigmentation	Mild-to-moderate, better with elevation
Arterial insufficiency	Toes, ankles, anterior tibia	Dry, necrotic, pale, fibrotic	Punched-out	Cool, cyanotic, delayed capillary refill	Moderate-to-severe claudication pain, rest pain, better with dependency
Neuropathic ulcers	Pressure sites, metatarsal heads, heels (Fig. 3)	Single or multiple well-defined ulcers Pink, moist, callus formation	Hyperkeratotic edges	Charcot's deformity, Architectural changes in foot, Amputation of toes (Fig. 4)	Painless because of neuropathy
Vasculitic ulcers	Variable	Single or multiple well-defined ulcers (Fig. 5) Size varies with caliber of vessel involved hemorrhagic, palpable purpura	Punched-out or jagged	Retiform purpura, livedo reticularis, atrophie blanche	Moderate-to-severe, not positional
Emboli	Typically unilateral toes, malleoli	Sloughy, devitalized tissue in the wound base and low levels of wound exudate	Punched-out	Cold leg, Decreased or no pulse in leg Toes and foot feel cool, Gangrene, cyanosis, livedo reticularis, nodules, and purpura	Sudden onset with severe pain
Pyoderma gangrenosum	Sites of trauma, common on lower legs, shin	Annular, cribriform, satellite pustules, multiple	Violaceous rolled margin (Fig. 6)	Stellate scarring	Severe, disproportionate to the size of ulcer

purpura or fibrosis, lipodermatosclerosis should also be noted if any. The skin changes, specific for various etiologies, have been tabulated in Table 2 (Figs. 7 to 9).

Examination in Suspected Venous Insufficiency as the Cause of Ulcer

Inspection

The location and distribution of all major subcutaneous varicosities should be noted. The findings should be recorded using charts or line diagrams. Large varicosities especially over the anatomical areas of perforators should be noted. Presence or absence of edema, vascular malformation should be noted. Spider veins, if any, should be recorded. Cutaneous changes like pigmentation, scars, atrophic blanche, lipodermatosclerosis, ulceration should be documented.

Palpation

All the inspectory findings should be confirmed by palpation. Palpation of the limbs may detect additional varicosities that are not readily appreciated by inspection, especially the terminal segments of the greater saphenous

History Taking and Examination in Chronic Leg Ulcers

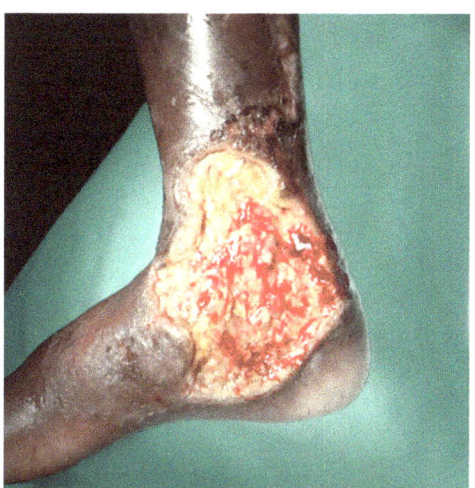

Fig. 2: An irregular large and deep ulcer in gaiter area due to venous insufficiency with secondary infection.

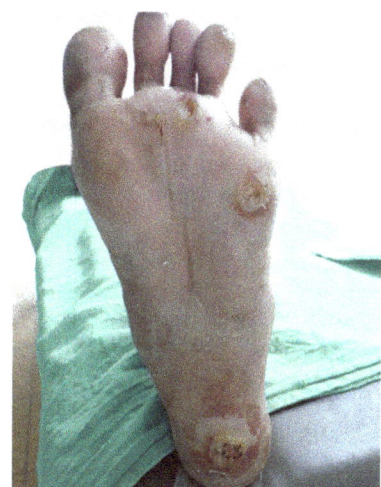

Fig. 3: Multiple well-defined ulcers with hyperkeratotic edges in pressure-bearing areas—neuropathic ulcers.

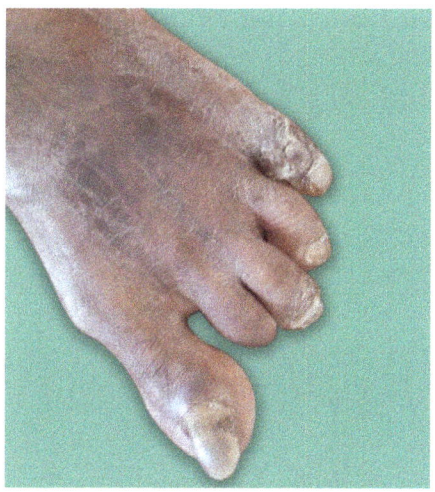

Fig. 4: Autoamputation of second toe in a Hansen's patient.

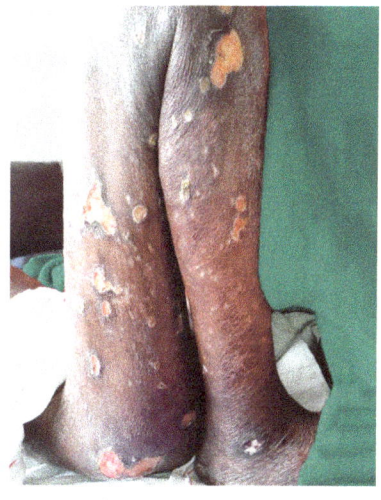

Fig. 5: Multiple well-defined ulcers with punched-out borders due to vasculitis.

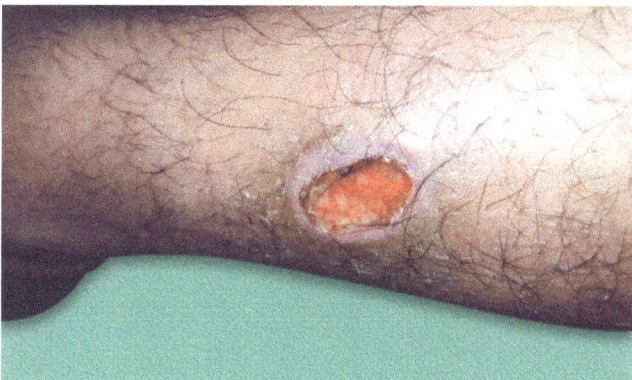

Fig. 6: Painful punched out ulcer with violaceous border due to pyoderma gangrenosum.

vein (GSV) (inner thigh) and lesser saphenous vein (LSV) (calf) where they join the femoral and popliteal veins, respectively. Palpation also throws light on presence of areas of induration, firm subcutaneous cords (due to previous episodes of thrombophlebitis), and presence of temperature difference between the legs.

Bedside Tests

- *Cough impulse test*: This test is performed while the patient is in standing position. Proximal part of the thigh at fossa ovalis (Fig. 10) is palpated and the patient is asked to cough. A palpable thrill at the saphenofemoral junction (SFJ), as a result of turbulent retrograde flow,

Table 2: The skin changes—specific for various etiologies.	
Surrounding skin changes	*Suggestive of:*
Indurated, inflamed, weeping, edema, varicose veins, hair loss, hyperpigmentation	Venous insufficiency
Cutaneous changes like pigmentation, eczema, scars, atrophic blanche, lipodermatosclerosis (Fig. 8), inverted champagne bottle (Fig. 8) appearance	
Cool, cyanotic, delayed capillary refill, disuse atrophy of surrounding structures	Arterial insufficiency
Charcot's deformity, architectural changes in foot	Neuropathic ulcers
Cold leg,	Emboli
Decreased or no pulsations in leg	
Toes and foot feel cool,	
Gangrene (Fig. 9), cyanosis, livedo reticularis, nodules, and purpura	
Stellate scarring	Pyoderma gangrenosum
Retiform purpura, livedo reticularis, atrophie blanche	Vasculitis

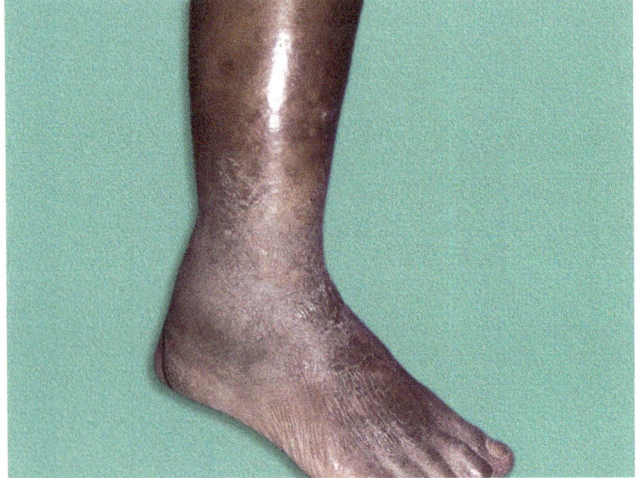

Fig. 7: Eczematous pigmented skin due to venous insufficiency.

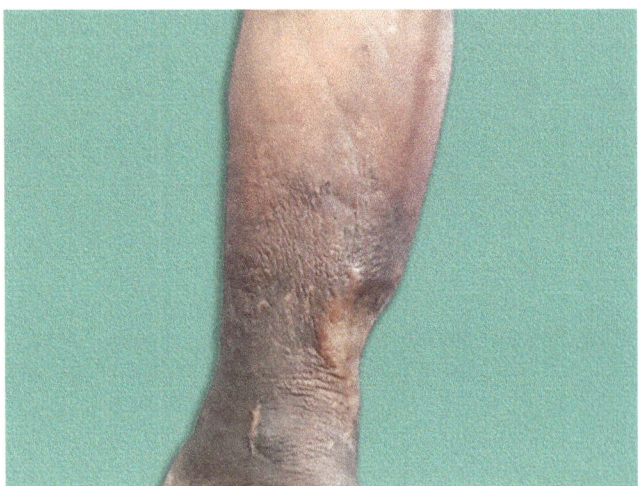

Fig. 8: Lipodermatosclerosis with inverted champagne bottle appearance.

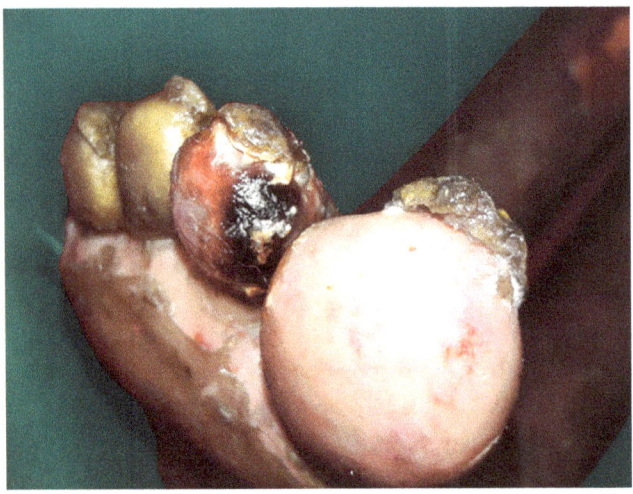

Fig. 9: Gangrenous changes due to arterial insufficiency.

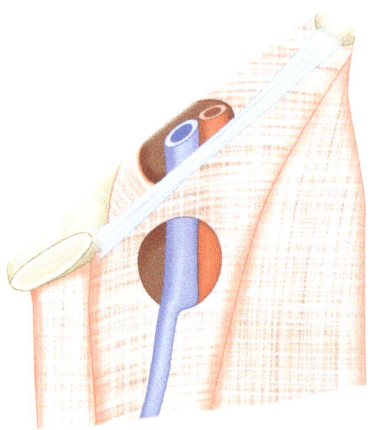

Fig. 10: Fossa ovalis.

indicates reflux at the SFJ. The drawback of the test is—it is difficult to perform in obese individuals.

- *The tap test or percussion test*: This test is also performed while palpating the SFJ in standing position. The GSV is tapped at the level of the knee. A palpable transmitted impulse at the SFJ suggests that the GSV is distended with blood. Conversely, the SFJ is then tapped while the GSV is palpated at the knee. A palpable transmitted pulse at the knee with this maneuver indicates incompetence of GSV valves between the SFJ and the knee.[1]
- *Brodie–Trendelenburg test*: Brodie–Trendelenburg test is done to differentiate between perforator and GSV incompetence. The Brodie–Trendelenburg test is highly sensitive for the identification of superficial veins and perforator reflux (91%), although poorly specific (15%).[1] The test is performed with patient in supine position. First, the superficial lower extremity veins are drained by raising the lower limbs to 45° and gently stroking the limb along the course of the major veins from foot toward thigh. A tourniquet is applied as close to the groin as possible and tight enough to prevent reflux in superficial veins. Then the patient is made to stand and leg is examined for refilling of veins (Figs. 11A to C). If the distal veins remain collapsed for 15–30 seconds after standing, the tourniquet is released.[2] Interpretation of the test is given in the Table 3.
- *Modified Trendelenburg test*: In this test firstly, the leg is elevated and the veins are emptied. The tourniquet is applied to control the saphenous vein near fossa ovalis. The patient then stands up and the tourniquet is removed at once. The sudden filling of varicose veins from above down indicates a reflux through a saphenous femoral valve and valvular incompetence.[3]

Table 3: Interpretation of Brodie–Trendelenburg test.

Observation	Inference
If the caudal veins fill rapidly when the patient stands with the tourniquet in place	Perforator incompetence is suggested
The location of the incompetent perforator can then be determined by varying the position of the tourniquet	
Rapid filling of the varices with a tourniquet in the suprapatellar position	Incompetent mid-thigh perforator
Rapid filling with the tourniquet below the knee	Incompetent lower leg perforators
If the distal veins fill rapidly upon release of the tourniquet	SFJ incompetence

(SFJ: saphenofemoral junction)

Table 4: Interpretation of Perthes test.

Observation	Inference
Emptying of the varicose veins	The site of reflux is cranial to the tourniquet, namely the SFJ, saphenopopliteal junction (SPJ), or thigh perforators
Persistence of distended varicose veins	The site of reflux caudal to the tourniquet, that is calf perforator
Pain associated with heel raising	It suggests the possibility of deep venous obstruction

(SFJ: saphenofemoral junction)

- *Perthes test*: Perthes test is highly sensitive but poorly specific similar to Trendelenburg test. It is performed with the patient in standing position with a tourniquet below the knee (Figs. 12A and B). The patient is asked to raise heel ten times to activate the calf muscle pump.[2] Interpretation of Perthes test is given in Table 4.
- *Modified Perthes test*: The leg is elevated and the veins are emptied. A tourniquet is applied to the upper thigh to constrict the saphenous vein return flow. The patient then walks around the room for 5 minutes. Absence of pain in the calf or definite swelling of the foot and ankle indicates patent deep veins.[3]

Evaluation for Arterial Insufficiency

Inspection

Clinical findings suggestive of arterial insufficiency include cyanosis/pallor, hair loss, shiny skin, ulcerations, dystrophic nails, edema, and gangrenous changes.

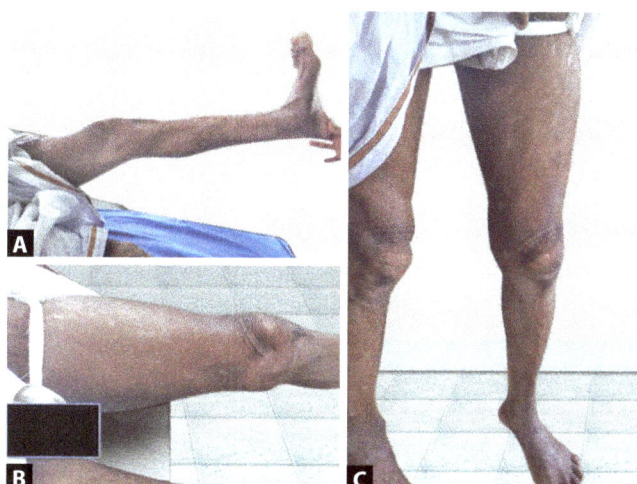

Figs. 11A to C: Demonstration of Brodie–Trendelenburg test.

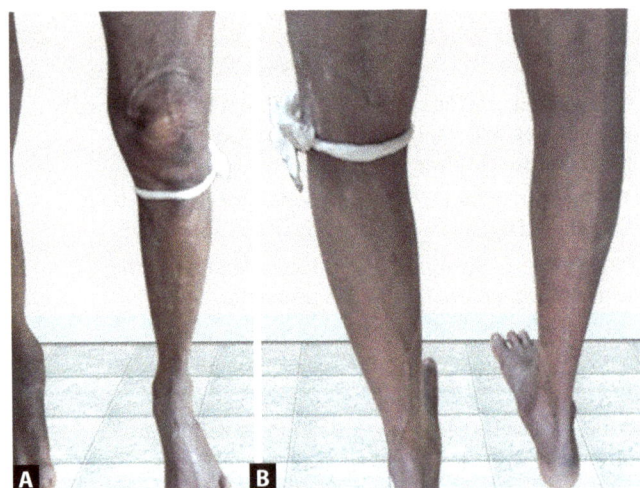

Figs. 12A and B: Demonstration of Perthes test.

Table 5: Anatomical landmark for lower limb vessels.

Artery	Anatomical land mark
Femoral	Midway between the pubis and ASIS (anterior–superior iliac spine)
Popliteal	Inferior lateral portion of the popliteal fossa (leg slightly flexed)
Posterior tibial	Inferior posterior border of medial malleolus
Dorsalis pedis	Upper one-third of dorsal foot, lateral to EHL (extensor hallucis longus)

Palpation

- Check for skin temperature and compare with the opposite side—the limb with arterial insufficiency will be cooler than the normal limb.
- Capillary refill time delayed in arterial insufficiency
- Check pulses (Table 5)
- Radiofemoral delay.

Auscultation

Check for bruit over femoral and popliteal arteries to rule out arteriovenous (AV) malformation.

Provocative tests

Systolic pressures can be taken at different locations in the lower extremities to help identify the location of arterial disease. Most commonly, pressures are taken at the high thigh, lower thigh, calf, and ankle.

A pressure gradient more than 20 mm Hg between cuffs is considered indicative of significant arterial disease. For example, a pressure difference of more than 20 mm Hg between the high and low thigh cuffs indicates the presence of a hemodynamically significant superficial femoral artery stenosis. Segmental pressures can give a general idea of the location of the disease, but cannot ascertain the exact site, extent, or severity of a lesion.[4]

Buerger's Test

Buerger's test is used to assess arterial sufficiency. The vascular angle, which is also called Buerger's angle, is the angle to which the leg has to be raised before it becomes pale, while in supine decubitus. In a limb with a normal circulation, the toes and sole of the foot stay pink, even when the limb is raised by 90°. In an ischemic leg, elevation to 15° or 30° for 30-60 seconds may cause pallor. (This part of the test checks for elevation pallor.) A vascular angle of less than 20° indicates severe ischemia.[5,6]

- *Check for rubor of dependency*: Raise the patient's legs to 45° for a minute. When a maximum blanching is seen, the patient is made to sit with both legs dangling down. In normal circulation, the foot will quickly return to pink color usually within 10 seconds. Whereas in peripheral artery disease, the leg will revert to the pink color more slowly than normal and also pass through the normal pink to red color, often known as sunset foot. This is due to the dilatation of the arterioles in an attempt to rid the metabolic waste that has built up in a reactive hyperemia. Finally, the foot will return to its normal color.

DeWeese's test

Disappearance of previously palpable distal pulses after walking.

Physical Examination in Suspected Neuropathic Ulcer

Sensory Test

The nylon monofilament test is performed to diagnose the presence of sensory neuropathy.[7] A 10-gauge monofilament nylon is pressed against each specific site of the foot with pressure just enough to bend the wire. If the patient does not feel the wire at 4 or more of these 10 sites, the test is positive for neuropathy. The clinician can also use professional Semmes-Weinstein filaments. In case of

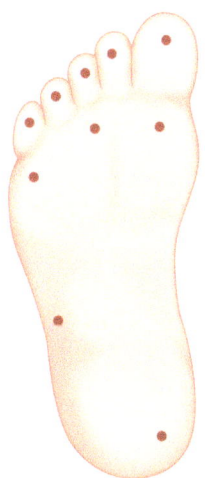

Fig. 13: WHO recommended sites for sensory examination of foot in Hansen's disease.

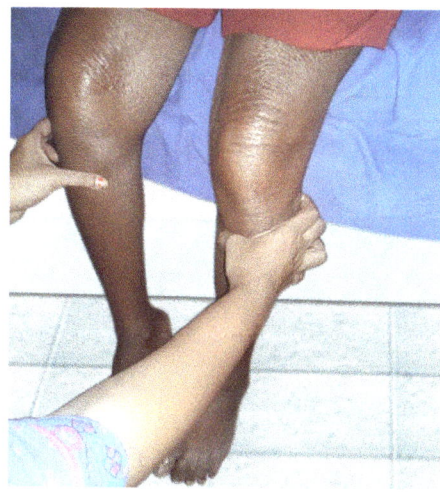

Fig. 14: Examination of lateral popliteal nerves.

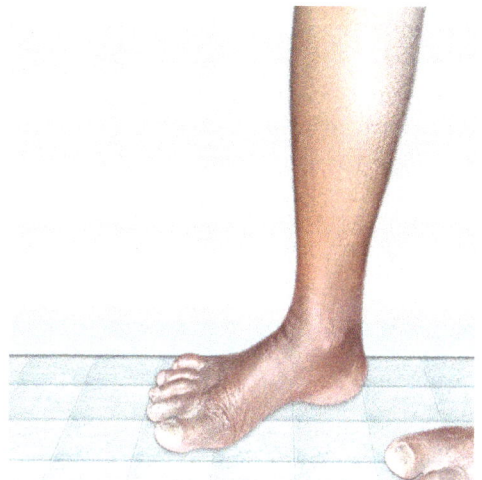

Fig. 15: Examination of superficial peroneal nerves.

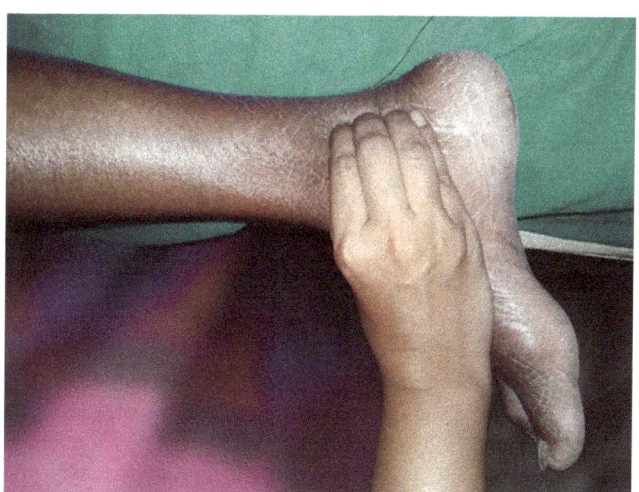

Fig. 16: Examination of posterior tibial nerve.

suspected Hansen's disease, sensation has to be checked on hypopigmented patches and glove-stocking distribution. The WHO recommended sites for sensory testing is given in Figure 13.

Examination of Peripheral Nerves

In suspected leprosy case, peripheral nerves have to be examined for thickening (regular/irregular), beading, tenderness, and fibrosis. The nerves to be examined in lower limb and their site has been tabulated in Table 6 (Figs. 14 to 17).

Examination of Motor Power of Lower Limbs

Clinical test to detect motor weakness of lower limbs have been tabulated in Table 7 (Figs. 18 and 19).

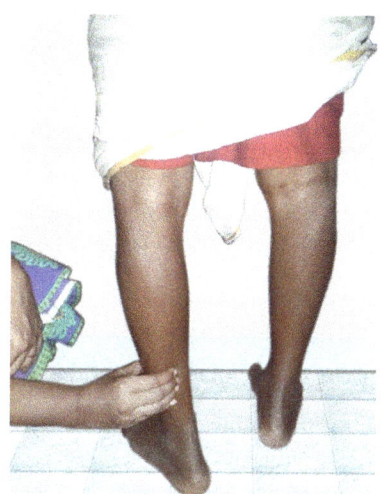

Fig. 17: Examination of sural nerve.

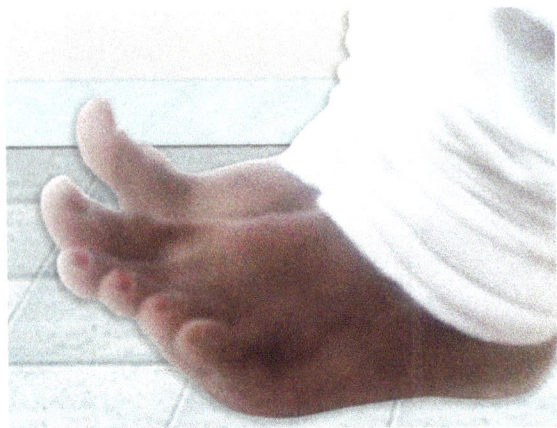

Fig. 18: Clinical test for dorsiflexors.

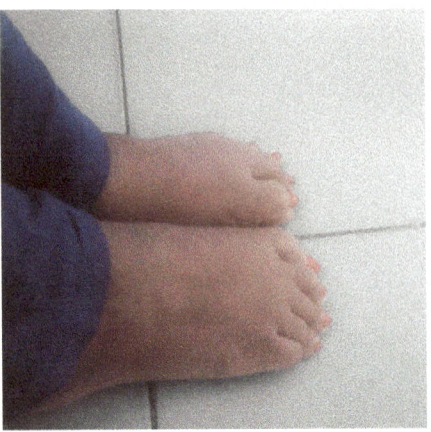

Fig. 19: Test for intrinsic muscles of foot.

Table 6: Anatomical site for lower limb nerve examination.

Nerve	Site
Lateral popliteal nerves	Make patient sit with legs hanging down with knee flexed. Palpate lateral popliteal nerve on the lateral part head of fibula as the nerve winds over it (Fig. 14).
Superficial peroneal nerves	Ankle should be gently internally rotated and plantar flexed. The nerve can be easily seen and palpated in front of the ankle coming toward second and third toe, if it is thickened (Fig. 15)
Posterior tibial nerve	Patient with sitting position, the nerve is palpated between posterior border of medial malleolus and Achilles tendon (Fig. 16).
Sural nerve	Patient in standing position, nerve is palpated between two bellies of gastrocnemius muscle (Fig. 17).

Table 7: Clinical test to detect motor weakness of lower limbs.

Clinical test	Interpretation	Nerve involved
Patient is made to stand on heels keeping all the toes lifted above the ground (Fig. 18)[8]	Normally a healthy individual can stand in that position for few seconds. Inability to stand indicates weakness of dorsiflexors	Common peroneal nerve
Patient is made to keep the feet firmly on ground and asked to retract the toes backwards (Fig. 19).[8]	Curling of toes rather than retraction indicates weakness of intrinsic muscles of feet	Tibial nerve

REFERENCES

1. Kim J, Richards S, Kent PJ. Clinical examination of varicose veins: a validation study. Ann R Coll Surg Engl. 2000;82:171-5.
2. Krishnan S, Nicholls SC. Chronic venous insufficiency: Clinical assessment and patient selection. Semin Intervent Radiol. 2005;22(3):169-77.
3. Pratt GH. Test for incompetent communicating branches in the surgical treatment of varicose veins. JAMA. 1941;117(2):100-1.
4. AbuRahma AF, Khan S, Robinson PA. Selective use of segmental Doppler pressures and color duplex imaging in the localization of arterial occlusive disease of the lower extremity. Surgery 1995;118:496-503.
5. Browse NL, Black J, Burnand KG, et al. Browse's introduction to the symptoms and signs of surgical disease, 4th edition/International student edition. Boca Raton, FL: CRC Press; 2005. p. 175.
6. Insall RL, Davies RJ, Prout WG. Significance of Buerger's test in the assessment of lower limb ischemia. J R Soc Med. 1989;82(12):729-31.
7. Mayfield JA, Sugarman JR. The use of Semmes-Weinstein filament and other threshold test for preventing foot ulceration and amputation in persons with Diabetes. J Fram Pract. 2000;49(11):517-29.
8. Srinivasan H. Guidelines for implementing disability prevention programme in the field. Indian J Lepr Rev. 1999;71:541-62.

CHAPTER 7

Venous Leg Ulcers

Amina Asfiya, Manjunath Shenoy

INTRODUCTION

Venous leg ulcers (VLU) are also known as "varicose ulcer", "gravitational ulcer", "stasis ulcer" or "hypo-static ulcer".[1] Venous ulcers account for approximately 60–80% of leg ulcers. Their prevalence is estimated to be between 0.18% and 1%. As the age increases above 65, the prevalence rises to 4%. They are called chronic leg ulcers if they last for more than 6 weeks, which is seen in 33–60%. Venous leg ulcers can be defined as open lesions between the knee and ankle joint that occur in the presence of venous disease.[2] Chronic venous leg ulcers cause significant morbidity and mortality leading to functional disability, emotional distress and increased financial burden.

ETIOPATHOGENESIS

The exact etiology of venous ulcers is uncertain. Many direct and indirect risk factors are associated with the development of venous ulceration (Table 1). Several of the recent hypothesis propose that microcirculatory abnormalities result in inflammatory response. (Table 1).

- *Fibrin cuff theory:*[3] Dilated capillaries in the epidermis lead to leakage of fibrinogen, which then forms a pericapillary fibrin cuff. This results in decreased diffusion of oxygenated blood to the surrounding tissues which results in ulceration.
- *Leukocyte entrapment theory*: The decreased pressure gradient between the capillary ends, causes slow movement of blood within capillaries and increases the cell adhesion to the endothelium. This releases inflammatory mediators [intercellular adhesion molecule-1 (ICAM-1), vascular cell adhesion molecule-1 (VCAM-1) and reactive oxygen species] causing obliteration of capillary loops and thus aggravates the existing ischemia and causes ulceration.
- *Microangiopathy theory*: According to this theory, capillaries are occluded by microthrombi or show capillary stasis. This cause reduced oxygenation and nutrition to the tissues, leading to ulceration.
- *Cytokine dysregulation*: Chronicity of ulcers is due to the cytokine and growth factor dysregulation which includes—transforming growth factor β (TGF-β), tumor necrosis factor-α (TNF-α) and matrix metalloproteinases.[2]
- *Miscellaneous*: Thrombophilic conditions including the following are also implicated:
  - Factor V Leiden mutation
  - Prothrombin mutation
  - Deficiency of antithrombin
  - Presence of antiphospholipid antibodies
  - Protein C and S deficiencies
  - Hyperhomocysteinemia[2]
- Venous hypertension

Table 1: Risk factors for venous ulceration.[4]

Direct	Indirect
Varicose veins	Risk factors causing deep vein thrombosis (protein-C, protein-S, and anti-thrombin III deficiency)
Deep vein thrombosis	Family history
Chronic venous insufficiency	Ulceration preceded by minor trauma
Insufficient calf muscle functioning	
Arteriovenous fistulae	
Increased body mass index (BMI)	
History of leg fracture	

CLASSIFICATION OF CHRONIC VENOUS INSUFFICIENCY

The CEAP classification consists of four parameters: the clinical manifestation (C), the etiologic factors (E), the anatomic distribution of disease (A), and the underlying pathophysiology (P)[5] (Table 2).

CLINICAL FEATURES

History[5]

- Typical symptoms include muscle ache, muscle cramps, pain, skin tautness, skin irritation, itching, heaviness, tingling, and the presence of dilated veins. Standing for long hours worsens the symptoms.
- Advanced stages of venous insufficiency may lead to edema, cutaneous changes, and ulceration.
- It is important to rule out arterial insufficiency, diabetes mellitus and neurotrophic causes by detailed history.

Physical Examination

- Always examine the patient in standing position and undressed from the groins to the toes to facilitate complete examination.
- A careful examination should be done to look for the presence of dilated veins, record the distribution and location of the varicosities.
- Palpation of the legs to look for rise in temperature, indurated areas, and presence of firm subcutaneous cords should be done.
- Several bedside tests may be performed to know the source of venous insufficiency. They include cough impulse test to know the saphenofemoral incompetence, Brodie-Trendelenburg test which helps to differentiate between perforator and great saphenofemoral vein incompetence and Perthe's test.[6]

Dermatological Manifestations

Cutaneous changes include:
- Ankle edema which progresses towards evening.
- Venous eczema (gravitational eczema, stasis dermatitis) occurs secondary to venous hypertension. It presents commonly around ankles and lower legs as pruritic, eczematous patches[6] (Fig. 1).
- Hemosiderin deposit[7] (reddish brown pigmentation) which occurs due to leakage of red blood cells from endothelium to the interstitium, resulting in conversion of hemoglobin to hemosiderin. It is usually seen in lower medial third of the leg.
- *Lipodermatosclerosis*: Chronic venous hypertension can lead to progressive fibrosis of skin and underlying subcutaneous tissues which is called as lipodermatosclerosis. It maybe acute or chronic. The acute form is painful with local rise of temperature in the affected

Table 2: CEAP classification system for chronic venous insufficiency.

C Class: Clinical Manifestation	E Class: Etiologic Factors	A Class: Anatomic Distribution	P Class: Pathophysiology
C0: No visible or palpable signs of venous disease	Ec: Congenital	As: Superficial veins	Pr: Reflux
C1: Telangiectasias or reticular veins	Ep: Primary	Ap: Perforator veins	Po: Obstruction
C2: Varicose veins, distinguished from reticular veins by a diameter ≥ 3 mm	Es: Secondary (post-thrombotic)	Ad: Deep veins	Pr,o: Reflux and obstruction
C3: Edema	En: No venous cause identified	An: No venous location identified	Pn: No venous pathophysiology identifiable
C4: Changes in skin and subcutaneous tissue			
C4a: Pigmentation or eczema			
C4b: Lipodermatosclerosis or atrophie blanche			
C5: Healed venous ulcer			
C6: Active venous ulcer			

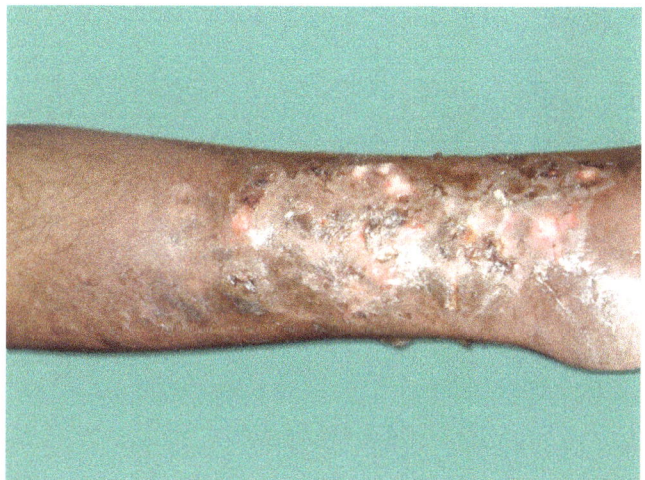

Fig. 1: Stasis Dermatitis.

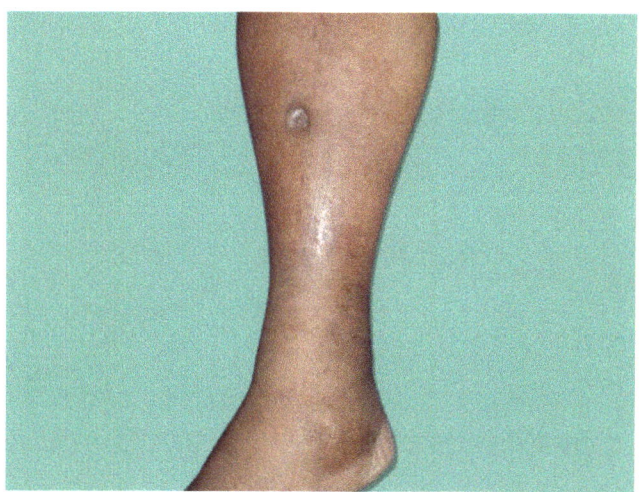

Fig. 2: Inverted champagne bottle appearance.

area. It presents as thickened raised red-brown area in the lower leg. It eventually progresses to become chronic which is characterized by stiff and shiny skin that is hard and indurated, due to contraction of the underlying subcutaneous tissues.

- *Altered shape*: Progressive contraction of skin and the underlying subcutaneous tissues leads to shrinking of the ankle region which along with edema in the calf above, gives the appearance of inverted "champagne bottle" (Fig. 2).
- *Atrophie blanche*: It clinically appears as atrophic porcelain white scars with hyperpigmentation and telangiectasia. It occurs after the ulcer has healed in venous disease and is commonly localized above the malleoli.
- *Ankle flare (corona phlebectatica or malleolar flare)*: presence of multiple small intradermal vessels around ankle or foot in a fan shaped manner, believed to be an early indicator of advanced venous insufficiency (Fig. 3).
- Healed ulcers in the surrounding skin.
- Dilated and tortuous superficial veins.

VENOUS ULCER

- The most common site of ulceration is anterior to medial malleolus, pretibial area, lower third of leg known as the gaiter region.[2] The margins are well defined with irregular edges, shallow depth and yellow white color exudates. The ulcer bed shows the presence of a fibrinous layer mixed with granulation tissue[8] (Figs. 4 and 5)
- Pain may be extreme, mild or absent. It is severe in the evenings and usually resolves by leg elevation.[2]

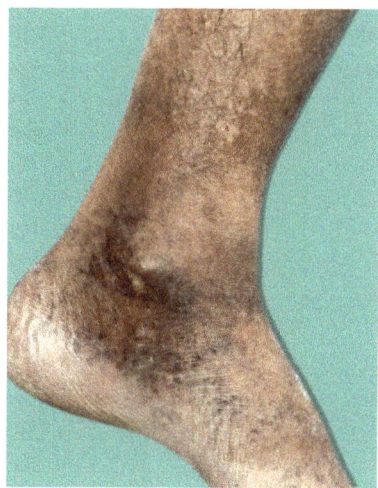

Fig. 3: Ankle flare.

Chronic venous ulcers can lead to osteomyelitis and rarely malignant transformation.

ARTERIAL DISEASE

The occurrence of mixed arterial-venous ulcers ranges from 10–18%. This knowledge becomes important while providing compression therapy, since in patients with chronic venous disease with ankle brachial pressure index (ABPI) less than 0.5, compression therapy is contraindicated. Also clinically, palpation of peripheral pulses becomes difficult in the presence of large venous ulcers. Hence, in the presence of persistent ulceration, intolerance to compression therapy, one has to keep in mind the possibility of mixed arterial-venous ulcers[9,10] (Table 3).

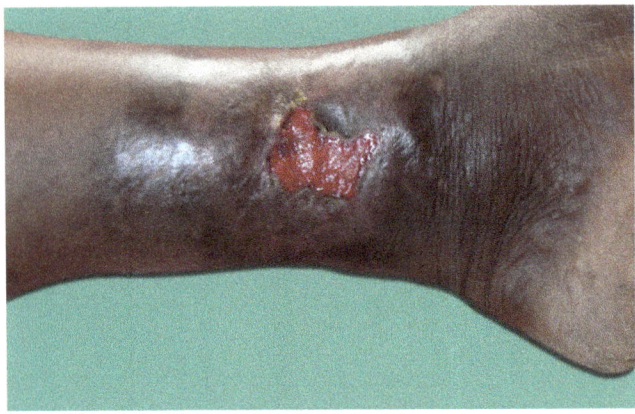

Fig. 4: Venous ulcer on medial malleolus with surrounding pigmentary changes.

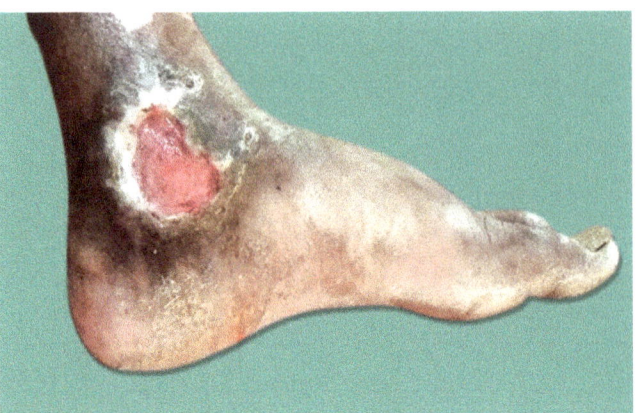

Fig. 5: Venous ulcer.

Table 3: Differential diagnosis: venous ulcers vs arterial ulcers.[10]

Assessment criteria	Venous disease	Arterial disease
Associated risk factors	• Varicose veins • Deep vein thrombosis • Reduced mobility • Trauma • Obesity, pregnancy • Recurrent phlebitis • Venous surgery in the past	• Diabetes mellitus • Hypertension • Smoking • Previous history of vascular disease • High body mass index (BMI)
Pain	• Throbbing, aching • Reduces with elevation and rest	• Intermittent claudication • Worsens at night, with rest • Dependency reduces pain
Common site	Medial aspect of ankle (Gaiter area)	Lateral malleolus, tibial area, toes and feet
Ulcer	• Shallow • Base: Slough with granulation tissue • Exudate: Moderate to heavy	• Punched out, maybe deep • Shape: Irregular • Base: Unhealthy with necrotic tissue/slough • Exudate: Mild, increases with infection
Surrounding skin	• Hemosiderin staining • Thickening and fibrosis • Varicosities • Dermatitis, itching • Peripheral pulses appreciated • Capillary refill—Normal • Limb edema	• Skin is dry, shiny and thin • No/absent hair on leg • Skin cold on touch • Pallor present on leg elevation • Pedal pulses: Feeble/absent • Capillary refill: Delayed • Gangrene

DIAGNOSTIC EVALUATION[2]

- *Duplex ultrasound*: It helps in the direct visualization of veins, potency and valvular reflux, influence of muscle contraction, valsalva maneuver, proximal and distal compression on the veins, and can identify the superficial and deep venous system. The technology combines ultrasound with Doppler ultrasonography to look for blood flow through arteries and veins.
- *Photoplethysmography*: It helps to determine efficiency of calf muscle pump and to detect abnormal venous reflux. It helps in assessing the decrease in skin blood flow following an exercise. Patients with superficial or

deep venous system involvement show abnormally rapid refilling (<25s) and poor emptying of veins.
- When planning for deep vein reconstruction, ascending and descending venography maybe considered.[8]
- In case of long standing ulcers, biopsy from ulcer edge can be done to rule out malignant transformation.
- *Patch testing*: Topically applied medications can cause allergic contact dermatitis as a complication of venous eczema, the incidence being as high as 40–90%. Patients not responding to standard therapy and those who are intolerant to a particular topical medication should be evaluated for contact sensitization by using patch test. The common allergens include fragrance mix, p-phenylendiamine, nickel, wool alcohol, chinoform, balsum of Peru, cobalt chloride, potassium dichromate, epoxy resin, thiuram mix and formaldehyde.[6]

MANAGEMENT

Treatment options for venous ulcers maybe divided into conservative management, mechanical treatment, medications, and surgery. The treatment goals include reduction of edema, to enhance ulcer healing, and to avoid recurrence.[11]

Conservative Management

Includes simple life style modifications such as weight reduction, regular exercise, and avoiding prolonged standing to improve the quality of living.

Compression Therapy

It is the standard of care for chronic venous insufficiency and venous ulcers. Compression maybe done by inelastic, elastic and intermittent pneumatic compression, and four layer bandage (providing compression pressure of 35–40 mm Hg comprising of orthopedic wool, crepe bandage, elastic bandage, and a cohesive retaining layer). It facilitates venous drainage, reduces pain and edema, and thus improves ulcer healing. Bandages should be applied from the base of the toes to just below the knee including the heel at 50% stretch and with 50% overlap providing a pressure of 20–30 mm Hg.

Leg Elevation

Leg elevation should be done above the level of the heart. It helps by reducing edema, increasing the microcirculation and oxygen delivery and thus promoting ulcer closure. It must be carried out for 30 minutes, three or four times each day.

Mechanical[11]

Vacuum assisted closure using negative pressure has been shown to decrease the ulcer depth and volume. However, there is lack of evidence for its use in venous ulcers.

Wound Dressing

Appropriate local wound care is of utmost importance. Elimination of infection, debridement of necrotic tissue and maintaining a proper moisture balance is important in wound healing. It is important to prevent maceration of the ulcer by using dressings that control the ulcer drainage.[12]

Medical[13] (Table 4)

Pentoxifylline

Inhibits platelet aggregation and thus reduces blood viscosity, thereby improving the microcirculation. It is given in a dose of 400 mg thrice a day. It is effective as an adjunct to compression therapy.

Aspirin[14]

Given in combination with compression therapy has been shown to reduce the ulcer healing time.

Antibiotics/Antiseptics

Wound infection can interfere with ulcer healing, however, regular antibiotic use (topical or systemic) is not recommended. Antibiotics maybe tried in case of cellulitis or osteomyelitis.

Apligraf[15]

Is a tissue-engineered biological dressing which is Food and Drug Administration (FDA) approved for treatment of venous ulcers. It acts by increasing the concentration of growth factors and cytokines.

Platelet Rich Plasma

Platelet rich plasma (PRP) releases various growth factors which help in wound healing. These growth factors promote proliferation and extra cellular matrix synthesis. They are safe and especially useful in chronic venous leg ulcers.[16]

Interventional

Sclerotherapy[17]

It refers to the introduction of a chemical solution into the vessel lumen, thus damaging the endothelium and leading to occlusion and ultimately fibrosis. It is highly effective in

Table 4: Mechanism of action of different drugs.

Class	Name	Mechanism of action
Alpha- benzopyrones	Coumarin	
Gamma- benzopyrones	Micronized purified flavonoid fraction Oxerutin, rutin, rutosides Diosmin	• Decreasing leucocyte adhesion, free radical formation, decreasing venous wall permeability, increasing venous tone, and protecting cells from hypoxia.
Saponins	Cuscus extract, escin (horse chestnut extract)	• Reduces symptoms and edema in CVI
Synthetic phlebotonics	Calcium dobesilate	• Synthetic venoactive drug with antioxidant properties, reduce capillary permeability, increase venous tone and reduce inflammation.
Other plant extract	Maritime pine tree extract	
Antibiotics		
Miscellaneous drugs	Pentoxifylline	• Increases microcirculatory blood flow, oxygenation of ischemic tissues, decrease whole blood viscosity, platelet aggregation.
	Aspirin	• Inhibition of platelet activation and reduction of pain and inflammation
	Stanozolol	• Anabolic steroid, fibrinolytic activity and decreases tissue plasminogen activator inhibitor
	Defibrotide	• Antithrombotic and profibrinolytic drug
	Zinc	• Antiinflammatory effect on phagocytes.

CVI: chronic venous insufficiency.

treating early small varicosities and for residual varicosities after surgery. Sclerotherapy of varicose veins/incompetent perforators improves the effectiveness of calf muscle pump, which helps in redistribution of extravascular fluid.

Sclerosants used (Table 5)

Can be divided into 3 groups on the basis of their mechanism:
1. Detergents
   - Act by protein theft mechanism
   - Alter the surface tension around the endothelial cells and cause vascular injury
   - *Examples*: Sodium tetradecyl sulfate (STS), polidocanol, sodium morrhuate, ethanolamine oleate.
2. Osmotic agents
   - Cause endothelial damage through dehydration
   - *Examples*: hypertonic saline, hypertonic saline dextrose.
3. Chemical irritants
   - Act by direct corrosive action
   - *Examples*: Chromate glycerine, polyiodinated iodine.
   - FDA approved sclerosis agents: STS, Sodium morrhuate, polidocanol, hypertonic saline.
   - Indications in varicose veins:[18]
     – Major tributaries of great saphenous vein (GSV), long saphenous vein (LSV)
     – Perforator reflux
     – Pain
     – Varicosities of lateral venous system
     – Cosmetic- spider webs/telangiectasia
     – Recurrent and residual veins following surgery
     – *Varicose veins complication*: venous ulcers/stasis dermatitis.
   - *Contraindications*:[19]
     – *Absolute contraindications*:
       ◆ Local infection
       ◆ Immobility
       ◆ Acute superficial or deep vein thrombosis
       ◆ Peripheral arterial occlusive disease (Stage 3 or 4)
       ◆ Hyperthyroidism
       ◆ Allergy to sclerosant
       ◆ Severe systemic disease
       ◆ Pregnancy- first trimester, more than 36 weeks
     – *Relative contraindications*:
       ◆ Saphenofemoral junction (SFJ) incompetence
       ◆ Edema
       ◆ Peripheral arterial occlusive disease (stage 2)
       ◆ Long standing diabetes

Table 5: Commonly used sclerosants: Comparison.[18]

Sclerosant	Concentration used	Maximum volume/dose	Size of vessels	Advantages	Disadvantages
Sodium tetradecyl sulfate (STS)	0.1–0.2%—telangiectasias 0.2–0.5%—reticular veins 0.5–1.0%—varicose veins 1.0–3.0%—axial varicose veins	10 cc of 3%	All sizes	Painless Painful only if injected extravascularly Food and Drug Administration (FDA) approved	Skin breakdown at higher concentrations
Sodium morrhuate	Undiluted-telangiecatsias, reticular veins	10 cc	Small	FDA approved	• Highest allergic reactions
Polidocanol	0.25–0.5%—telangiectasias 0.5–1.0%—reticular veins 1.0–3.0%—varicose	20 cc of 3%, not to exceed 2 mg/kg	Small to medium	Painless FDA approved	• Can cause ulceration
Hypertonic saline	23.4–11.7% telangiectasias 23.4% reticular veins	20 cc per session, restrict volume in salt restricted diet	Small	Risk of allergic reactions-low	• Painful • Ulcerogenic

- Thrombophilia with history of deep venous thrombosis (DVT)
- Myocardial decompensation
- Allergic diathesis
- Poor general health
- Asthma
- Known hyper coagulability
- Migraine

Patient Evaluation

- *History*: Patients likely to benefit:
  - Those with overt signs of chronic venous insufficiency
  - Symptoms reduced after wearing compression stockings.
- *Medical history*:
  - General medical condition, smoking, drugs (oral contraceptives, aspirin, anticoagulants), physical activity
  - History of Raynaud's phenomenon, vascular insufficiencies
  - Systemic diseases: Diabetes mellitus, hypertension, ischemic heart disease.
- *Examination*:
  - Skin at site of injection: Look for eczema, infection and ulceration.
  - Peripheral arterial pulses
  - Evidence of previous DVT
  - Doppler study

- *Procedure*[18]: Area is cleaned with spirit and povidone iodine. Sclerosant is diluted to the required concentration and loaded into the syringe and labeled. Anesthesia is usually not required.
- *Reticular veins*:
  - Subdermal reticular veins are treated only after eliminating all sources of reflux either by surgery or sclerotherapy.
  - Usually STS in concentrations of 0.2-0.5% is used.
  - With the patient in recumbent position, 3 mL syringe attached to a 30 G needle is inserted into the reticular vein (which is superficial and visible as bluish color).
  - After the sensation of entering the vein is felt, the plunger is gradually pulled back until visible blood is seen. Volume injected is no more than 0.5 mL per injected site.
  - Treatment interval varies from 4-8 weeks.
- *Varicose veins*: 2 techniques employed: Fegan's technique and Sigg's technique

Fegan's Technique

Position: patient sitting at the end of the table with leg in dependant position.

The visible varicosity is cannulized with butterfly, needle or angiocatheter. Following this, the leg is elevated above the heart level for 1-2 minutes so as to drain the blood. Make sure that the syringe is in the lumen by drawing small amount of blood into the syringe. While injecting the sclerosant, apply finger pressure above and below the

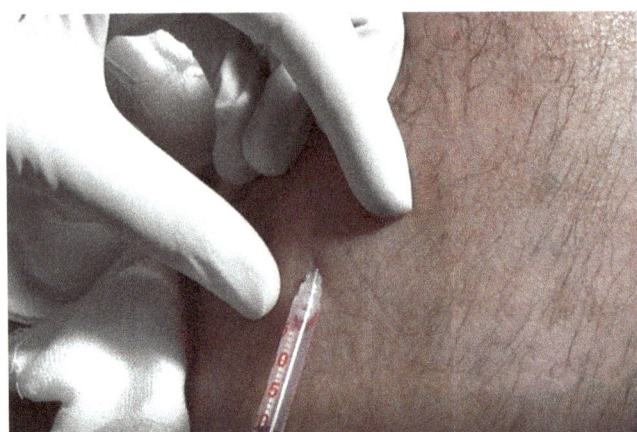

Fig. 6: Technique of sclerotherapy injection.

injection site for 30–60 seconds (Fig. 6). This is followed by immediate application of compression with foam pad which is then secured in place with foam elastic tape or inelastic wrap so as to maintain the compression.

Sigg's Technique

It is used for sclerosing saphenous junctions.

An open needle is introduced into the skin and manipulated till blood drips from the needle hub. The sclerosant is then injected into the needle.

Post Sclerotherapy Compression

Immediate, quick and sufficient compression after injection is advised. Either cotton balls with elastocrepe or graduated compression hoses maybe used.

Sclerotherapy for Varicose Veins

- Always inject proximal to distal
- Empty the vein of blood by different maneuvers
- Inject the larger vein before the smaller ones
- After injection, apply direct finger pressure in spreading and compressing motion.

Complications of sclerotherapy[20]

- *Transient complications*: Erythema, edema
- Rarely—hematoma, bleeding, superficial thrombophlebitis, nausea, post sclerotherapy hyperpigmentation, matting
- Allergic reactions in the form of allergic dermatitis, contact erythema, urticaria
- *Anaphylactic shock*: extremely rare.
- Extravasation of sclerosant causes skin necrosis.
- Dreaded complications include pulmonary embolism, arterial injection.

Foam Sclerotherapy[21]

Sclerosing foam contains a mixture of gas bubbles in a liquid solution which contains surface-active molecules. Only detergent sclerosants such as STS, POL produce foam. Foam sclerotherapy is believed to have higher efficacy than classic sclerotherapy.

- *Procedure*: Most commonly employed method is that of Lorenzo Tessari's Tourbillon technique for preparing the microfoam. It requires two plastic disposable syringes connected by a three-way stopcock. Here the sclerosant is mixed with air in the ratio of 4–5:1, by vigorously mixing them by multiple passages between the two syringes with hub at 30 degree rotation. (Figs. 7 and 8)
- *Types of foam*:[18]
    - *Wet foam*: Here the relative volume fraction of the liquid is more than 5%. Example: Tessari's foam. It has maximum stability
    - *Dry foam*: When the relative volume fraction of the liquid is less than 5%.
- *Advantages of foam sclerotherapy*:
    - Foams produce displacement of blood from the treated vein which causes prolonged undiluted intimal contact.
    - Smaller volume and concentration needed
    - Increase in effective surface area of foams
    - Increased sclerosis and vasospasm at a greater distance from injection site
    - Echogenicity of foams produces enhanced visibility on duplex.
- *Disadvantages of foam sclerotherapy*:
    - Difficulty in standardization
    - Dislodgement of foam to lungs in patients with patent ductus arteriosus.
    - Deep vein thrombosis, superficial thrombophlebitis
    - Pain and pigmentation relatively more common.

Sclerotherapy can be aided by sonography especially in difficult veins such as saphenous junctions, perforating veins and truncal veins next to saphenous junctions. This helps in increased efficiency and lower complications.

Laser Therapy[18]

Indications: telangiectasia/venulectasia or reticular veins of less than 3 mm in diameter.

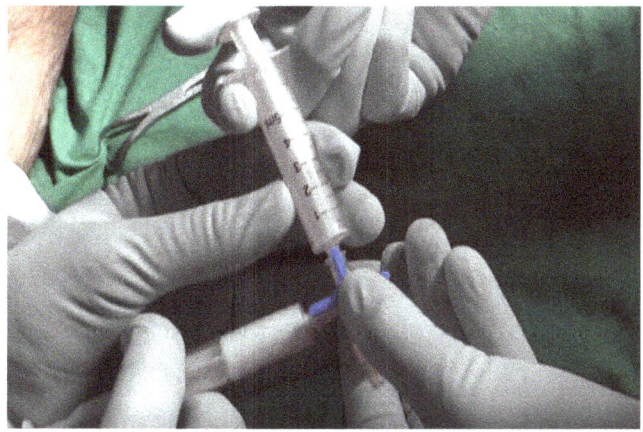
Fig. 7: Foam preparation.

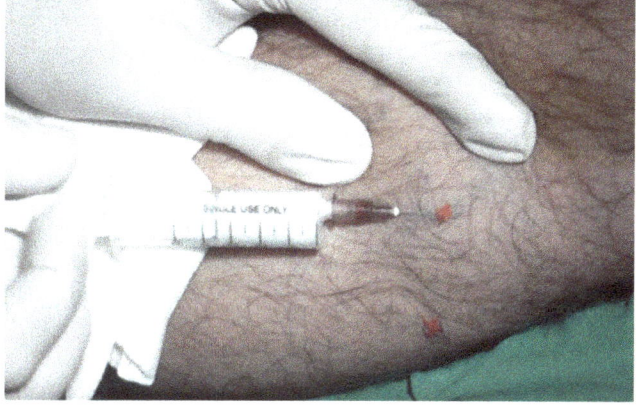
Fig. 8: Injection of foam preparation.

Various lasers used include pulsed dye (585–605 nm), KTP (532 nm), Alexandrite (755 nm), diode (810 nm), Nd:YAG (1064 nm) and intense pulse light.

Surgery for Venous Ulcers[22]

Endovenous Ablation
Includes thermal or chemical (sclerotherapy) techniques. It aims to ablate the incompetent vein so as to reduce complications associated with surgical procedures.

Open Venous Surgery
Includes high ligation, division and stripping (HL/S) of the great saphenous vein (GSV) or short saphenous vein (SSV), combined with excision of segments of varicose veins.

Perforator Incompetence
Can be tried using subfascial endoscopic perforator vein surgery, percutaneous ablation of perforators (PAPs), radiofrequency ablation and endovenous laser ablation.

Skin Grafting
The skin grafts used are pinch grafts and split-thickness skin, or meshed grafts. It may be done on refractory or large ulcers with normal venous pressure and ulcers covered with healthy, granulation tissue.

VENOUS ULCER RECURRENCE[23]
- Venous leg ulcers can recur after healing, with recurrence rates being as high as 37%. Recurrence rates are higher in those with deep venous insufficiency and those who have not been treated with surgery. Reduction in venous pressure is very important both in treatment as well as in avoiding recurrence of ulceration.
- The various measures that can help in preventing venous ulcer recurrence include progressive resistance exercises, elevation of lower limbs while sitting and avoiding prolonged standing. Diet modifications, weight reduction, avoidance of smoking, maintaining good cardiac status reduce the venous load on the legs. Use of compression stockings for a long period should be advised in patients treated surgically or conservatively. Studies indicate that venous surgery, sclerotherapy, phlebotonics can reduce the risk of ulcer recurrence.

CRITERIA FOR SPECIALIST REFERRAL FOR APPROPRIATE MANAGEMENT

Includes the following:
- Less than 25% reduction in ulcer size in 4 weeks
- Uncontrolled pain
- Atypical distribution of ulcers
- Suspicion of malignancy
- Ulcers that have not healed within 3 months
- Peripheral arterial disease (ABPI <0.8)
- ABPI above 1.2
- Diabetes mellitus
- Rheumatoid arthritis/vasculitis
- Healed ulcers with a view to venous surgery.

REFERENCES
1. Aydin A, Shenbagamurthi S, Brem H. Lower extremity ulcers: venous, arterial, or diabetic? Emergency Medicine. 2009; 41(8):18-24.

2. Biju Vasudevan. Venous leg ulcers: Pathophysiology and Classification. Indian Dermatol Online J. 2014;5(3):366-70.
3. Agile VS. Chronic leg ulcers: Epidemiology, aetiopathogenesis, and management. Ulcers. 2013:9.
4. Grey JE, Harding KG, Enoch S. Venous and arterial leg ulcers. BMJ. 2006;332:347-50.
5. Nicholls CS, Krishnan S. Chronic venous insufficiency: Clinical assessment and patient selection. Semin Intervent Radiol. 2005;22:169-77.
6. Jindal R, Sharma NL, Mahajan VK, et al. Contact sensitization in venous eczema: Preliminary results of patch testing with Indian standard series and topical medicaments. Indian J Dermatol Venereol Leprol. 2009;75:136-41.
7. Nicholls SC. Sequelae of untreated venous insufficiency. Semin Intervent Radiol. 2005;22:162-8.
8. Chatterjee SS. Venous ulcers of the lower limb: Where do we stand? Indian J Plast Surg. 2012;45:266-74.
9. Matic M, Matic A, Djuran V, et al. Frequency of peripheral arterial disease in patients with chronic venous insufficiency. Iran Red Crescent Med J. 2016;18:1-6.
10. Newton H. Leg ulcers: Differences between venous and arterial. Wound Essentials. 2011;6:20-8.
11. Prakash S, Tiwary SK, Mishra M, et al. Venous ulcer: Review article. Surgical Science. 2013;4:144-50.
12. Caprini JA, Partsch H, Simman R. Venous Ulcers. J Am Coll Clin Wound Spec. 2012;4:54-60.
13. Nair B. Venous leg ulcer: Systemic therapy. Indian Dermatol Online J. 2014; 5:374-7.
14. Kirsner SR, Nole KL, Fox JD, et al. Healing refractory venous ulcers: New treatments offer hope. J Investig Dermatol. 2015;135:19-23.
15. Zaulyanov L, Kirsner RS. A review of a bi-layered living cell treatment (Apligraf®) in the treatment of venous leg ulcers and diabetic foot ulcers. Clin Interv Aging. 2007;2(1):93-8.
16. Sarvajnamurthy S, Suryanarayan S, Budamakuntala L, et al. Autologous platelet rich plasma in chronic venous ulcers: Study of 17 cases. J Cutan Aesthet Surg. 2013;6:97-9.
17. Subbarao NT, Aradhya SS, Veerabhadrappa NH. Sclerotherapy in the management of varicose veins and its dermatological complications. Indian J Dermatol Venereol Leprol. 2013;79:383-8
18. Sacchidanand S, Nagesh TS, Sujala S. Sclerotherapy. In: Venkataram M (Ed). Textbook of Cutaneous & Aesthetic Surgery. New Delhi: Jaypee Brothers Medical Publishers (P) Ltd; 2017. p 559-68.
19. Khunger N, Sacchidanand S. Standard guidelines for care: Sclerotherapy in dermatology. Indian J Dermatol Venereol Leprol. 2011;77:222-31
20. Gupte J, Udare S. Basic Dermatosurgery Procedures. In: Viswanath V, Gopalani V (Eds). Cosmetic Dermatology: A practical and evidence Based Approach. New Delhi: Wiley India Pvt. Ltd; 2016. p 511-4.
21. Worthington-Kirsch RL. Injection Sclerotherapy. Semin Intervent Radiol. 2005; 22(3): 209–217.
22. Sarma N. Guidelines and recommendation on surgery for venous incompetence and leg ulcer. Indian Dermatol Online J. 2014;5:390-5.
23. Shenoy MM. Prevention of venous leg ulcer recurrence. Indian Dermatol Online J. 2014;5:386-9.

CHAPTER

Diabetic Foot Ulcers

Vivekanand, Vaibhav Lende, Sravan CPS

INTRODUCTION

Diabetic foot disease poses a growing global public health challenge and a major financial burden on healthcare systems worldwide. The prevalence of diabetes is exploding worldwide and is expected to involve more than 500 million people in the next 10-15 years. Diabetes is the leading cause of foot pathology, causing foot ulcerations from neuropathy, infection, and ischemia. According to an estimate by International Diabetes Federation (IDF), 80% of people with diabetes live in low- to middle-income countries including India, a country with the second largest number of diabetic patients in the world after China. India is home to 69.1 million patients with diabetes mellitus with an overall prevalence of 9.3%.[1] Lower extremity diseases, including peripheral neuropathy, peripheral arterial disease (PAD), and foot ulceration, is twice as common in diabetic subjects as compared with non diabetic persons and affects 30% of diabetic people older than 40 years. The annual incidence of diabetic foot ulcer (DFU) in population-based studies is 1.0-4.1% and prevalence of 4.5-10%, with an overall lifetime incidence of up to 25%.[2,3] The age-adjusted annual incidence for nontraumatic lower limb amputations in persons with diabetes ranges from 2.1 to 13.7 per 1,000 persons. Therefore, it is believed that in every 30 seconds a lower limb is lost somewhere in the world as a consequence of diabetes.[3] After a unilateral amputation, rates for mortality are also very high, ranging from 13 to 40% in 1 year, 35 to 65% in 3 years, and 39 to 80% in 5 years, which is worse than most malignancies.[4]

EPIDEMIOLOGY

There is a dearth of countrywide data for the prevalence of risk factors for DFU and diabetic foot infections (DFIs) among patients with diabetes in India. There have been various single-center and few multicenter reports with heterogeneous study population (hospitalized, outpatients, or community based), as well as use of varying assessment tools for the diagnosis of DFI. In a multicentric study from India, on patients with diabetes, the prevalence of neuropathy was found to be 15% and peripheral vascular disease (PVD) as 5%. The prevalence of DFIs is estimated to be 6-11%, and neuropathy is considered to be the most important determinant for occurrence of infection in diabetic foot wound.[5] Among newly diagnosed patients of diabetes with DFU, almost half of the ulcers were neuropathic, 19.7% ischemic, 34.2% neuroischemic, and nearly 3% of subjects had history of minor or major amputation of extremities.[6] Beyond their devastating complications, such as amputation, DFUs have also been associated with poor quality of life outcomes and a significant financial burden, both to the patient and to the economy through direct costs and lost productivity. The reduced mobility, multiple and prolonged hospitalizations and clinic visits, and the deteriorating quality of life lead to cardiovascular stress and an increased risk of mortality compared with the general population.

PATHOPHYSIOLOGY

The etiology of diabetic foot ulceration is a well-understood, but multifactorial and complex process (Fig. 1). Major risk factors associated with DFU formation are diabetic peripheral neuropathy and PAD, which act either in isolation or concurrently. Other important risk factors include soft tissue infection, biomechanical abnormalities, peripheral edema, plantar callus formation, nephropathy, poor glucose control, age, and a prolonged diabetic course.[7] Abnormal foot biomechanics often results from structural foot deformities combined with the limited joint mobility and bony abnormalities found in diabetic patients. Trauma

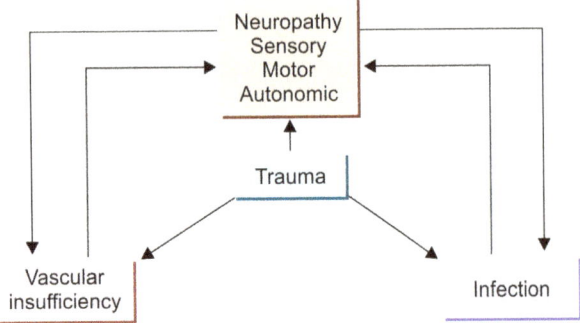

Fig. 1: Multifactorial etiology of diabetic foot pathology.

due to poorly fitting footwear also frequently plays a major role and ulcer formation. Ulceration of the heel often combines decubitus or pressure forces with ischemia, resulting in a difficult management issue.

Neuropathy

Hyperglycemia is the trigger that starts the cascade of neuropathy. The sensory neuropathy can cause loss of a variety of sensation like touch, pressure, temperature, vibration, position and pain. When the sensation of pain is lost it gives rise to an insensate foot and makes vulnerable to trivial trauma. It can become a portal of entry for the bacteria to enter. As many as 81% amputations have been found to be due to initial minor trauma.[8]

Persons with diabetes loose proprioception, i.e. the sense of foot position with loss of pain. This does not allow the patient to know how he places his feet. That results in abnormal foot positions, and pressure ulcers. The heat and cold sensations are carried by C fibers. Some authors have considered C fibers to be the first to be affected in diabetic neuropathy.[9] Diabetes affects rhythmic vasomotion of small arterioles due to sympathetic damage early in disease. Loss of warm thermal threshold also occurs early with C fiber damage and correlates significantly to reduced vasomotion.[9] Since these deficits may occur as a part of sensory neuropathy a patient is not likely to be aware if his feet come in contact with a hot object. This causes necrosis of the skin leading to ulcers.

Motor neuropathy and some components of autonomic neuropathy cause change in the shape of the foot. Motor neuropathy leads to the weakness and/or atrophy of the interosseous muscles of the foot, resulting in the loss of ability of the small or the intrinsic muscles to hold the foot in normal shape and place it in the correct position. This leads to the deformity of foot. The repetitive pressure leads to keratosis and callus formation. The high pressure at the callus results in the damage to the tissues of the foot and can start the formation of ulcer below the callus that later on, breaks through. The common deformities due to motor neuropathy are crowding of toes, cock up toes, hallux valgus, clawing of toes. The diabetic state is known to give rise to the glycation of long lasting collagen fibers of the ligaments that hold various joints. The subsequent inflammatory changes leading to advanced glycated end products make the ligaments inflexible resulting in various abnormal postures of feet and toes making them susceptible to ulceration.

Autonomic neuropathy results in two distinct mechanisms that contribute to diabetic foot ulceration, i.e. sudomotor dysfunction and arteriovenous shunting in the foot. Sudomotor dysfunction is the dysfunction of the sympathetic nerves supplying the sweat glands in the foot. This results in the reduction or absence of sweating which normally keeps the feet moist. Feet become dry and the skin cracks more easily.[10] This neuropathy can also result in arterial-venous shunting and impaired microvascular regulation of the skin.[11] As such, the insensitive diabetic foot may appear warm and well perfused, resulting in a false sense of security by both the patient and the provider as to the risk of diabetic ulcer formation.[12]

Vascular Insufficiency

Arterial disease contributes to the development of 50% of (DFUs) and plays a role in 70% of the mortality among diabetic patients.[13] Arterial occlusive disease may be present in isolation or in combination with neuropathic disease in up to 45% of lower extremity ulcerations. Infrapopliteal occlusive disease with heavy calcification is the classic picture of diabetic arterial disease. In addition, despite the basement membrane affected at the capillary level in those with diabetes, microvascular disease precluding revascularization in diabetic patients has been disproved. Diabetic patients are at a higher risk of digital artery disease with palpable pedal pulses that nonetheless can result in digital ulceration and subsequent impaired healing and gangrene. Despite the relatively common occurrence of an incomplete pedal arch in diabetic patients, tibial revascularization, especially to the angiosome in which the ulceration is located, is possible in the vast majority of diabetic patients to overcome foot ischemia.[14]

Infections

Diabetic foot ulcers may present with or without infection with a classification proposed by the Infectious Diseases Society of America (Table 1), including a PEDIS (perfusion,

Table 1: Infectious Diseases Society of America (IDSA) classification system of diabetic foot infection.

Clinical presentation	IDSA infection severity	Threatened limb class
Wound without purulence or inflammation	Uninfected	N/A
Presence of >2 manifestations of inflammation, cellulitis <2 cm surrounding ulcer, no systemic symptoms	Mild infection	Non–limb threatening
Infection with >2 cm of surrounding cellulitis; any infection with the presence of gangrene, abscess, deep involvement, or gas in the tissue; no systemic signs or symptoms	Moderate infection	Limb threatening
Infection as above with the presence of systemic signs or symptoms	Severe infection	Life and limb threatening

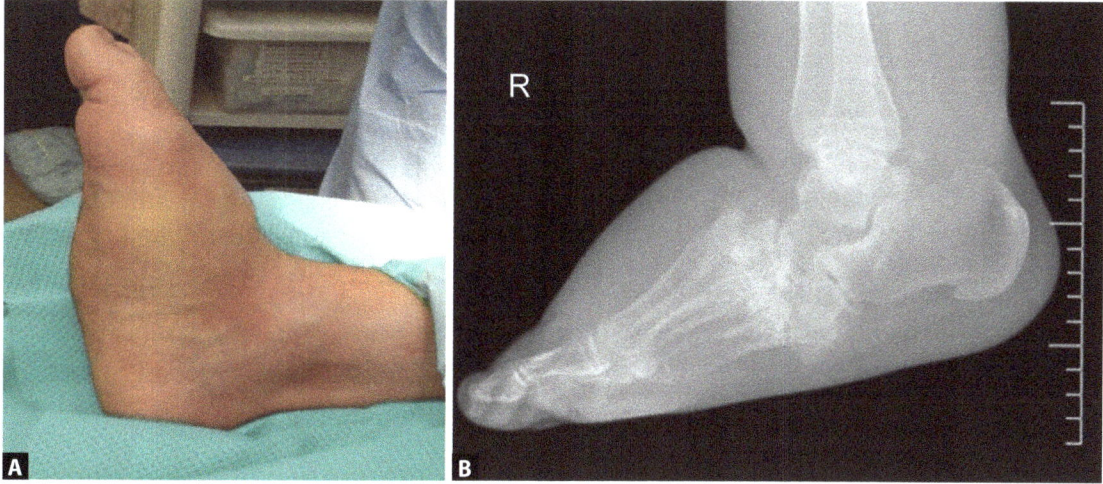

Figs. 2A and B: Charcot foot; typical "rocker bottom appearance (A) characteristic X-ray (B) with neuroarthropathy stage 1.

extent, depth, infection and sensation) score to guide assessment of severity and subsequent therapy. A wound culture should be obtained when signs of an infection, such as purulence, cellulitis in the adjacent skin, malodor, and tissue necrosis, are present. However, ulcers that are otherwise clean and free from any local or systemic signs of infection should not be swabbed or cultured.[15] In addition, diabetics have elevated serologic concentrations of adhesion molecules that bind monocytes, leukocytes, and platelets to the endothelium and impair its function, leading to diminished skin perfusion and healing, thus reducing the ability to deliver antibiotics to sites of infection.[15]

Charcot Neuroarthropathy

Charcot neuroarthropathy (CN) can be considered end stage sequela of a pathologic diabetic foot process with devastating economic and clinical consequences. CN has been reported to increase healthcare costs by 17.2% and results in an increase of hospital length of stay.[17] CN classically presents with edema, erythema, and calor with fractures and/or dislocations across joints of the foot or ankle. The prevailing theory involves demineralization of the bone, causing instability. CN progresses through four stages: Stage 0—clinical stage presenting with warm, swollen, often painful foot; Stage 1—fragmentation/destruction, bony cysts, and erosion; Stage 2—joint subluxations; Stage 3—arch collapse and coalescence; and Stage 4—consolidation.[18] The key to the treatment of CN is early recognition and immobilization with non–weight-bearing (Figs 2A and B).

As compared to the West, which has predominant Gram-positive infections, centers throughout India have reported a consistent Gram-negative bacterial preponderance in DFI.[13] The common bacterial isolates in various studies from different parts of India is shown in Table 1. *Pseudomonas aeruginosa* has been consistently shown to be the most common organism isolated form diabetic foot wounds in our country.[19] However, few others have shown *Escherichia coli* as the most common organism followed by *Staphylococcus aureus*.[13]

BIOMECHANICS AND FOOT PRESSURES

Altered biomechanics of the diabetic foot are major contributors to ulcer development and chronicity. Foot biomechanics encompass the dynamics involved in ambulation. The foot must be both flexible and rigid, depending on the demands of the phase in the gait cycle. This intrinsic adaptability is maintained by the underlying bony architecture, as well the soft tissue attachments. Structural changes occur in the diabetic foot that alters the underlying biomechanics. Stiffening of soft tissue structures, including tendons, ligaments, and joint capsules, leads to a limitation of range of motion across joints and joint subluxation, and dislocation.[20] The principal forces experienced by the foot that can lead to ulceration are abnormal plantar pressures (sagittal plane) and shear. These forces are experienced between the bone-overlying soft tissue envelope, foot-ground, and foot-shoe. Both sagittal plane and shear forces are typically minimized in the sensate foot through compensation by subtle or overt changes in postural stance or positioning, but in the environment of peripheral neuropathy, compensation is compromised, leading to prolonged periods during which abnormal forces are applied until the skin and subcutaneous tissue fail. Joint deviations and subluxations caused by the loss of structural integrity lead to further malalignment of the pull of the tendons further exacerbating biomechanical faults. Alterations in lower extremity biomechanics are appreciated through gait analysis and biomechanical examination of the lower extremity on physical examination. Alterations in gait pattern (i.e., shuffling, antalgic, wide base, unsteady) imply an underlying abnormality.[21] Limited joint mobility (LJM) (i.e., limitation of range of motion in the joints of the foot and ankle) and structural deformities (i.e., bony prominences or joint contractures) are signs of malalignment.

PRESENTATION AND DIAGNOSIS

The assessment of the diabetic foot broadly falls into:
- Detail history
- Clinical assessment
- Investigation

History

A detailed medical and surgical history should be obtained from every diabetic patient with a foot ulcer to determine how the patient's diabetes is managed, whether the ulcer appeared suddenly or secondary to a traumatic incident, whether the patient traveled recently or acquired new footwear, and to determine the wound's duration and any noticeable changes in its appearance and character. Any previous wounds should also be documented, as well as any wound care treatments that the patient has received. Wounds that are accompanied by systemic symptoms suggestive of infection, such as malaise or cold sweats, should be treated without delay.

Clinical Assessment

The diabetic foot physical examination must include dermatologic, neurologic, vascular, and musculoskeletal assessments (Table 2). The skin of patients with advanced diabetic disease is usually dry and brittle because of peripheral neuropathy. Areas of hyperkeratosis indicate pressure points that are often accompanied by pre ulcerative or ulcerative changes. Preulcerative changes may be subtle and can appear as pinpoint hemorrhages or shallow hematomas within the dermis.

Inspection of the foot may reveal the sequelae of motor neuropathy, such as atrophy of the intermetatarsal musculature and hollowing of tissue between the metatarsals and arch of the foot.

The patient should also be examined for Charcot neuropathic osteoarthropathy, also known as "Charcot foot." The classic, but late, presentation of a "rocker bottom foot" in these patients creates severe mid-foot plantar pressures and subsequent ulceration.[22] A unilateral, hot, swollen foot should be considered an acute presentation of Charcot foot until proven otherwise.[23] Early offloading and immobilization can prevent further damage and prevent a rocker bottom foot. Sensory testing using a Semmes-Weinstein monofilament (10 g) is a predictive and easily reproducible test to assess the neuropathic risk of foot ulceration and amputation in diabetic patients.[24] Failure of the patient to perceive more than four or more of the 10 test sites has been associated with a 15-fold increase in the risk of plantar ulceration.[25] Testing perception of vibration with a 128-mHz tuning fork is also predicative of ulceration risk, although this test is less reliable than the Semmes-Weinstein test.[26] Lower extremity arteries, including the femoral, popliteal, and tibial arteries, should be palpated to detect a pulse. However, palpation is affected by factors

Table 2: Essential components of diabetic foot examination.			
Vascular	*Neurologic*	*Dermatologic*	*Musculoskeletal*
Palpate pedal and lower extremity pulses. Look for distal hair growth on feet, toes Assess capillary filling time in the toes	Test for loss of protective sensation by Semmes-Weinstein monofilament, biothesiometry, or electronic tuning fork Look for muscle atrophy of the feet	Note the ulcer depth, tissue in the wound bed, if bone is palpable Look for signs of infection around a wound (erythema, purulence) Inspect for other preulcerative lesions (blisters, calluses, corns)	Inspect for deformities Look for signs of Charcot foot (collapsed arch or hot, red swollen foot Check the dorsiflexion of the ankle and the great toe joint

Source: Miller JD, Carter E, Shih J, et al. How to do a 3-minute diabetic foot exam. J Fam Pract. 2014;63:646-56.

Table 3: Wagner and Texas classification systems of diabetic foot ulcers.			
Wagner method		**University of texas method**	
Grade	Details	Grade	Details
0	No open foot lesion	0	Presence of preulcer
1	Presence of superficial ulcer, partial or full thickness	1	Superficial ulcer not penetrating tendon, bone or joint
2	Ulcer extends to ligaments, tendon, joint capsule or deep fascia without abscess or osteomyelitis	2	Ulcer penetrating through to tendon or capsule
3	Presence of deep ulcer with abscess, osteomyelitis	3	Ulcer penetrating to bone or joint
4	Gangrene localized to the forefoot or heel	A	Noninfected and nonischemic ulcer
5	Extensive	B	Infection present
		C	Ischemia Present
		D	Both Infection and ischemia present

such as the patient's body habitus, peripheral edema, and blood pressure fluctuations, as well as the examiner's level of experience. As such, clinical decision-making should not be based solely on the presence or absence of palpable pulses without further noninvasive vascular testing. An ankle brachial index (ABI) measurement is often obtained at the time of initial clinical evaluation but may be falsely elevated due to the prevalence of medial arterial calcinosis in the tibial arteries of the diabetic foot.[27]

Diabetic Ulcer Classification

Numerous diabetic foot ulcer classification systems have been developed, and used for clinical and research purposes. The Wagner Classification is the first such system and was initially developed for pressure wounds rather than diabetic ulcers. The University of Texas Classification System and the PEDIS ulcer classification were subsequently developed to correlate wound characteristics with clinical outcomes (Table 3).[27] The wound, ischemia, foot infection (WIfI) classification system as advocated by the Society for Vascular Surgery is the most recent foot ulcer staging system that has been clinically validated by several investigators.[28]

Investigation

Apart from routine investigation i.e. Hb gm%, HbA1c, total count, the culture sensitivity of infected tissue to be sent. Numerous imaging modalities are available for the workup of diabetic foot ulcers. Foot X-rays should be obtained to rule out bony deformities, and, if infection is suspected, evaluate for subcutaneous gas. When ulcer healing does not progress at a satisfactory rate, other imaging studies that should be considered include computed tomography (CT), magnetic resonance imaging (MRI), labeled white blood cell scans, single-photon emission computed tomography (SPECT), and positive emission tomography (PET) scans to rule out osteomyelitis or soft tissue infections. Although PET and labeled white blood cell scans have been shown to have the highest diagnostic accuracy in confirming or excluding the diagnosis of osteomyelitis, they are time-consuming and expensive tests and many clinicians will preferentially order MRIs first for the workup of osteomyelitis.[29]

MANAGEMENT

General Principles

The decision to treat a diabetic foot ulcer in an outpatient setting or as an inpatient in the hospital often hinges on the patient's presenting clinical status. The integration of knowledge and experience through a multidisciplinary team approach promotes more effective treatment, thereby improving outcomes and limiting the risk of lower extremity amputation.[30]

Wound Debridement

The purpose of debriding a diabetic foot ulcer is to alter the environment of the wound and to promote healing by removing abnormal tissue, such as hyperkeratotic epidermis and necrotic dermal tissue, foreign debris, and bacteria.[31] In addition to removing nonviable tissue, debridement converts a stagnant wound into an acute healing wound by releasing platelet growth factors, inhibiting proteinases, and limiting the action of bacterial biofilm.[32] Different modalities for debriding a wound include sharp, surgical, enzymatic, autolytic, mechanical, and intraoperative with ultrasonic and hydrosurgical devices. Because the majority of these patients are neuropathic, aggressive debridement can usually be carried out with minimal discomfort. If the patient is anxious or an extensive debridement is required, a local anesthetic block or sedation in an operating room setting may be helpful. Exposed bone needs to be debrided to stippled punctate bleeding, and bone cultures should be obtained. The bacteria most likely to be involved in diabetic osteomyelitis are skin organisms, frequently *Staphylococcus aureus* and sometimes resistant strains.[33] Copious pulse lavage irrigation should be performed at the end of each debridement.

Diabetic patients with foot ulceration and tracking abscesses, wet gangrenous changes, gas in the tissue on plain film radiographs, or systemic signs of sepsis require urgent surgical attention. A thorough incision and drainage of any abscesses or infectious tracks must be aggressively performed in the operating room, along with an appropriate exploration of fascial compartments and layers of the foot, because abscesses originating from a forefoot ulcer can track up to the ankle or lower leg. Amputation of digits or portions of the foot may be necessary due to gangrene or to limit the advancement of infection. If the viability of any of the patient's foot tissue is questionable, then one might consider limiting the amount of tissue that is resected, to preserve later closure options. Any resected tissue or bone should be cultured and sent for a pathology evaluation. Patients will often subsequently require multiple procedures to resect necrotic wound edges and debride the wound to promote granulation. After treating the foot infection, the focus of care should be directed towards the need for revascularization and primary or secondary wound closure. Because of the complex altered physiology of these wounds, as well as additional systemic issues in diabetic patients, wound closure is slow and multiple interventions are frequently required. However, with meticulous attention to detail, closure rates of up to 80% have been reported.[34] Defining principles of successful wound closure include infection control, wound debridement, adequate perfusion, offloading of pressure, and moisture balance. Antibiotic-impregnated bone beads might also be used to enhance the treatment of any residual osteomyelitis.[35]

Dressing

Wound healing is a complex process involving highly regulated responses of specified cell types, which harbor locally secreted growth factors that play a key role in wound healing.[36] Wound healing can be enhanced by the appropriate choice of a topical regime. However, before choosing a regime one should consider factors such as the general health of the patient, the process of tissue repair, assessment of the wound by means of grading, description and classification of the wound, local environment of the wound, knowledge on specific properties of the dressing materials and devices as well as their availability, affordability, and accessibility.

Antibiotic Use

Use of anti-infectives/antibiotics must be guided by appropriate cultures. Inappropriate use of antibiotics could lead to resistance and adverse effects. Oral and parenteral antibiotics are prescribed for mild soft tissue infections and moderate to severe infections, respectively (Table 4).[15] Every hospital should develop an institutional antibiotic policy containing guidelines and protocols for antibiotic use.

Choice of Topical Regimen

Wet to dry dressing or simple saline: Wet-to-dry dressings are described in the literature as a means of mechanical

Table 4: Guidelines on antibiotic therapy.

Severity	Route of administration	Duration
Soft tissue infections		
Mild	Topical or oral	1–2 weeks
Moderate	Initial parenteral then oral	1–3 weeks
Severe	Initial parenteral, switch to oral when improvement noted	2–4 weeks
Bone or joint		
No residual infected tissue (eg. Postamputation)	Parenteral or oral	2–5 days
Residual infected soft tissue	Parenteral or oral	1–3 weeks
Minimally infected (but viable) bone	Initial parenteral, then switch to oral	4–5 weeks
Residual dead bone	Initial parenteral, then switch to oral	≥3 months

debridement.[37] This dressing has a good debriding action and helps in wound bed preparation. It is very absorptive as well as adherent and one of the cheapest dressings used throughout the world, but requires frequent dressing change (twice or thrice a day) based on wound severity

Antibacterial agents: Metronidazole gel has good anaerobic coverage and helps in maintaining a moist wound healing environment.[38] Antibiotics such as neomycin, gentamycin, and mupirocin have good antibacterial coverage when used topically. Silver containing dressings come in different formulations and have very good antibacterial coverage. Povidone iodine solution dressings are toxic.[39] It should not be used on granulating or epithelizing wounds because it slows down the healing process and is cytotoxic to keratinocytes and fibroblasts.

Tulle dressings: These are gauze dressings impregnated with paraffin, which lowers the dressing adherence, but this property is lost if the dressing dries out. Tulle dressings are mainly indicated for superficial clean wounds and skin grafts.

Polyurethane films: These are vapor-permeable films which allow diffusion of gases and water vapor which helps in maintaining a moist wound healing environment. Their transparency allows for wound monitoring without dressing removal, but there is a chance of maceration of surrounding skin. They can be used for low exudating wounds.

Polyurethane foam: These dressings are extremely absorbent, non-adherent, and have a semi-permeable backing which allows moisture to escape. They are capable of absorbing light to heavy amounts of exudate, thereby preventing maceration, facilitating removal of slough, and promoting the proliferative stage of wound healing.[40] They are also used as outer dressings after application of topical antibiotics, such as metronidazole, or hydrogels.

Hydrogel dressings: These dressings consist of cross-linked insoluble starch or carboxymethyl cellulose polymers and water (96%). Hydrogels donate fluid to dry necrotic and slough wounds and promote autolysis. They apparently debride by rehydrating the wound. These dressings are the best choice for the treatment of dry wounds with necrotic eschar, and the hydrogel reaches a 50% debridement level more quickly than wet-to-dry dressings and are more cost-effective.[41]

Hydrocolloid dressing: These dressings are a combination of polymers such as gelatin, pectin and cellulose which form a waterproof adhesive dressing. Exudates produced by the wound are absorbed into the dressing and form a gel. Hydrocolloid dressings are capable of absorbing low to moderate levels of exudate and can be used to promote autolytic debridement of dry, sloughy, or necrotic wounds.[42] Hydrocolloid dressings should be avoided on plantar ulcers of the foot, as the periwound skin is susceptible to maceration.

Alginate dressings: The alginate forms a gel when it comes into contact with the wound surface. It can be used in granulating, epithelializing, and cavity wounds. Cochrane reviews detail the role of alginate dressings in the treatment of diabetic foot ulcers.[43]

Growth factors: Diabetic wounds are enriched in proteases and supports the premise that impaired growth factor availability may act as a rate limiting factor in diabetic wound healing.[44] A recombinant human (rh)-platelet derived growth factor (PDGF) dressing is an effective modality for facilitating wound healing in patients suffering from diabetes and can be used as an adjunct to the conventional mode of treatment for healing diabetic wounds.[45] It can be used in the granulating stage of the wound.

Honey-impregnated dressings: Proposed to have antimicrobial and anti-inflammatory properties, these dressings can be used for acute or chronic wounds. The antimicrobial properties of honey have been demonstrated in the laboratory, however, *in vivo* evidence is scant, particularly in comparison to the literature on silver antimicrobial dressings.[46,47]

Topical enzymes: Collagenase, fibrinolysin, or papain containing ointments help in the enzymatic debridement of sloughy tissues and thus promote granulation formation. Papain-urea (89.2%) is a better enzymatic debriding agent than collagenase (82.2%).[48]

Vacuum therapy: Vacuum-assisted closure generates a topical negative pressure over the wound bed. Pressure of 125 mm Hg is the ideal pressure. Vacuum-assisted closure is extremely effective in removing exudate and reducing edema, while leaving the surface of the wound moist. It is contraindicated in avascular wounds or exposed tendons or bones. Some of the contraindications include untreated osteomyelitis, non-enteric and unexplored fistula, presence of necrotic tissue, exposed organs or blood vessels, and malignancy in the wound.[49]

Hyperbaric oxygen: Treatment with hyperbaric oxygen therapy involves the intermittent administration of 100% oxygen at a pressure greater than that at sea level. A small amount of data suggests significant reduction of the ulcer area[50] as well as reduction of the risk for major amputation.[51] Hyperbaric oxygen can be applied as an adjunctive therapy for patients with severe soft-tissue foot infections and osteomyelitis who have not responded to conventional treatment. A systematic review by the National Institute for Health and Clinical Excellence (NICE) Guidelines Development Group in the UK concluded that the available data are insufficient to demonstrate that hyperbaric oxygen therapy is cost-effective.[52]

Human skin equivalents: Apligraf (Organogenesis, Canton, Massachusetts) is a cultured bilayer cellular construct (BLCC) originating from neonatal foreskin. A bovine collagen lattice is used as a base to support the organization of dermal fibroblasts and epithelial cells. A layer of allogeneic keratinocytes is cultured over the fibroblast layer to form a stratified epidermis. The bilayer has a structure similar to human skin, with the absence of hair follicles or sweat glands. The product requires a well-granulated wound bed in which exudate and bacterial levels have been controlled to yield positive results. The BLCC is easily applied in a clinic or operating room setting after aggressive wound debridement and hemostasis.[53] Porcine small intestine submucosa (OASIS wound matrix, Healthpoint Ltd., Fort Worth, Texas) has been shown in a prospective RCT to accelerate healing.[54] Dermagraft (DG, Advanced BioHealing Inc., La Jolla, California) is an allogeneic dermal fibroblast culture derived from human neonatal foreskin samples and grown on a biodegradable scaffold.[55] The resulting three-dimensional matrix can be implanted into chronic nonhealing wounds to supply functional fibroblasts and their corresponding expressed proteins. Integra dermal regeneration template (IDRT) is an acellular bilayer matrix designed to assist with dermal regeneration in multiple types of problem wounds. The bottom layer that is applied to the wound surface consists of a three-dimensional matrix of collagen and chondroitin-6-sulfate, a glycosaminoglycan. The top layer is a temporary layer made of silicone. This construct has been employed for years in burns, traumatic wounds, and other types of wounds with some success. The bottom layer is designed to incorporate into the wound and support tissue regeneration while the top layer provided a mechanical barrier to bacterial contamination. It is critical that the construct is applied to a clean wound that is free of bacteria that might lead to infection over time. This wound matrix has been adapted for use in diabetic foot ulcers in the outpatient clinic.[56]

Growth factors: Although multiple growth factors have been studied in clinical trials, to date, only PDGF has been approved by the FDA for the treatment of diabetic foot ulcers. Becaplermin (Regranex, Ortho- McNeil, Raritan, New Jersey) is a recombinant human BB isoform of PDGF suspended in a gel designed for topical application. Becaplermin is applied daily to the diabetic foot ulcer and covered with saline-moistened gauze. It has been studied clinically in four prospective, randomized, placebo-controlled trials. Adverse events were rare, and the only medication-related event was local tissue sensitivity in 2%.[57]

Biomechanical Correction

Altered biomechanics can be addressed through a combination of conservative and surgical methods.

Offloading

Conservative methods focus on the concept of offloading focal areas of pressure and distributing pressure across a wider surface area. Offloading can be achieved through padding, multidensity orthotics, and braces, which may

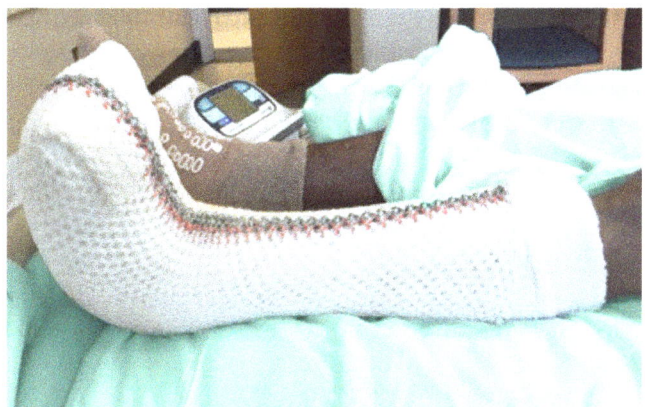

Fig. 3: Total contact cast.

be helpful in ulcer prevention or recurrence.[58] Foot ulcer recurrence can be dramatically reduced when inexpensive, low-tech approaches are employed.[59,60] A multidensity accommodative insert, seamless inner, extra-depth, rocker-bottom shoe is ideal for the at-risk foot. A functional/accommodative device can also, depending on the degree of reducibility, realign the foot in a more anatomical position. Offloading is also used to treat an active ulcer. The total contact cast (TCC) (Fig. 3) is one such effective method of healing plantar forefoot ulcerations.[61] Although level one evidence for these individual modalities is sparse, a meta-analysis showed greater wound healing efficacy with the use of total contact casting and irremovable cast walkers.[62] Multilayer customized offloading orthoses and fillers at sites of partial foot amputation are available to stabilize the position of the foot within the shoe. Other methods, including a walker boot or healing shoe, are also utilized with a lesser degree of success.[63] Decubitus ulcers of the posterior heel should also be offloaded, especially when the patient is supine, utilizing a foam or airbladder filled device with complete relief of the posterior heel. It is necessary to balance and offload pressure from both prior and potential ulceration sites.[64] Offloading is the single most important treatment for the DFU.

Surgical Methods

The goal of surgical biomechanical correction, whether it be a soft tissue or bony procedure, is to produce a rectus, balanced foot. Soft tissue corrections largely focus on tendon lengthening and rerouting and should be reserved for reducible or semi-reducible deformities. Once the biomechanical abnormality has been addressed, not only is the ulcer healing rate high, but the incidence of reulceration is significantly less compared with patients treated with TCC alone. For the latter patients, the pressure and shear which caused the ulcer are only modified during the period of TCC therapy, remaining as pathologic forces to cause reulceration after TTC removal if no other means of offloading is utilized. Digital flexor tendon releases have also been utilized as a simple method of relieving the pressure at the dorsal aspect of the interphalangeal joints or the distal aspects of toes.[65] Bony procedures include exostectomies (simple removal of bony prominences) and joint realignment through arthrodesis and/or osteotomies. Surgical correction can be conducted prophylactically (to prevent ulceration) or therapeutically (to heal an ulceration).[66,67] These surgical techniques are typically reserved for nonreducible deformities. Tendon balancing and skeletal reconstruction (e.g., TAL and mid-foot arthrodesis) are often done in combination. Conservative offloading is still necessary after the surgical incisions have healed. The goal of all of these options is to optimize function while minimizing new ulcer formation or ulcer recurrence.

Diabetes-related Amputations

The greatest area of overlap in which podiatrists and vascular surgeons collaborate is the foot complications of diabetes and amputation prevention. When a patient is referred to a multidisciplinary team, the vascular team treats wounds that are profoundly ischemic, with the goal of improving flow and when flow is adequate, the podiatry team manages wound healing, off-loading, reconstruction, and prevention.

Armstrong and Frykberg proposed classifying non-vascular diabetic foot surgery into four categories based on indications and perceived risk: elective, prophylactic, curative, and emergency (Fig. 4). This system, which focuses on historical variables such as neuropathy, presence of ulceration, and limb-threatening infection,[68] was validated in a study we reported in 2006.[69]

Diabetic foot	Description
Class IV: Emergency	Limit progression of acute local and generalized sepsis
Class III: Curative	Surgery to help healing with secondary intention
Class II: Prophylactic	Reduce risk of ulceration of reulceration in an insensate foot with open wound
Class I: Elective	Reduce pain or limitation of motion in an insensate foot

(Risk for high level amputation ↑)

Fig. 4: Diabetic foot surgery classification.

Amputation prevention

The prevention of amputations can be placed in three broad categories: primary prevention, secondary prevention, and post– secondary prevention (Fig. 5 and Flowchart 1).

THE CHARCOT FOOT

The charcot foot ulcer can be particularly troublesome to off-load and deserves special mention. Charcot arthropathy or neuroarthropathy is a fracture and dislocation process of the foot and ankle that occurs in patients with sensory and autonomic neuropathy. Fracture is often associated with unrecognized injury or minor trauma that might otherwise appear innocuous.[70,71] Charcot arthropathy patients classically present with a painless, hot, swollen foot. Others may present with what initially seems to be a unilateral flatfoot deformity, with the arch of the foot "suddenly" collapsing. Patients generally have excellent

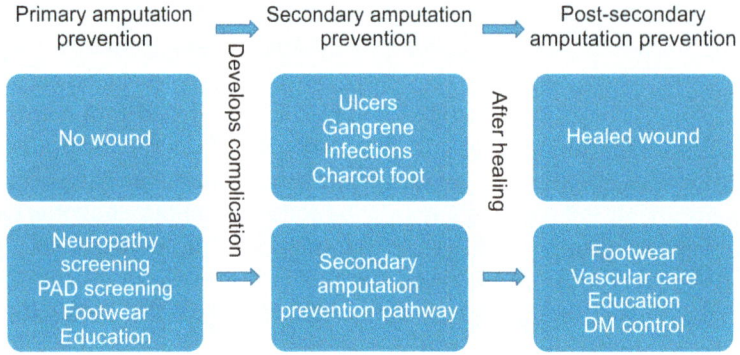

Fig. 5: Amputation prevention pathways.
(PAD: peripheral arterial disease)

Flowchart 1: Secondary amputation prevention pathway.

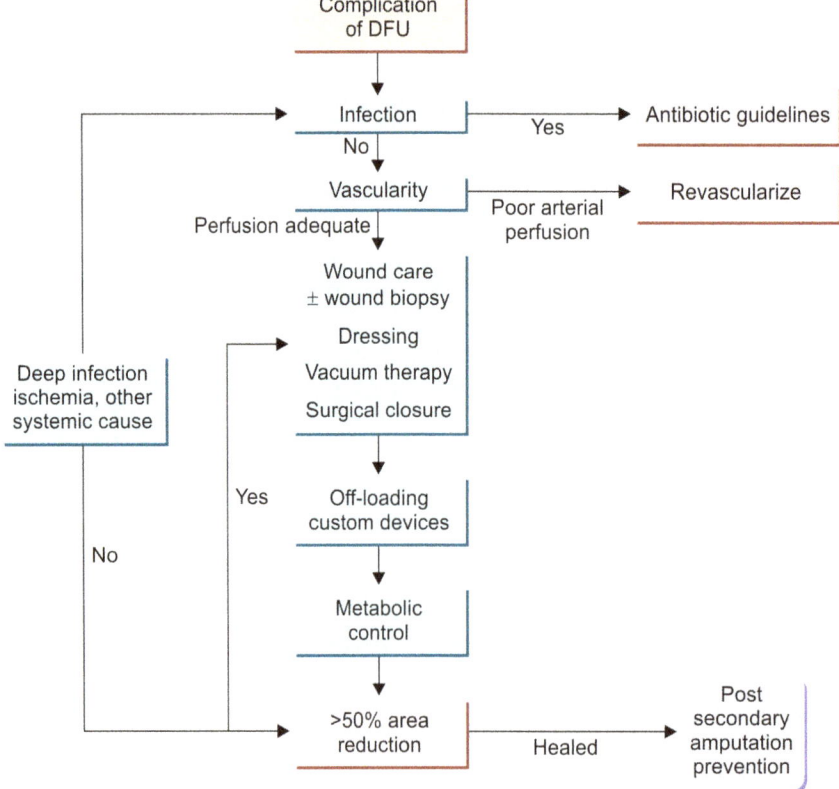

(DFU: diabetic foot ulcer)

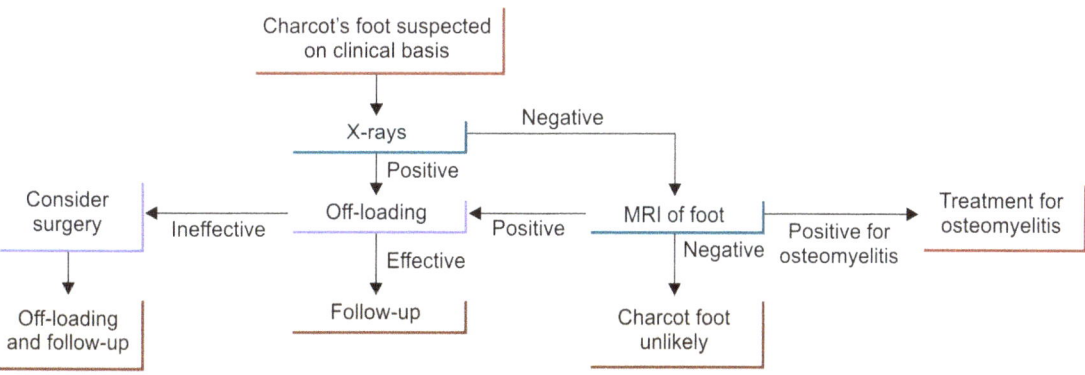

Flowchart 2: The Charcot Foot basic treatment algorithm.

arterial pulses and severe sensory neuropathy. Diabetic patients with sensory neuropathy and ischemia have been reported to develop Charcot arthropathy following in situ pedal bypass, after perfusion to the foot has been restored. Certain cases require surgical reconstruction and arthrodesis. In some cases, a simple exostosectomy can reduce pressure enough to heal an ulcer;[72] many others require complete foot reconstruction.[73]

Charcot arthropathy is often misdiagnosed as an infectious process unless the treating physician has a high index of suspicion. The differential diagnosis includes infection, osteomyelitis, deep venous thrombosis, posterior tibialis tendon dysfunction, and even bone tumor. Imaging studies can be misleading, especially early in the course of the disease. Plain film radiographs often show periosteal elevation, multiple fractures, and, in some instances, osteopenia that may be misinterpreted as osteomyelitis by an inexperienced radiologist or surgeon. Many patients are treated for osteomyelitis even though they have never had a wound or injury. Bone scanning and magnetic resonance imaging are usually not reliable for differentiating bone infection, trauma, fracture, and postsurgical inflammation. The surgeon should have a clear diagnosis of bone infection before planning an amputation, especially in the absence of a wound. A bone biopsy is the "gold standard" to diagnose bone infection. A Jamshidi needle used under fluoroscopy permits the surgeon to obtain a bone specimen for a definitive diagnosis and minimizes the ambiguity associated with more expensive imaging techniques. The mid-foot is the most common site of a Charcot fracture. The result is often a convex arch, with the head of the talus and navicular bones or the cuboid projecting from the bottom of the foot; in some cases, the talus bone may be destroyed, with the weight of the extremity borne by the malleolus, which easily ulcerates. Ulcers often occur because of the abnormal pressure and shear forces created by the collapse of the arch. When these wounds fail to heal, it is usually not due to ischemia but rather to a combination of neuropathy, bony abnormality, pressure, shear, and repetitive local trauma. The treatment for both ulcers and active Charcot arthropathy is cast immobilization. Charcot fractures may take 2–3 times longer to heal than fractures at the same site in persons without diabetes.

The American Diabetes Association and the American Pediatric Medical Association have created a joint task force on the Charcot foot which resulted in a consensus document publication in 2011[74] and the generation of a treatment algorithm (Flowchart 2).

Diabetic Revascularization

An appropriate revascularization strategy should be customized for diabetic patients according to their anatomy and comorbidities. The Bypass versus Angioplasty in Severe Ischemia of the Leg (BASIL) trial attempted to compare endovascular intervention with surgical bypass.[75] Among the 452 patients randomized to bypass or endovascular intervention, perioperative morbidity was higher with surgery, but amputation-free and overall survivals were similar in both groups at 1 year. However, at the 2-year interval, surgery was associated with a reduced risk of amputation and death. The authors concluded that angioplasty should be used first for patients with a life expectancy of 2 or fewer years and that bypass is preferred when a vein conduit is available. However, the generalizability of these results to diabetic patients is limited because only 42% of the patients in the study were diabetic. Ongoing trials like BEST-CLI and BASIL 2 would shed more light on the optimal revascularization strategy for diabetic patients.

Box 1: Organizational structure of a multidisciplinary team.

```
Multidisciplinary team

Physician team
Staff
Diagnostic imaging
Vascular therapy
    Endovascular
    Open surgery
Soft tissue therapy
    Wound care
    Reconstruction and amputation
Hyperbaric O₂
Rehabilitation
Education
Research
Marketing
Financial analysis
```

Multidisciplinary Limb Preservation Programs

The Society for Vascular Surgery and the American Podiatric Medical Association have stressed the importance and prospective benefits of multidisciplinary care for diabetic foot ulcer patients.[76] Evidence is available that a multidisciplinary program can bestow these advantages, including a significant reduction in the incidence of major leg amputations (Box 1).[77]

CONCLUSION

Unfortunately, many complications of diabetes are manifested in the foot. The management of these complications follows a predictable course of multiple hospitalizations, operations, and progressive limb loss. Early recognition and identification of the at-risk diabetic foot can curtail this downward spiral by a specialized and dedicated diabetic foot team.

REFERENCES

1. International Diabetes Federation. IDF Diabetes Atlas, 7th edition. Brussels, Belgium: International Diabetes Federation; 2015.
2. Armstrong DG, Wrobel J, Robbins JM. Guest editorial: are diabetes-related wounds and amputation worse than cancer? Int Wound J. 2007;4:286-7.
3. Singh N, Armstrong DG, Lipsky BA. Preventing foot ulcers in patients with diabetes. JAMA. 2005;293(2):217-28.
4. Reiber GE. Epidemiology of foot ulcers and amputations in the diabetic foot. In: Bowker, JH, Pfeifer, MA (Eds). Levin and O'Neal's: The diabetic foot, 6th edition. St Louis: Mosby; 2001. pp. 13-32.
5. Vishwanathan V, Thomas N, Tandon N, et al. Profile of diabetic foot complications and its associated complications—A multicentric study from India. J Assoc Physicians India. 2005;53: 933-6.
6. Sinahary K, Paul UK, Bhattacharyya AK, et al. Prevalence of diabetic foot ulcers in newly diagnosed diabetes mellitus patients. J Indian Med Assoc. 2012;110:608-11.
7. Noor S, Zubair M, Ahmad J. Diabetic foot ulcer—a review on pathophysiology, classification and microbial etiology. Diabetes Metab Syndr. 2015;9:192-9.
8. Pecoraro RE, Rieber GE, Burgess EM. Pathways to diabetic limb amputation: basis for prevention. Diabetes Care. 1990;13: 513-21.
9. Sentochnik DE, Eliopoulos GM. Infection and Diabetes. In Kahn CR, Weir GC, (Eds). Joslin's Diabetes Mellitus, 13th edition. Philadelphia: Lea and Febiger; 1994. pp 867-88.
10. Bowker JH, Pfeifer MA. Levin and O'Neal's: The Diabetic Foot, 6th Edition. St. Louis: Mosby; 2001. pp. 219.
11. Flynn MD, Tooke JE. Aetiology of diabetic foot ulceration: a role for the microcirculation? Diabet Med. 1992;9:320-9.
12. Shaw JE, Boulton AJ. The pathogenesis of diabetic foot problems: an overview. Diabetes. 1997;46:S58-61.
13. Janka HU, Standl E, Mehnert H. Peripheral vascular disease in diabetes mellitus and its relation to cardiovascular risk factors: screening with the Doppler ultrasonic technique. Diabetes Care. 1980;3:207-13.
14. Neville RF, Attinger CE, Bulan EJ, et al. Revascularization of a specific angiosome for limb salvage: does the target artery matter? Ann Vasc Surg. 2009;23:367-73.
15. Lipsky BA, Berendt AR, Cornia PB, et al. 2012 Infectious Diseases Society of America clinical practice guideline for the diagnosis and treatment of diabetic foot infections. Clin Infect Dis. 2012;54:e132-73.
16. Fasching P, Waldhausl W, Wagner OF. Elevated circulating adhesion molecules in NIDDM–potential mediators in diabetic macroangiopathy. Diabetologia. 1996;39:1242-4.
17. Labovitz JM, Shofler DW, Ragothaman KK. The impact of comorbidities on inpatient Charcot neuroarthropathy cost and utilization. J Diabetes Complications. 2016; 30:710-5.
18. Rosenbaum AJ, DiPreta JA. Classifications in brief: Eichenholtz classification of Charcot arthropathy. Clin Orthop Relat Res. 2015;473:1168-71.
19. Elamurgan TP, Jagadish S, Kate V, et al. Role of bone biopsy specimen culture in the management of diabetic foot osteomyelitis. Int J Surg. 2011;9:214-6.
20. Grant WP, Foreman EJ, Wilson AS, et al. Evaluation of Young's modulus in Achilles tendons with diabetic neuroarthropathy. J Am Podiatr Med Assoc. 2005;95:242-6.
21. Hsu WC, Liu MW, Lu TW. Biomechanical risk factors for tripping during obstacle—Crossing with the trailing limb in patients with type II diabetes mellitus. Gait Posture. 2016;45:103-9.
22. Lipsky BA, Berendt AR, Deery HG, et al. Diagnosis and treatment of diabetic foot infections. Clin Infect Dis. 2004;39:885-910.
23. Rogers LC, Frykberg RG, Armstrong DG, et al. The Charcot foot in diabetes. Diabetes Care. 2011;34:2123-9.
24. Feng Y, Schlosser FJ, Sumpio BE. The Semmes Weinstein monofilament examination is a significant predictor of the risk

24. of foot ulceration and amputation in patients with diabetes mellitus. J Vasc Surg. 2011;53:220-6.
25. Kumar S, Fernando DJ, Veves A, et al. Semmes-Weinstein monofilaments: a simple, effective and inexpensive screening device for identifying diabetic patients at risk of foot ulceration. Diabetes Res Clin Pract. 1991;13:63-7.
26. Young MJ, Breddy JL, Veves A, et al. The prediction of diabetic neuropathic foot ulceration using vibration perception thresholds. A prospective study. Diabetes Care. 1994;17:557-60.
27. Armstrong DG, Lavery LA, Harkless LB. Validation of a diabetic wound classification system. The contribution of depth, infection, and ischemia to risk of amputation. Diabetes Care. 1998;21:855-9.
28. Mills JL Sr, Conte MS, Armstrong DG, et al. The Society for Vascular Surgery Lower Extremity Threatened Limb Classification System: risk stratification based on wound, ischemia, and foot infection (WIfI). J Vasc Surg. 2014;59:220-34.
29. Termaat MF, Raijmakers PG, Scholten HJ, et al. The accuracy of diagnostic imaging for the assessment of chronic osteomyelitis: a systematic review and meta-analysis. J Bone Joint Surg Am. 2005;87:2464-71.
30. Sumpio BE, Aruny J, Blume PA. The multidisciplinary approach to limb salvage. Acta Chir Belg. 2004;104:647-53.
31. Lebrun E, Tomic-Canic M, Kirsner RS. The role of surgical debridement in healing of diabetic foot ulcers. Wound Repair Regen. 2010;18:433-8.
32. Falanga V. Wound healing and its impairment in the diabetic foot. Lancet. 2005;366:1736-43.
33. Rao N, Ziran BH, Lipsky BA. Treating osteomyelitis: antibiotics and surgery. Plast Reconstr Surg. 2011;127:177S-87S.
34. Blume PA, Paragas LK, Sumpio BE, et al. Single-stage surgical treatment of noninfected diabetic foot ulcers. Plast Reconstr Surg. 2002;109:601-9.
35. Eneroth M, Apelqvist J, Stenstrom A. Clinical characteristics and outcome in 223 diabetic patients with deep foot infections. Foot Ankle Int. 1997;18:716-22.
36. Bennett NT, Schultz GS. Growth factors and wound healing: biochemical properties of growth factors and their receptors. Am J Surg. 1993;165:728-37.
37. Bryant RA. Acute and chronic wounds, 2nd edition. St. Louis: Mosby; 2000. pp. 189-96.
38. Kalinski C, Schnepf M, Laboy D, et al. Effectiveness of a topical formulation containing metronidazole for wound odor and exudates control. Wounds. 2005;17:84-90.
39. Kashyap A, Beezhold D, Wiseman J, et al. Effect of povidone iodine dermatologic ointment on wound healing. Am Surg. 1995;61:486-91.
40. Karlsmark T, Agerslev RH, Bendz SH, et al. Clinical performance of a new silver dressing, Contreet Foam, for chronic exuding venous leg ulcers. J Wound Care. 2003;12:351-4.
41. Schultz GS, Sibbald RG, Falanga V, et al. Wound bed preparation: a systematic approach to wound management. Wound Repair Regen. 2003;11:S1-28.
42. British National Formulary (2011). British National Formulary for advanced wound dressing. [online] Available from https://www.bnf.org/ [Accessed December 2018].
43. Dumville JC, O'Meara S, Deshpande S, et al. Alginate dressings for healing diabetic foot ulcers. Cochrane Database Syst Rev. 2012;2:CD009110.
44. Burrow JW, Koch JA, Chuang HH, et al. Nitric oxide donors selectively reduce the expression of matrix metalloproteinases-8 and -9 by human diabetic skin fibroblasts. J Surg Res. 2007;140:90-8.
45. Basavaraj GV, Uppin IV, Raghavendra BYP. Chronic diabetic wound healing: recombinant PDGF v/s normal saline dressing. J Pharm Biomed Sci. 2012;24:118-20.
46. Molan PC, Betts JA. Using honey to heal diabetic foot ulcers. Adv Skin Wound Care. 2008;21:313-6.
47. Molan PC. The evidence supporting the use of honey as a wound dressing. Int J Low Extrem Wounds. 2006;5:40-54.
48. Vijaykumar H, Pai SA, Pandey V, et al. Comparative study of collagenase and papain-urea based preparations in the management of chronic nonhealing limb ulcers. Indian J Sci Technol. 2011;4:1096-100.
49. Andros G, Armstrong DG, Attinger CE, et al. Consensus statement on negative pressure wound therapy (V.A.C. Therapy) for the management of diabetic foot wounds. Ostomy Wound Manage. 2006;(Suppl):1-32.
50. Kessler L, Bilbault P, Ortéga F, et al. Hyperbaric oxygenation accelerates the healing rate of nonischemic chronic diabetic foot ulcers: a prospective randomized study. Diabetes Care. 2003;26:2378-82.
51. Faglia E, Favales F, Aldeghi A, et al. Adjunctive systemic hyperbaric oxygen therapy in treatment of severe prevalently ischemic diabetic foot ulcer. A randomized study. Diabetes Care. 1996;19:1338-43.
52. Tan T, Shaw EJ, Siddiqui F, et al. Inpatient management of diabetic foot problems: summary of NICE guidance. BMJ. 2011;342:d1280.
53. Streit M, Braathen LR. Apligraf—a living human skin equivalent for the treatment of chronic wounds. Int J Artif Organs. 2000;23:831.
54. Mostow EN, Haraway GD, Dalsing M, et al. Effectiveness of an extracellular matrix graft (OASIS Wound Matrix) in the treatment of chronic leg ulcers: a randomized clinical trial. J Vasc Surg. 2005;41:837-43.
55. Naughton G, Mansbridge J, Gentzkow G. A metabolically active human dermal replacement for the treatment of diabetic foot ulcers. Artif Organs. 1997;21:1203-10.
56. Driver VR, LAvery LA, Reyzelman AM, et al. A clinical trial of Integra Template for diabetic foot ulcer treatment. Wound Repair Regen. 2015;23:891-900.
57. Smiell JM, Wieman TJ, Steed DL, et al. Efficacy and safety of becaplermin (recombinant human platelet-derived growth factor-BB) in patients with nonhealing, lower extremity diabetic ulcers: a combined analysis of four randomized studies. Wound Repair Regen. 1999;7:335-46.
58. Bus SA, van Deursen RW, Armstrong DG, et al. Footwear and offloading interventions to prevent and heal foot ulcers and reduce plantar pressure in patients with diabetes: a systematic review. Diabetes Metab Res Rev. 2016;32:99-118.

59. Bus SA, van Netten JJ. A shift in priority in diabetic foot care and research: 75% of foot ulcers are preventable. Diabetes Metab Res Rev. 2016;32:195-200.
60. van Netten JJ, Price PE, Lavery LA, et al. Prevention of foot ulcers in the at-risk patient with diabetes: a systematic review. Diabetes Metab Res Rev. 2016;32:84-98.
61. Elraiyah T, Prutsky G, Domecq JP, et al. A systematic review and meta-analysis of off-loading methods for diabetic foot ulcers. J Vasc Surg. 2016;63:59S-68S.
62. Armstrong DG, Nguyen HC, Lavery LA, et al. Off-loading the diabetic foot wound: a randomized clinical trial. Diabetes Care. 2001;24:1019-22.
63. Driver VR, Madsen J, Goodman RA. Reducing amputation rates in patients with diabetes at a military medical center: the limb preservation service model. Diabetes Care. 2005;28:248-53.
64. Rasmussen A, Bjerre-Christensen U, Almdal TP, et al. Percutaneous flexor tenotomy for preventing and treating toe ulcers in people with diabetes mellitus. J Tissue Viability. 2013;22:68-73.
65. Armstrong DG, Lavery LA, Stern S, et al. Is prophylactic diabetic foot surgery dangerous? J Foot Ankle Surg. 1996;35:585-9.
66. Catanzariti AR, Blitch EL, Karlock LG. Elective foot and ankle surgery in the diabetic patient. J Foot Ankle Surg. 1995;34:23-41.
67. Rogers LC, Armstrong DG. Podiatric Care. In: Sidway AN, Perler BA (Eds). Rutherford's Vascular Surgery and Endovascular Therapy, 9th edition. New York: Elsevier; 2018. pp. 1557.
68. Armstrong DG, Frykberg RG. Classifying diabetic foot surgery: toward a rational definition. Diabet Med. 2003;20:329-31.
69. Armstrong DG, Lavery LA, Frykberg RG, et al. Validation of a diabetic foot surgery classification. Int Wound J. 2006;3:240-6.
70. Nielson DL, Armstrong DG. The natural history of Charcot's neuroarthropathy. Clin Podiatr Med Surg. 2008;25:53-62.
71. Armstrong DG, Todd WF, Lavery LA, et al. The natural history of acute Charcot's arthropathy in a diabetic foot specialty clinic. J Am Podiatr Med Assoc. 1997;87:272-8.
72. Catanzariti AR, Mendicino R, Haverstock B. Ostectomy for diabetic neuroarthropathy involving the midfoot. J Foot Ankle Surg. 2000;39:291-300.
73. Bevilacqua NJ, Rogers LC. Surgical management of Charcot midfoot deformities. Clin Podiatr Med Surg. 2008;25:81-94.
74. Rogers LC, Frykberg RG, Armstrong DG, et al. The Charcot foot in diabetes. J Am Podiatr Med Assoc. 2011;101:437-46.
75. Adam DJ, Beard JD, Cleveland T, et al. Bypass versus angioplasty in severe ischaemia of the leg (BASIL): multicentre, randomised controlled trial. Lancet. 2005;366:1925-34.
76. Sumpio BE, Armstrong DG, Lavery LA, et al. The role of interdisciplinary team approach in the management of the diabetic foot: a joint statement from the Society for Vascular Surgery and the American Podiatric Medical Association. J Vasc Surg. 2010;51:1504-6.
77. Krishnan S, Nash F, Baker N, et al. Reduction in diabetic amputations over 11 years in a defined U.K. population: benefits of multidisciplinary team work and continuous prospective audit. Diabetes Care. 2008;31:99-101.

CHAPTER 9

Neuropathic Ulcers

Savitha AS, S Sacchidanand

INTRODUCTION

Neuropathic ulcer is a common complication, which may occur secondary to an anesthetic foot. These are also called plantar or trophic ulcers. Lack of sensation over the pressure points leads to cumulative microtrauma, minor wounds or scratches and cuts, which go unnoticed and eventually developing into ulcers. Neuropathic ulcer is usually a secondary complication, which results from the triad of disorders namely peripheral neuropathy, peripheral vascular disease, and infection.

CAUSES OF NEUROPATHIC ULCERS

The most common cause of neuropathic ulceration to the lower limb is diabetes mellitus.[1]

Other causes are shown in Table 1.

Table 1: Causes of neuropathic ulcers.

Primary neurological conditions	Multiple sclerosis
	Paraplegia
	Spina bifida
	Syringomyelia
	Hereditary sensory motor neuropathy
Systemic causes	Diabetes mellitus
	Renal failure
	Chronic liver failure
	Alcoholism
Nutritional deficiencies	
Infections	Leprosy
	HIV
	Syphilis
	Poliomyelitis
Trauma, surgery	

ETIOPATHOGENESIS

Peripheral neuropathy affects both sensory and motor nerves.

Involvement of Sensory Nerves

An anesthetic foot is "ulcer liable" and ulceration makes it "ulcer prone" producing a cycle of ulcer scar ulcer.[2] When the sensory nerves are affected, the protective sensations like pain, pressure, proprioception, and temperature are lost. Foot injuries go unnoticed by the patients. A foreign body, which may be lodged in the footwear, or a sharp object like a nail, which has penetrated the shoe or slipper goes unnoticed by the patient, causing repeated trauma. Small cuts or punctures on skin due to mechanical and thermal damage go unnoticed, progressing to ulcers over time. As the affected foot has less discomfort, the patient exerts more weight on the same foot, causing repetitive mechanical trauma and callous formation, followed by tissue breakdown, and eventually chronic ulceration.[3] The callus, which is present at the margins of the ulcer prevent the ulcer healing by blocking the epidermal cell migration during the healing process. Loss of pain prevents the patient from altering his gait to prevent further injury when there is wound formation. "Holiday ulcers" are reported where people have walked barefoot on hot sandy beaches and developed blisters and ulcers due to lack of temperature sensation.[4]

The mechanisms of plantar ulceration is summarized in Box 1.[5]

Involvement of Motor Nerves

Wasting and weakness of intrinsic muscles of the foot is caused by motor nerve involvement, leading to an

> **Box 1:** The mechanisms of plantar ulceration.
>
> The five mechanisms by which plantar ulcer is caused in an anesthetic foot are:
> 1. Continuous pressure, causing necrosis due to poor blood supply
> 2. High pressure causing injury by mechanical violence
> 3. *Thermal injuries*: Burns or frostbite
> 4. Repetitive mechanical stress causing inflammation and autolysis
> 5. Pressure causing spread of infection

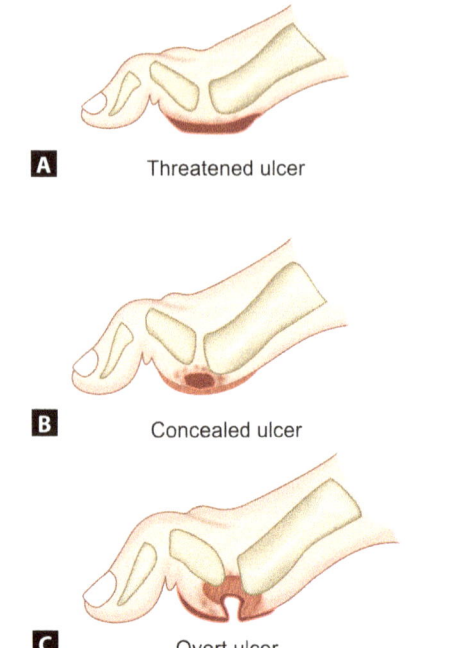

Figs. 1A to C: Schematic representation of stages of ulcer.

imbalance between the flexor and extensor muscles. This further causes deformities and creates additional pressure points, which are prone to ulceration.[6] The plantar intrinsic muscles are active maximally during the push off stage of walking, where the front portion of the foot pushes the ground backward to propel the body forward. Maximum forces are generated at the metatarsophalangeal joints at this stage of walking which is countered by these intrinsic muscles. When these muscles are paralyzed, this protective effect is lost causing the toes to claw during the push off stage causing momentary increase in stress and strain over the metatarsophalangeal joints during each step, even small increase in stress when repeated long enough results in ulceration.[7]

Another consequence of muscle wasting is the reduction of soft tissue padding to the skin. As the skin is closer to the bone, the skin is exposed to higher mechanical force between the bone and walking surface.

Involvement of Autonomic Nerves

Reduction of sweating and sebaceous secretion causes dryness of the skin. Dry skin has less elasticity and is more prone to mechanical stress. Fissuring of the skin is more common following autonomic neuropathy.

STAGES OF ULCER FORMATION[8] (FIGS. 1A TO C)

Stage of Threatened Ulcer

This is called the preulcerative stage of aseptic inflammation. Increased stress exerted over prolonged time causes traumatic (aseptic) inflammation in the subcutaneous layer of the sole, which is most vulnerable to mechanical stress. This usually occurs under a joint or a bony prominence just distal to the head of a metatarsal. The affected site is edematous. Clinically, this is visible as mild or obvious splaying of a toe, which stands apart from other toes. Tenderness on deep digital pressure can be elicited at the affected site.

Stage of Concealed Ulcer

In this stage, a necrotic blister is formed. The tissue undergoes necrosis due to inflammation and the stress of continued walking. The liquefied tissue mixed with blood is forced to the surface by continued walking to present as a blister. This usually overlies the area of necrosis, but sometimes the overlying tissue is too tough that it may track along a path of least resistance and emerge to the surface at a distance, at the side of the toe or in the interdigital web. This stage may go unnoticed. With the formation of the necrotic blister, the destruction of the subcutaneous tissue is complete, except that the "ulcer" is not seen or obvious because it is still covered with skin.

Stage of Overt or Open Ulcer

This is the stage where necrotic area becomes exteriorized as the skin overlying the blister breaks open.

CLINICAL FEATURES

The sequence of chronic ulcer formation is shown in Flowchart 1.

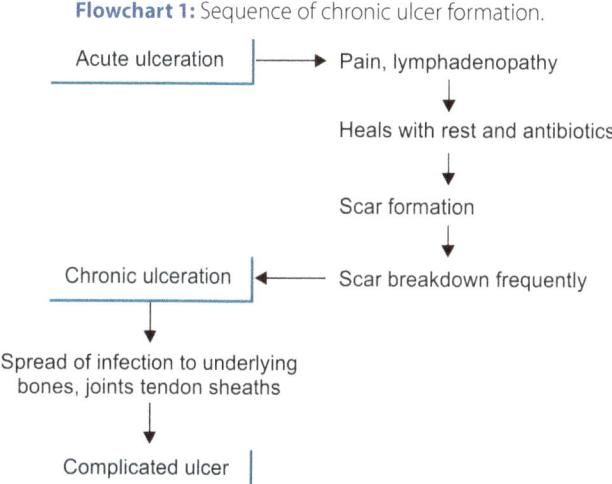

Flowchart 1: Sequence of chronic ulcer formation.

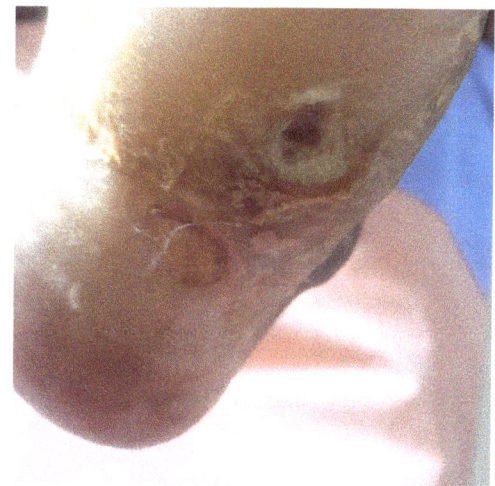

Fig. 2: Typical chronic neuropathic ulcer with punched out edges and callus formation.

Site

Neuropathic ulcers occur commonly at the site of repeated trauma, as in the area at the metatarsal heads, dorsal surface of hammer toes and distal most portion of hammer toes where there is flexion at the interphalangeal joints.[4] Leprosy trophic ulcers are seen more in the front portion. Medial aspect is more vulnerable than the lateral part. The proximal phalanx of the great toe is the most common site for leprosy trophic ulcer.[2]

Symptoms

Neuropathic ulcers are usually painless. Presence of pain indicates either associated arterial component or secondary infection. Due to the absence of pain, patients have unaltered gait despite having large ulcers.

Signs

The ulcers are usually small with sharp punched out edges. The wound margins of neuropathic ulcers have callus build-up, which is a clue to the constant pressure load (Fig. 2). There may be scanty discharge. The floor of the ulcer is fibrosed, hard, and covered with unhealthy granulation tissue. When the ulcer is infected, the edges are swollen, with edema of the feet. There is copious pus discharge, and floor is covered with necrotic tissue. Associated tender lymphadenopathy and fever may be present. Initially when the inflammation is limited to subcutaneous tissue, it is called simple or uncomplicated ulcer. At this stage, it heals easily with scarring, but recurrences occur due to underlying pathogenic factors.

The peripheral pulses are bounding and normal unless there is a vascular component. Skin is warm and nontender on the foot and may appear dry due to loss of autonomic sensation.

Associated findings include limited joint mobility (LJM), and deformities (pes cavus, flattened plantar arch, hallux rigidus, hammer toes, claw toes, etc.).[9]

APPROACH TO PATIENT WITH NEUROPATHIC ULCER

Points to be considered during history taking:
- Elicit the cause for underlying neuropathy, medical history, medications, diabetes
- Smoking, alcohol habits
- Previous ulcers
- Onset, duration, progression of the ulcer, pain and discharge, preceding trauma
- Occupation and lifestyle
- Type of footwear.

Management of neuropathic ulcers involves multiple disciplinarians like physicians, surgeons, orthopedicians, vascular surgeons, and trained nurses.

MANAGEMENT OF ULCER

Two main components of ulcer management are:
1. Wound closure with healing
2. Prevention of further ulcer developments.

Various measures in neuropathic ulcer management are given in Figure 3.

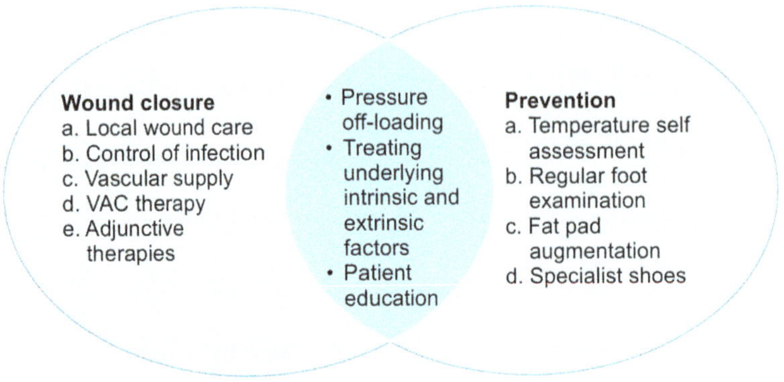

Fig. 3: Schematic of management of neuropathic ulcers. (VAC: vacuum-assisted closure).

Debridement

Wound management begins with proper debridement. Debridement involves removal of callus, hyperkeratotic skin, devitalized and infected tissue to aid the healing process, to assess the depth of the ulcer and reduce the risk of infection. Debridement may be done once, or it may need to be ongoing for maintenance of a clean wound bed.[10] Deep tissue culture samples should be taken during debridement.

- Sharp debridement can be performed in an outpatient setting with forceps, scissors, and scalpel. If extensive debridement is required, it should be performed surgically under adequate anesthesia. Sharp debridement is avoided in patients requiring revascularization due to the risk of trauma to tissues that are vascularly compromised.
- Autolytic debridement is a process by which the body attempts to shed devitalized tissue using moisture. If tissue is kept moist, it will degrade naturally and deslough from the underlying healthy tissues. The presence of matrix metalloproteinases (MMPs) enhances this process. It is a slow process, which increases the risk of infection and maceration. A moist wound environment also facilitates the migration of keratinocytes to wound bed.
- Maggot debridement therapy involves applying sterile larvae of the green bottle fly to a neuropathic ulcer. Maggots have the ability to provide antimicrobial activity, debride wound beds, and also stimulate wound healing. Larval therapy is not recommended to be used as the only method of debridement in neuropathic ulcers as calluses cannot be removed by the larvae. It is also not recommended for use in ulcers with an ischemic component as the process can cause or aggravate severe pain.[11]
- *Hydrosurgical debridement*: A high-energy saline beam is used as a cutting implement to remove devitalized tissue here. The benefits of this technique include a short treatment time and the ability to remove most, if not all, dead tissue from the wound bed. Disadvantages include the need for specialist and expensive equipment.[12]

Management of Secondary Infections

Presence of infection should be detected and treated urgently with appropriate systemic antibiotics. Evidence for use of topical antibiotics is weak. Infection may go unnoticed in the early stages due to lack of pain. Diagnosing infection at an early stage although challenging, is crucial in preventing progression of the infection and thereby preventing necrosis, gangrene, and amputation. Systemic signs may only be present in severe infections such as osteomyelitis or septicemia.[13] Box 2 enumerates the risk factors for infection[14] and Box 3 the investigations required.

Advanced moist wound therapy is given with hydrogels and alginates. The silver barrier dressings destroy bacteria in the wound. The antimicrobial barrier is effective for up to 3 days. Exudative wounds are dressed with hydrocolloid dressings, which can absorb the exudate. Dressing selection should be reassessed at regular intervals.[15]

Adjuvant Therapies

- *Vacuum-assisted closure therapy*:[16] Vacuum-assisted closure (VAC) therapy is a technique to accelerate the

Box 2: Risk factors for infection in neuropathic ulcers.

- Walking barefoot
- Presence of diabetes
- Positive probe to bone test
- Chronic ulcers > 30 days
- Presence of previous recurrent ulcers
- Associated peripheral arterial disease
- Complete loss of pain sensation
- Associated renal failure

> **Box 3:** Investigations in suspected infected ulcer.
>
> - Microbial culture: As the open wounds are colonized with pathogens, superficial swabs for culture are not adequate
> - Complete blood count
> - Random blood sugar
> - C-reactive protein
> - Renal function tests
> - X-ray of the foot for osteomyelitis—signs are focal destruction of cortical bone, periosteal new bone formation, soft tissue swelling, focal osteoporosis
> - MRI when there is high clinical suspicion of osteomyelitis in spite of normal radiograph

(MRI: magnetic resonance imaging)

healing of nonhealing ulcers that fail to heal on their own (primary healing). VAC uses controlled negative pressure (–125 mm Hg) using vacuum-assisted drainage to remove blood or serous fluid from wound site, to provide a drier surgical field and control blood flow. It also promotes increased angiogenesis and granulation tissue.

- *Platelet-derived fibrin*: Platelet-derived growth factor (PDGF) is a protein involved with regulating cell growth and division. It has a significant role in angiogenesis. The reader is referred to the chapter 17 for further reading.
- *Granulocyte colony-stimulating factor (G-CSF)* is a hematopoietic growth factor required for the proliferation and differentiation of hematopoietic precursors of neutrophil granulocytes. G-CSF also enhances the antimicrobial functions of mature neutrophils. Addition of G-CSF was associated with fewer surgical interventions, including amputations. Addition of G-CSF was also found to reduce length of hospital stay, but it did not affect the length of systemic antibiotic therapy.[4]
- *Honey* has been used in the healing of leg ulcers for centuries. One theory is that honey may facilitate autolytic debridement; another theory proposes antimicrobial properties. However, there is a lack of data to support the routine use of honey in the management of neuropathic ulcers.
- *Phenytoin sodium* fine powder zinc paste has been used to treat leprosy ulcers.[17]
- *Low-level laser therapy*.[18]

Management of Underlying Causes

- *Reducing pressure on the foot*: Reducing and redistributing pressures from high-risk areas to an even share throughout the foot are important step in the management of neuropathic ulcers. This can be achieved through complete bed rest. The gold standard method for pressure offloading is a total contact cast (TCC). This is a minimally padded cast, which is molded to the foot and lower leg. It redistributes pressure evenly across the whole of the plantar surface of the foot. It is not easy for the patient to remove so the TCC has much higher compliance rates, and in turn higher success rates. The application and removal of TCCs require specially trained personnel. If fitted by unskilled staff, ulcers can develop inside the cast. TCCs are not suitable for patients with infected ulcers or osteomyelitis as wounds cannot be inspected regularly. A modification has been developed to circumvent this problem. Here, a plaster casing with window and a walking iron for weight bearing is used. Regular dressing can be accomplished through the window and patient can be ambulatory with walking iron. This helps in early mobilization and prevents secondary complications like foul-smelling discharge and decalcification of bone.[19]

  Other devices used, if a TCC is either contraindicated or not tolerated by the patient include removable cast walkers, Scotchcast boots, healing sandals, crutches, walkers, air cushions, water beds, wheelchairs.[20]

  Injectable silicone oil has been used in attempts to increase the thickness of tissue on the plantar surface of the foot and reduce peak foot pressures. There is currently no evidence to prove that fat pad augmentation improves outcomes such as ulceration or amputation.[1]

- *Deformities*: Deformities result from neuropathic changes and these can predispose to ulcerations. Feet should be inspected for common deformities including hammer toes (a fixed flexion deformity of the proximal interphalangeal joint), claw toes (flexion at the distal and proximal interphalangeal joints with dorsiflexion at the metatarsophalangeal joint), prominent metatarsal heads, and pes cavus (high arch).
- *Dealing with vascular compromise*: Poor blood supply impairs healing. If there is a vascular compromise, patient is referred to vascular surgeon for its correction.
- Strict glycemic control in diabetics
- *Avoidance of smoking*: Cigarette smoking reduces the rate of oxygen intake and delivery to the wound site and retards wound repair. Nicotine, carbon monoxide, and hydrogen cyanide in the smoke also have a toxic effect on platelets and inhibit normal cellular metabolism, which may affect healing. Smoking may cause vasoconstriction and accelerate the development of atherosclerosis.

- Malnutrition, anemia to be corrected
- Dialysis in patients with renal failure.

Surgical Management

Surgical management of complicated foot ulcers are tried mainly in cases of leprosy when the ulcer is nonhealing even after conservative management for 2 months. Skin grafts, plantar artery fascia flap, advancement flaps, rotation flap, and island flaps have been described.[15]

Patient Education

Patient education plays a prominent role in preventing further ulcerations. Self-care can be defined as "the range of behavior undertaken by the individuals to promote or restore health", or "the process of enabling people to increase control over, and to improve, their health".

The patient must be educated about the origin of neuropathic ulcers.

- Daily foot checks should be part of the patient's routine from a preventive aspect.
- Fungal and bacterial infections of the toenails should be looked for and treated accordingly. Routine grooming of the nails and feet should be performed in all cases of neuropathic feet. This includes regular trimming of nails, treatment of ingrown toenails, and application of skin creams to keep the skin and nails soft.
- Patients should also be advised regarding safe limits of walking and the distance in which the patient can walk without damaging the foot. After walking for some known distance, the patient should rest for about 20 minutes and examine the feet for signs of internal damage, persistent warmth, swelling or blistering, burning sensation, or tenderness. The presence of some or all of these signs indicates that the foot has been damaged and that the distance walked has exceeded the safe limit for that foot. Patients should be advised not to walk beyond a safe limit.[7]
- Patients should be advised to check the temperature of bath water with their elbow before stepping in to avoid thermal trauma to their feet.
- Avoiding close proximity to fire, heated objects to prevent thermal burns.
- Patients are advised not to walk barefoot in the house or outside.
- In patients with diabetes, the importance of glycemic control needs to be highlighted.
- High-temperature gradients between feet have been shown to precede the onset of neuropathic ulceration.

The incidence of ulceration can be significantly reduced by daily at-home patient self-monitoring of foot temperatures.[1]

Footwear

Without proper footwear, anesthetic feet are vulnerable to repetitive pressures, which result in inflammation, ulcers, and infection causing partial to complete foot destruction. The prime step in prevention of trophic ulcers is even distribution of pressure over the plantar surface of the foot. A metatarsal bar over the arch helps in pressure distribution. The sole of the shoe is molded to fit in the curvature of the foot to distribute the pressure equally. The most effective way to reduce pressure under the forefoot of shortened, deformed feet is to wear a shoe with a rigid sole pivoting on a rocker near the center of the foot. The use of insoles made of microcellular rubber (MCR) is recommended. The MCR sheets manufactured with a shore hardness of 15' Shore 'A' help to prevent high-pressure points and thus avoid plantar ulcers in anesthetic feet. Natural rubber along with several other chemicals is used in optimum quantities to manufacture MCR. The unique manufacturing process gives MCR the ability to spring back to original shape when pressure is released while walking.[21] MCR is lightweight, flexible, shock absorbent, and highly durable. It is important to fit each shoe to the patient with a pressure indicating footprint for guidance. The shoes should not have metallic buckles or nails. Inspection of shoes for small pebbles or nails stuck in them is important.

CONCLUSION

The presence of peripheral neuropathy reduces the protective sensations of the feet, leading to neglecting minor trauma, which further progresses to ulcers. These ulcers are slow to heal and occur commonly over the pressure points. Optimal management is achieved by multidisciplinary approach and patient involvement. Secondary infection should be treated effectively. Educating the patient about self-care goes a long way in preventing and early detection of the ulcers.

REFERENCES

1. Ndip A, Ebah L, Mbako A. Neuropathic diabetic foot ulcers. Evidence to practice. Int J Gen Med. 2012;5:129-34.
2. Gahalaut P, Pinto J, Pai G, et al. A novel treatment of plantar ulcers in leprosy: local superficial flaps. Lepr Rev. 2005;76: 220-31.
3. Edmonds ME, Foster AVM. ABC of wound healing, diabetic foot ulcers. BMJ. 2006;332:407-10.

4. Ndip A, Sadler K, Lower N. Neuropathic ulcers. In: Khanna AK, Tiwary SK (Eds). Ulcers of lower extremity. New Delhi: Springer; 2016. pp. 237-47.
5. Sabato S, Yosipovitch Z, Simkin A, et al. Plantar trophic ulcers in patients with leprosy. A correlative study of sensation, pressure and mobility. Int Orthop. 1982;6:203-8.
6. Shaw JE, Boulton A. The pathogenesis of diabetic foot problems: an overview. Diabet Med. 1996;13 Suppl 1:812-6.
7. Srinivasan H. Management of ulcers in neurologically impaired feet in leprosy affected persons. In: Schwarz R, Brandsma W (Eds). Surgical Reconstruction and Rehabilitation in Leprosy and Others Neuropathies. Kathmandu: Ekta Books; 2004: 193-226.
8. Riyaz N, Sehgal VN. Leprosy: Trophic Skin Ulcers. Skinmed. 2017;15:45-51.
9. Boulton AJ, Armstrong DG, Albert SF, et al. Comprehensive foot examination and risk assessment. Diabetes Care. 2008;31: 1679-85.
10. Wounds UK. (2013). Effective debridement in a changing NHS: a UK consensus. [online] Available from www.wounds-uk.com. [Accessed December, 2018].
11. Gottrup F, Jorgensen B. Maggot debridement: an alternative method for debridement. Eplasty. 2011;11:e33.
12. Haycock S, Chadwick P. Debridement of diabetic foot wounds. Nurs Stand. 2012;26(24):51-8.
13. Wounds International. (2013). International Best Practice Guidelines. Wound management in diabetic foot ulcers. [online] Available from www.woundsinternational.com. [Accessed December, 2018].
14. Lipsky BA, Berendt AR, Cornia PB. Infectious Diseases Society of America clinical practice guideline for the diagnosis and treatment of diabetic foot infections. IDSA guidelines. Clin Infect Dis. 2012;54(12):132-73.
15. Puri V, Venkateshwaran N, Khare N. Trophic ulcers—Practical management guidelines. Indian J Plastic Surg. 2012;45:340-51.
16. Ali Z, Anjum A, Khurshid L, et al. Evaluation of low-cost custom made VAC therapy compared with conventional wound dressings in the treatment of non-healing lower limb ulcers in lower socio-economic group patients of Kashmir valley. J Orth Surg Re. 2015;10:183.
17. Sehgal VN, Prasad PVS, Kaviarasan PK, et al. Trophic skin ulceration of leprosy: evaluation of efficacy of topical phenytoin sodium zinc paste. Int J Dermatol. 2014;53:873-8.
18. Tunér J, Hode L. The Laser Therapy Handbook. Gränsgesberg, Sweden: Prima Books AB; 2004.
19. Chaudhury AR. Chronic planter ulcer: a new technique of management. IJPMR. 2004;15:45-7.
20. Cavanagh PR, Bus SA. Off-loading the diabetic foot for ulcer prevention and healing. J Vasc Surg. 2010;52:37s-43s.
21. Paul SK, Rajkumar E, Mendis T. Microcellular rubber (MCR)—a boon for leprosy affected patients with anesthetic feet in preventing secondary impairments. J Foot Ankle Res. 2014;7(Suppl 1):A92.

CHAPTER 10

Ischemic Ulcers, Pyoderma Gangrenosum and Vasculitic Ulcers

Biju Vasudevan, Gayatri Gupta

ISCHEMIC (ARTERIAL) ULCERS

INTRODUCTION

Ischemic or arterial leg ulcers are caused by reduction in arterial blood flow that leads to insufficient tissue perfusion. The commonest cause in younger age group is thromboangitis obliterans (TAO) while in old age atherosclerosis is the causative factor. Other common causes which predispose to ischemic arterial ulcers are thromboangiitis, vasculitis, pyoderma gangrenosum (PG), thalassemia and sickle cell disease as given in Box 1.[1-3] They are classified as acute and chronic (Table 1). For chronic ulcers, atherosclerosis is the commonest cause with peripheral arterial disease (PAD) as the most common manifestation affecting medium and large sized arteries.

RISK FACTORS[4]

Peripheral vascular disease is most common in men older than 45 years and women older than 55 years, and patients may have a family history of premature atherosclerotic disease. Patients may also have a history of generalized vascular problems, such as myocardial infarction, angina, stroke and intermittent claudication.[4] Common risk factors for the development of atherosclerosis are given in Box 2.[4,6]

Box 1: Etiology of ischemic leg ulcer.

Arterial disease
- Arteriosclerosis obliterans
- Thromboangiitis obliterans
- Arteriovenous malformation
- Aortic coarctation
- Endofibrosis of external iliac artery (iliac artery syndrome in cyclists)
- Popliteal entrapment
- Persistent sciatic artery

Microthrombotic disease
- Antiphospholipid syndrome
- Cholesterol emboli
- Cryofibrinogenemia

Others
- Sickle cell anemia
- Polycythemia vera:
  – Acute trauma (arterial ulcer treatment)
  – Acute thrombosis
  – Primary vascular tumors
  – Pseudoxanthoma elasticum

Table 1: Classification of ischemic ulcers.

Types	Etiology
Acute	Thrombosis and trauma
Chronic	Atherosclerosis—peripheral arterial disease

Box 2: Risk factors for ischemic ulcers.

- Race and ethnicity (African Americans and those of Hispanic origin)
- Elderly age
- Male gender
- Smoking
- Diabetes mellitus
- Hypertension
- Dyslipidemia
- Obesity, and sedentary lifestyle
- Hypercoagulable and hyperviscous states
- Hyperhomocysteinemia
- Chronic renal insufficiency
- C-reactive protein, β2-microglobulin, cystatin C, lipoprotein (a)

Ischemic Ulcers, Pyoderma Gangrenosum and Vasculitic Ulcers

In population with age less than 70 years, the incidence of PAD ranges from 3–10% while in above 70 years age group it rises to 15–20%.[6] There are multiple modifiable risk factors associated with PAD as follows:[6]

- Smokers are at 4 times higher risk as compared to non-smokers
- Diabetics having 1.5–4 times increased risk especially in females
- Hypertensives having 50–92% association with PAD
- Dyslipidemia increasing the risk of PAD by 10% for every 10 mg/dL rise in total cholesterol.

PATHOGENESIS[5,7]

Atherosclerosis is a complex process and involves myriad of events like endothelial dysfunction, lipid deposition, oxidative stress and genetic factors as described in Flowchart 1 and Figure 1.

CLINICAL FEATURES

Almost 65–75% PAD patients are asymptomatic.[5] Those who are symptomatic have varied presentations like acute limb ischemia (Table 2) or critical limb ischemia.[5,8]

Critical Limb Ischemia[5]

Defined by European Society of Vascular Surgeons as recurring ischemic rest pain requiring analgesia for more

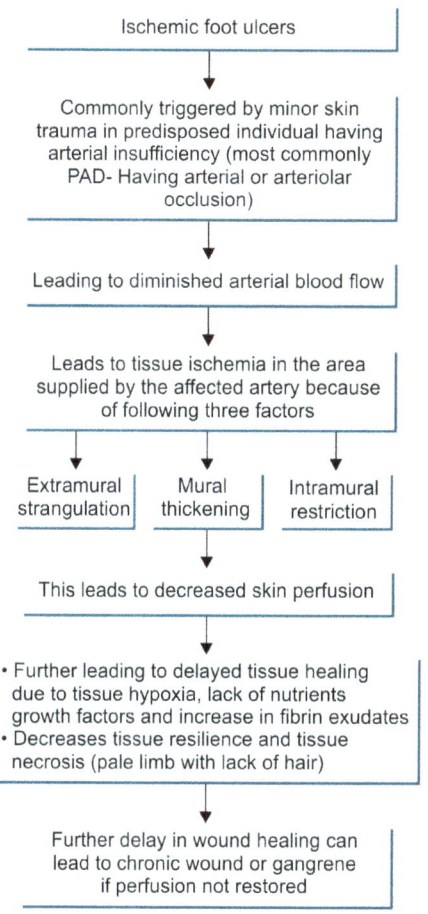

Flowchart 1: Pathogenesis of ischemic ulcer.

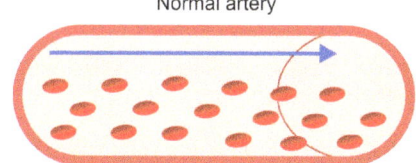
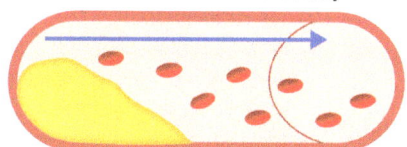

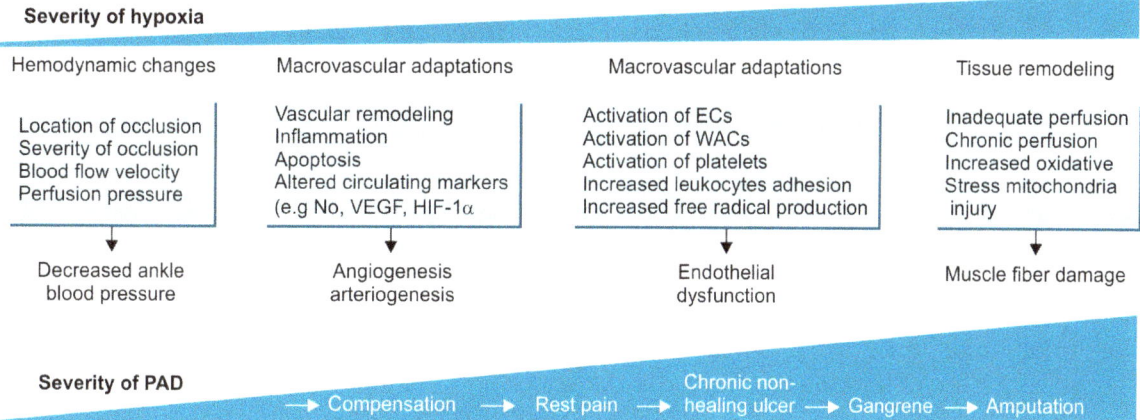

Fig. 1: Pathophysiology of atherosclerosis leading to chronic leg ulcer formation.[5]

than 2 weeks or presence of ulceration or gangrene of foot or toes with ankle systolic pressure less than 50 mm Hg or toe systolic pressure lower than 30 mm Hg (Fontaines III or IV). It commonly manifests as rest pain, ulceration and gangrene. Fontaines classification (Table 3) is a well known clinical classification for staging PAD.

The clinical symptoms and signs are presented in Tables 4 and 5.

The differentiating features with other ulcers are discussed in Table 6.

Also the differentiating features between intermittent claudication of PAD from pseudoclaudication caused by musculoskeletal, neurologic and venous cases is presented in Table 7.

The Edinburgh claudication questionnaire (91% specificity and 99% sensitivity) is used for diagnosing intermittent claudication in symptomatic patients. It is a self-answered questionnaire having made series of six questions in relation to the type of pain (Table 8).[8]

Table 2: Acute limb ischemia.

Definition	Sudden reduction in the blood supply of a previously stable leg of <2 weeks duration, causing rest pain and shows features of severe ischemia and threatening limb viability.
Subdivisions	Acute (onset <24 h) and sub-acute (onset 24 h–2 weeks)
Etiology	Emboli most common cause Thrombus formation at the site of stenosis
Clinical features	Symptoms: pain, paralysis and paraesthesia. Signs: pallor, pulselessness and cold extremities. Grades of severity: viable/ threatened /non- viable limb depends on following factors: • The presence or absence of sensory and motor function • Mottling (blanching or non-blanching) • Muscle tenderness
Treatment	Aim: immediate revascularization (within 06 hrs to prevent irreversible muscle damage) needs vascular surgery intervention. Immediate anticoagulant therapy with intravenous heparin is mandatory in all patients. (The 30-day mortality rates are 15–20% and amputation rates are 10–30%)

Table 3: Fontaines classification of critical ischemia.

Fontaines classification of critical ischemia

Stage	Clinical presentation
I	Asymptomatic
II	Intermittent claudication IIA: on walking >200 m IIB: on walking <200 m
III	Rest pain
IV	Ulceration or gangrene

Table 4: Symptoms of critical limb ischemia (CLI).

Symptoms[5,6,8]

Pain	Common *Typical description* • Muscle cramps • Fatigue or pain in the lower legs caused by exercise/exertion • Relieves rapidly by rest *Less commonly* Patients may present with CLI
Rest pain	• Indicates "CLI" • It is caused by reduced blood supply to leg presenting as 'night pains' • Felt in the most distal part of the toes and foot present as 'burning sensation or numbness' • H/o Patient getting relief by dangling leg by the bed side, or sleeping in a chair in an attempt to improve the blood supply to the foot. • And further this progress to paresthesias, coldness of the extremity, muscular weakness, and stiffness of the foot and ankle joints.
Intermittent claudication	The patient gives a classic history of inability to walk as the symptoms develop (because of lactic acid accumulation in the muscles) which relieves after resting for 15 or 20 minutes (reversible muscle ischemia) Evaluate the degree of limitation i.e. claudication distance The symptom indicates levels of arterial involvement Claudication Level of obstruction • Calf Superficial femoral or popliteal • Thigh, hip, buttock Aorto-iliac disease

Contd...

Contd...

Symptoms[5,6,8]

	Look for clinical features of atherosclerosis in other vascular beds (coronary, cerebrovascular and renal). Important to distinguish from non-vascular causes like lumbar stenosis
General examination	
Blood pressure	Blood pressure of each arm should be noted and compared to rule out associated subclavian or axillary artery disease.
	If blood pressure difference is more than 20 mm Hg it indicates arterial disease.
	Also look for bruits by auscultating the carotid and subclavian arteries; if present they may indicate stenosis as it has greater risk for myocardial infarction (MI) and cerebrovascular accident (CVA).
Systemic examination	
Cardiovascular system (CVS)	To look for any arrhythmias
Abdomen	To exclude an abdominal aortic aneurysm and if present abdominal ultrasound advised.

Table 5: Clinical signs of critical limb ischemia (CLI).

Signs[3-6,8]

Ulcers	*Sites*: commonly toes, heel, anterior surface of tibia
	Acute presentation: Affects smaller arteries which leads to sudden appearance of bluish red indurated plaque with fluid filled bleb over it. This plaque becomes black and later sloughs to form ulcer
	Chronic presentation: It has insidious onset occurring after infection or trivial trauma to toes or foot having other signs of arterial disease. These are small, indolent and painful (Fig. 2).
	Martorell's ulcer (hypertensive) presents with very painful wounds on the lateral-dorsal aspect of the calf or in the Achilles tendon region with bilateral involvement in 50% of cases (Fig. 3).
Skin condition	Inspect the feet should look for any associated calluses or tinea infection
	Look for surrounding skin erythema/cool to touch, hair loss, thin and brittle with a shiny texture
	Dry or wet gangrene: Indicates 'CLI'
Pulsations	The common femoral, popliteal, dorsalis pedis and posterior tibial pulses should all be assessed in both legs.
	The peripheral pulsation should be assessed in common femoral, popliteal, dorsalis pedis and posterior tibial in both legs. Further the pulsation is graded as:
	• Normal [2+]
	• Diminished [1+]
	• Absent [0].
	In 12% cases dorsalis pedis pulse can be absent and is considered to be normal, whereas absence of posterior tibial pulse is never normal.
	The femoral or popliteal aneurysms if any should be noted.
Capillary refill time	In individuals with normal capillary refill, after compression of the dorsum of the foot or great toe for a few seconds, the skin color returns to normal in less than two to three seconds. In case of delay in return of the normal color, it indicates vascular compromise
Buerger's test	A delay of more than 10–15 seconds in return of color after raising an ischemic leg to 45° for one minute (Buerger's test) indicates vascular compromise.
Ankle brachial pressure index (ABI) (ABI is the ratio of the ankle systolic pressure to the arm systolic pressure) (Fig. 4)	ABI is an objective and reproducible measure of vascular status of lower limbs.
	The normal range is 0.9–1.3 (100% specificity in identifying healthy individuals)
	ABI ≤0.9 in patients with symptoms has 95% sensitivity in detecting peripheral arterial disease (PAD).
	If there are palpable pulses at rest but there is drop in the pressure by 20% following exercise— suggestive of significant arterial disease.
	A low ABI has been shown to be an independent predictor of increased mortality.
	False positive ABI—in the presence of arterial calcification, (as heavily calcified vessels may be incompressible).
	Methods used when ABI is not reliable:
	• Toe–Brachial index
	• Ischemic angle (pole test).
Toe–Brachial index	The normal value is >0.70. In cases of arterial calcification where ABI is inaccurate, the 'toe–brachial index' is used in diagnosing PAD because digital vessels are spared from calcification.
Ischemic angle (pole test)	Evaluated by the level at which a pedal Doppler signal disappears on elevating the foot.

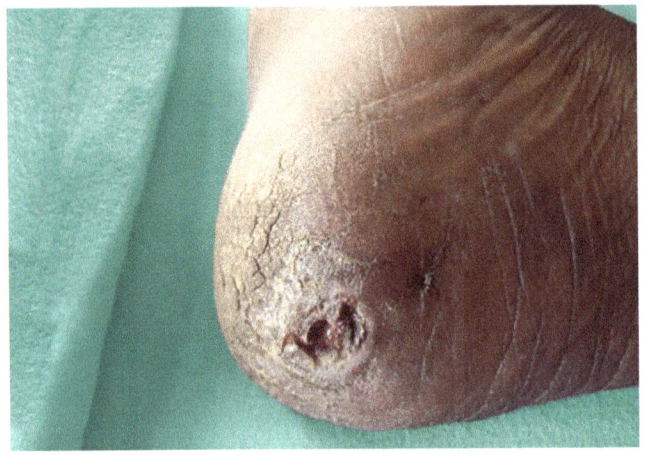

Fig. 2: Chronic ulcer.

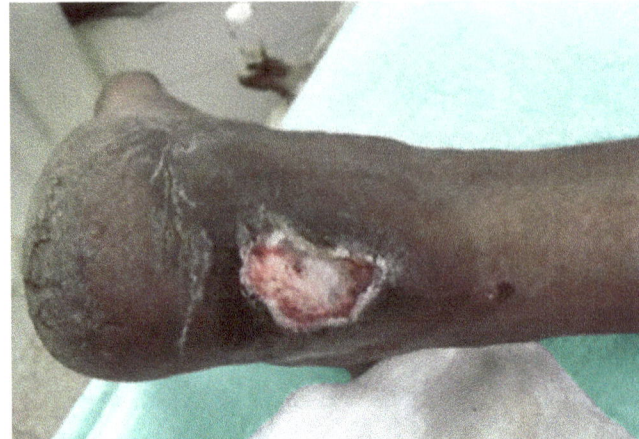

Fig. 3: Martorell's ulcer.

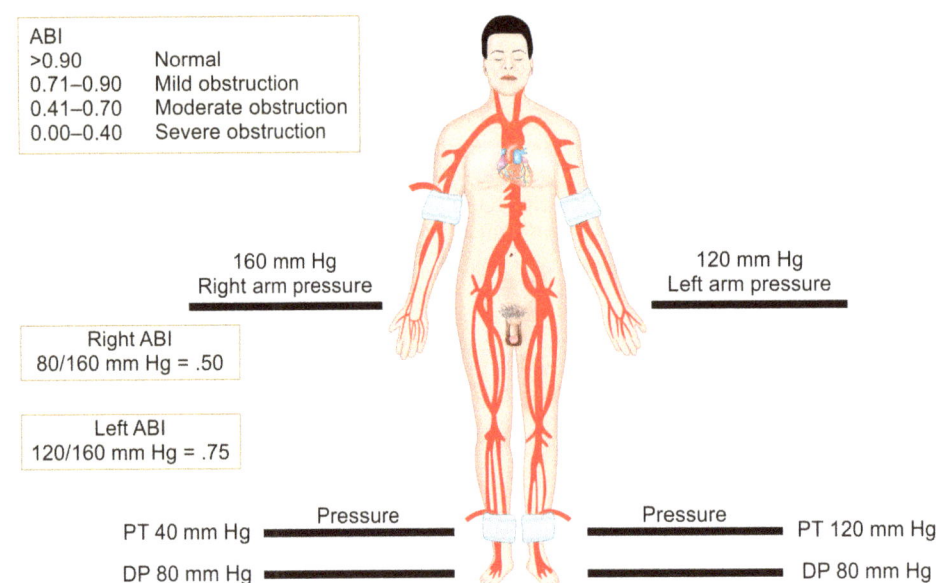

Fig. 4: Ankle brachial pressure index at various sites.

Table 6: Local examination of arterial ulcer and difference with other ulcers.[3,4,6,9]					
	Arterial ulcers	**Pyoderma gangrenosum**	**Vasculitic**	**Venous ulcers**	**Neuropathic**
Site	Commonly over toes, foot and lateral malleoli	More commonly legs pretibial area	Often distally, Usually bilateral	Medial graiter region of leg (Fig. 5)	Pressure points, toes
Size	Small and round	Start as a papule/pustule		Large, shallow and vertically oval	Variable
Border	smooth, well-demarcated borders	Bluish raised and rolled margin		serpiginous	Regular
Edges	Punched out	Violaceous undermined		Sloping and edematous	Punched out/callus

Contd...

Contd...

	Arterial ulcers	Pyoderma gangrenosum	Vasculitic	Venous ulcers	Neuropathic
Base	Shallow with slough and necrotic granulation tissue (typically pale)	Cribriform base		Covered with slough and red granulation tissue	Slough
Depth	Shallow or deep			shallow	
Surrounding skin	Thin, shiny, dry, cold and lack of hair Pallor on leg elevation	Halo of erythema		Hemosiderin staining associated with dry skin eczema and varicose veins	Callosity, Loss of sensation and warm foot
Peripheral pulses	Decreased capillary refill decreased	Present	Present	Present	Present
Pain	+++	+++	++	Commonly painless	-

Table 7: Differentiating features of intermittent claudication of peripheral arterial disease (PAD) from pseudo-claudication caused by musculoskeletal, neurologic and venous cases.

Intermittent claudication		Pseudoclaudication		
	PVD	Neurologic	Venous	Chronic compartment syndrome
Causes	Younger: thromboangitis obliterans (TAO) Older: Atherosclerosis	Spinal stenosis (most common cause) pseudoclaudication.	Deep venous thrombosis (DVT) (iliac)	Muscular cause
Type of pain	Cramping, pain, tightness, heaviness, burning localized in the legs	Back pain that radiates down the legs. Tightness of buttocks > calf paresthesia	Bursting pain in leg usually thigh	Bursting pain in muscle compartment
Effect of rest	Pain subsides immediately with rest	Pain does not subside immediately with rest	Delayed relief with rest	Delayed relief with rest
Onset of pain	After walking or exercise	After walking or standing	Increases on walking	Increases with heavy periods of exertion
Relief of pain	Stopping walk and standing relieves pain	After sitting or stooping rather standing	Improves on leg elevation	Improves on leg elevation

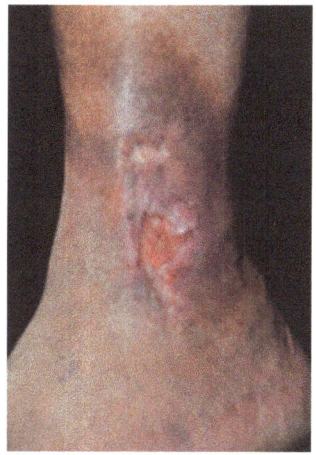

Fig. 5: Venous ulcer.

MANAGEMENT[3,5,6,8]

Management comprises of investigating the etiology by means of various laboratory and other parameters (Table 9).

A deep biopsy is indicated and it can help in differentiating various ulcers (Table 10).

Treatment includes management of associated co-morbidities, life style modification with local management of ulcer and surgical intervention if required (Tables 11 and 12).

Table 8: Edinburgh claudication questionnaire.

Edinburgh Claudication Questionnaire

Question	Response	Sensitivity (%)	Specificity (%)
Do you get pain or discomfort in your leg(s) when you walk?	Yes (If patient answers no. then stop here)	99.3	'13.1
Does this pain ever begin when you are standing still or sitting?	No	99.3	80.3
Do you get pain if you walk uphill or hurry?	Yes	98.8	13.1
Do you get pain if you walk at an ordinary pace on level ground?	Yes or no. dependent on severity of claudication	—	—
What happens if you stand still?	Pain gone in 10 minutes or less	90.6	63.9
Where do you get this pain?	Calf,* thigh. or buttock[†] marked	—	—

NOTE : A positive classification for peripheral vascular disease requires tile indicated responses for all questions.
*Definite claudicant = pain in calf.
[†]Atypical claudication = pain in thigh or buttock (in the absence of calf pain).

Table 9: Investigations in arterial ulcer.

	Investigations
	Hematological
Complete blood	Anemia, polycythamia and thrombocythemia
Biochemical profile	(Diabetes mellitus and renal dysfunction) and fasting lipid profile can all guide medical therapy
Miscellaneous	(With unusual presentation or patients <50 years) • Thrombophilia screen • Vasculitis screen • Homocysteine levels
	Radiological
Duplex ultrasound scan	Duplex ultrasound scan will give further information—on arterial occlusion, stenosis, and areas of diffuse and continuous atheromatous disease.
Arteriography	Arteriography is the ideal investigation in preoperative planning, allowing direct assessment of the vascular anatomy of the lower limb

Color-assisted duplex ultrasound scan	• Advantages:
	  – Safe, non-invasive and non-expensive.
	  – Provide anatomical as well as functional information.
	  – It is often used in surveillance following angioplasty or reconstruction.
	• Disadvantages:
	  – Accuracy is highly operator dependent
	  – Length of examination
	  – Difficulty in imaging crural arteries.
	  – National Institute for Health and Clinical Excellence (NICE) guidelines recommends—duplex ultrasound as 'first-line imaging' to all patients with peripheral arterial disease (PAD) for whom revascularization is being considered. It further recommends to do contrast-enhanced magnetic resonance angiography (MRA) [or computed tomography angiography (CTA) if MRA is contraindicated] to patients with PAD before revascularization is undertaken.

Contd...

Contd...

	Investigations Hematological

MRA and CTA	• Both are more sensitive and specific to confirm and localize PAD especially in cases where intervention is being considered.
	• Both are similar in terms of diagnostic accuracy, clinical outcome and ease of use.
	• MRA advantages:
	  – Avoiding the nephrotoxic iodinated contrast material and radiation
	  – Ability to provide rapid high-resolution 3D images of the abdomen, pelvis and lower limbs in one setting
	• MRA disadvantages:
	  – MRA is a more expensive
	  – MRA is contraindicated in patients with implanted devices such as metallic clips and pacemakers and in those with claustrophobia
	  – Previous arterial stents—causes difficulty in assessment of patency/in-stent stenosis because of signal dropout
	  – Association of gadolinium (the contrast agent used for MRA) with nephrogenic systemic fibrosis has been seen

Digital subtraction angiography	• 'Gold standard' investigation for PAD • Invasive procedure, hence only performed when a simultaneous endovascular intervention is anticipated. • Complications: Nephrotoxicity and allergic reaction induced by the iodinated contrast, arterial dissection and spasm; hematoma, pseudoaneurysm and arteriovenous fistula at the access site.

Table 10: Importance of ulcer biopsy in diagnosis.

Ulcer/Deep wound biopsy[9]

Indication: to confirm diagnosis and to rule out other etiologies

Criteria of deep wound biopsy:
- Preferably elliptical biopsy
- Should include all skin levels down to fascia
- It should be taken across the ulcer edge and necrosis

4 types of painful ulcers associated with ischemic subcutaneous arteriolosclerosis : (Hafner et al)
1. Martorell hypertensive ischemic leg ulcer (HYTILU)
2. Calciphylaxis with distal skin necrosis in chronic renal insufficiency
3. Nonuremic calciphylaxis in morbid obesity with proximal skin necrosis
4. Pyoderma gangrenosum

Association of various arterial ulcers

Associated factors	Martorell HYTILU	Calciphylaxis with distal skin necrosis in chronic renal insufficiency	Nonuremic calciphylaxis in morbid obesity with proximal skin necrosis	Pyoderma gangrenosum
Hypertension	Present	-	Present	-
Diabetes	Present	-	Present	-
Ischemic subcutaneous arteriolosclerosis	Present (hallmark finding)	-	Present (hallmark finding)	Not found
Chronic failure/kidney transplant	-	Present	-	-
Histopathology	All 3 layers involved	All 3 layers involved	All 3 layers involved	Superficial skin involvement

Contd...

Contd...

Ulcer/Deep wound biopsy[9]

Inflammatory bowel disease	-	-	-	Present
Hematoproliferative disorders	-	-	-	Present
Rheumatoid arthritis	-	-	-	Present
Smoking	-	-	-	Risk factor
Idiopathic	-	-	-	50% cases
Response to immunosuppression	-	-	-	Present

Hypertensive ischemic ulcer histology: Typical necrosis or necrobiosis (death of cells within the tissue) of all 3 skin layers (epidermis, dermis, and subcutis).

HPE hallmark—presence of arteriosclerotic arterioles with a thickened vessel wall having a narrow vessel lumen most consistently seen in the subcutaneous fat layer. In two-thirds of cases, arterioles show a significant medial calcinosis that is associated with intimal hyperplasia.

Table 11: Management of arterial ulcers.

Management of arterial ulcers[3,9]

Find out the etiology of arterial ulcer	
Bed rest	
Local care of ulcer	Cleaning of ulcer with EuSOL or normal saline (NS) followed by stretch dressing
	Local debridement of slough and excision of the hanging edges
Antibiotics	Local antibiotics are better than injectables as the concentration is maintained higher by local antibiotic use
Vacuum compression therapy	Increase capillary filling time
Curettage	Arterial ulcers should not be debrided as this may cause further ischemia and lead to the formation of a larger ulcer
	However there are studies with extensive necrosis where after checking the perfusion, extensive curettage under local anesthesia was done followed by the use of intravenous sodium thiosulfate
Lumbar sympathectomy	Improve vascularity by opening collateral pathways of the skin and aids in healing of the ulcer
Skin grafting	New treatment approach
	Grafts most effectively alleviate the intractable pain from the skin infarction
Becaplermin	Recombinant platelet-derived growth factor with some evidence to facilitate wound healing
Vitamin K antagonists	Known to inhibit vitamin K-dependent calcification-protecting protein
Advanced therapies	Hyperbaric oxygen
	Prostaglandin E1 intravenous infusions
Amputation	No response to conservative treatment and severe rest pain
	Persist
Arterial reconstruction surgery	
Associated venous ulceration	High saphenous ligation with modified stripping of veins (only in or above the upper quadrant of leg) is advised. Once the ulcer is healed treat as pure arterial disease
New omental transfer surgery	Good results found in case of end stage vascular disease in thromboangitis obliterans (TAO)

Ischemic Ulcers, Pyoderma Gangrenosum and Vasculitic Ulcers

Table 12: Management of peripheral arterial disease associated with ulcers.

Management of peripheral vascular disease (PVD) associated with ulcers[5,6,8]

Aim	• To increase the peripheral blood flow • To affect the healing process in arterial ulceration
Lifestyle modification	
Exercise therapy	• 30 min walking sessions (to near maximum pain) thrice weekly for minimum 06 months- leads to 50–200% overall improvement in walking ability. • Sleeping in a bed raised at the head end is beneficial.
Smoking cessation	• Recommended by 'transatlantic inter-society consensus' for the management of peripheral arterial disease (TASC II). • No significant effect in improving overall walking distance. • It slows the progression to CLI and reduces the risk of cardiovascular events. • Multimodality approach i.e, behavioral therapy, nicotine replacement and medication has better effect in stopping smoking than a single modality approach.
Modification of risk factors	
Lipid control	• 'Heart Protection Study'—Simvastatin reduces vascular mortality by 17%, coronary artery events by 24% and strokes by 27% in patients with PAD at 5 years. • Statins should be prescribed for all PAD patients irrespective of cholesterol level of >3 mmol/l • Bezafibrate—no effect on total fatal and non-fatal cardiovascular events.
Hypertension control	• The target blood pressure in patients with PAD is <140/90 mm Hg (<130/80 mm Hg in diabetic or renal failure patients). • PAD patients will require more than one type of anti-hypertensive to control their blood pressure. The Heart Outcomes Prevention Evaluation (HOPE) study showed- in patients with ankle-brachial index (ABI) <0.90, blood pressure modification was twice as effective in preventing major adverse cardiovascular events as compared with those with ABI >0.90. Angiotensin-converting enzyme (ACE) inhibitors—there is not enough evidence to support their routine use and further research is required. Ramipril treatment was associated with a 25% reduction in the primary combined outcome of cardiovascular mortality, myocardial infarction or stroke in patients with PAD, independent of blood pressure lowering. Beta blockers—can be safely used in claudicants, especially in the presence of coronary arterial disease (Cochrane review refuted earlier presumption that beta blockers are ineffective).
Diabetic control	Diabetes mellitus: PAD risk increases by three to four times, and diabetes doubles the risk of claudication. Strict glycemic control reduces the risk of microvascular complications i.e. reduces myocardial infarction, stroke and vascular death (does not reduce the PAD complications which are mediated by dyslipidemia). Target levels- HbA1c level of <7%
Antiplatelets and anticoagulants	Antiplatelet therapy—no improvement in claudication but is important in reducing the adverse cardiovascular outcomes and PAD by 23% (the Antithrombotic Trialists' Collaboration). 'There is no strong evidence to support superiority of any one antiplatelet agent. CAPRIE study (patients at risk of ischaemic events)—long-term use of 'clopidogrel is more effective than aspirin' in reducing the risk of myocardial infarction, stroke or vascular-related death in PAD patients. Conversely, the CHARISMA trial—showed no benefit for 'clopidogrel + aspirin over aspirin alone' in reducing this risk. WAVE trial—added oral anticoagulants (warfarin or acenocoumarol) to antiplatelet therapy in patients with PAD and concluded that 'combination therapy had no benefit over antiplatelet therapy alone' but caused higher rates of bleeding. Current recommendation—'long-term low- dose aspirin or clopidogrel' in patients with symptomatic PAD to minimize the rate of serious vascular events.
Homocysteine	Hyperhomocysteinemia is implicated in both PAD and coronary artery disease but no evidence suggests improvement in walking distance or vascular risk by lowering its levels with folate therapy. Ramipril treatment was associated with a 25% reduction in the primary combined outcome of cardiovascular mortality, myocardial infarction or stroke in patients with PAD, independent of blood pressure lowering. Beta blockers—can be safely used in claudicants, especially in the presence of coronary arterial disease (Cochrane review refuted earlier presumption that beta blockers are ineffective).

Contd...

Contd...

Management of peripheral vascular disease (PVD) associated with ulcers[5,6,8]

Other pharmaceutical therapies	Following 4 drugs have randomized controlled evidence showing improvement in walking distance in patients with intermittent claudication. 1. Naftidrofuryl oxalate, a 5-hydroxytryptamine type 2 antagonist 2. Cilostazol, a phosphodiesterase III inhibitor 3. Pentoxifylline, a vasodilator 4. Inositol nictonate, a vasodilator (Naftidrofuryl oxalate and cilostazol both are effective treatments for intermittent claudication with minimal adverse effects with naftidrofuryl being cost-effective too). 5. Other drugs and therapies: • Carnitine and Propionyl-L-carnitine interact with the skeletal muscle oxidative metabolism to improve treadmill walking distance in claudicants. • Iloprost, a prostacycline analogue showed a reduction in death and major amputation at 6 months (35 versus 55% in controls). • Spinal cord stimulation and Lumbar chemical sympathectomy- new therapies with limited evidence for use in CLI.

Surgical intervention

Methods	• Revascularization e.g. angioplasty (for localized stenosis) • Reconstructive surgery (for diffuse disease)

Revascularization

Indication of revascularization	• Intermittent claudication affecting quality of life or preventing employment, causing rest pain and tissue loss.
	• The outcomes of revascularization are dependent on:
	   – Site and extent (length and number of lesions) of disease
	   – Quality of inflow and run-off vessels
	   – Patient comorbidities
	   – Type of procedure performed.

Types of revascularization procedure	Based on technique: • Endovascular (percutaneous balloon angioplasty and/or stent) • Surgical (bypass using autologous vein or synthetic graft) Based on site of intervention: • Supra-inguinal revascularization • Infra-inguinal revascularization for claudication

Supra-Inguinal revascularization

Endovascular	• First-line treatment for most patients with supra-inguinal disease. • Aorto-iliac angioplasty—reported to have an initial clinical success rate of >90% with 5-year primary patency rates ranging from 72 to 79%. • Use of a stent in aorto-iliac occlusive disease improves technical success rates and reduces the risk of long-term failure by almost 39%.
Aorto-bifemoral bypass	• Indications: Diffuse aorto-iliac disease or where an endovascular intervention has failed. • Advantages: Better long-term patency than the endovascular strategy with reported 5-year primary patency rates of up to 94%. • Disadvantages: Significant morbidity and mortality related to this surgery.

Infra-inguinal revascularization

• Medical therapy and supervised exercise is better than any infra-inguinal endovascular intervention for claudication.
• Despite this there are increasing numbers of endovascular interventions being performed worldwide.
• Standard angioplasty of superficial femoral artery disease has patency rates of 50–60% at 3 years; Femoro-AK popliteal bypass with vein (75% at 4 years) and with PTFE (50–55% at 4 years).

Contd...

Contd...

Management of peripheral vascular disease (PVD) associated with ulcers[5,6,8]

Stent insertion	The FAST trial showed no difference in re-stenosis and clinical outcomes at 1 year in both short and long superficial femoral artery (SFA) lesions patients between percutaneous angioplasty (PTA) and stent.
	ABSOLUTE trial involving longer lesions showed improved walking distance at 1 year in the primary stent group and with lower rate of re-stenosis but clinical benefit was lost in the stent arm by 2 years (49%)- suggesting bare stents do not provide long-term patency of endovascular interventions.
	RESILIENT study (a multi-center prospective randomized trial of PTA versus Nitinol stent for claudicants with moderate length disease) showed sustained benefits in both radiological patency and symptomatic relief with stenting at 3 years follow up suggesting that the newer generation stents with improved flexibility and reduced fracture rates may increase stent longevity.
Drug-eluting stents	Need of drug eluting stent: The problem of both angioplasty and bare metal stents (BMSs) is the development of neo-intimal hyperplasia causing re-stenoses and subsequent thrombosis.
	SOROCCO trial: Compared sirolimus-eluting stents and bare stents in claudicants with moderate length SFA disease. Clinical improvement and re-stenosis rates were similar between groups at 2 years.
	(The lack of additional benefit with drug-eluting stents may be explained by the much lower re-stenosis rates i.e. 21% in the bare stent arm of this trial than in the previously discussed BMS trials (49% in ABSOLUTE trial at 2 years).
	Zilver PTX trial: Compared a paclitaxel-coated nitinol drug-eluting stent with PTA and provisional BMS placement in patients with femoro-popliteal disease. The study suggested that treatment with the paclitaxel-eluting stent was associated with a better primary patency (83.1 versus 32.8%; $P < 0.001$) and 12-month event-free survival (90.4 versus 82.6%; $P = 0.004$) compared with PTA and provisional BMS placement.
Covered stents	e-polytetrafluoroethylene (ePTFE) covered stents have been proposed to improve patency over non-covered stents.
	Useful in patients with no vein available for bypass, as patency rates equate to PTFE bypasses with reduced morbidity and length of hospital stay.
Atherectomy	An alternative to standard endovascular techniques is the removal of the obstructing thrombus.

Treatment for CLI

Amputation	Indications: • Tissue is beyond salvage or there is extensive tissue death. • In the presence of non-reconstructible PAD with significant infection or severe pain. • When amputation can help improve the quality of life. • There is significant morbidity (30% of amputees will end up losing the other leg in 2 years) and mortality (50% of them die within 5 years) after amputation.
New endovascular techniques	• Developed for treating long and complex infra-inguinal arterial lesions causing CLI whose treatment is not clearly understood. • The addition of 'cryoplasty' to balloon angioplasty was tried but studies suggest poor patency rates and poor relief from claudication at 1 year. • 'Pharmacomodulation' is a new stream which uses knowledge of pathophysiology of neointimal hyperplasia. • In open surgery, 'tissue-engineered grafts' and 'prosthetic grafts' are being tried which are closer to biomechanics of human arteries. Thus concerns regarding reduced patency rates and increased infection risk with present prosthetic graft materials will be taken care of. • For CLI there is ongoing research for new modalities in view of existing treatment options being ineffective. • 'Gene therapy and therapeutic angiogenesis': The knowledge that development of collateral vessels leads to improvement in clinical condition led many studies to determine the mechanism which regulates new vessel formation. Treatments including gene therapy and therapeutic angiogenesis regulate the fine balance between pro- and antiangiogenic pathways by the manipulation of local inflammatory pathways. Presently, there are no clinical studies that show a significant benefit of gene therapy when compared with placebo therapy hence more research needs to be done before using angiogenesis as a treatment modality in CLI.

PYODERMA GANGRENOSUM

DEFINITION

Pyoderma gangrenosum was primarily known as "Phagedenisme geometrique" introduced by Brocq in 1916, it was further modified by Brunsting, et al, in 1930 as PG and Greenstein et al in 1976 reported its association with inflammatory bowel disease.[10,11] Currently PG is contemplated as a rare non-infectious inflammatory neutrophilic dermatosis commonly associated with underlying systemic diseases.[11] The diagnosis is based on the classic hallmark features of PG with exclusion of other ulcerative dermatosis.[11]

EPIDEMIOLOGY

The incidence of PG reported from a UK based study is 0.63% per 100,000 persons- years whereas an Indian study estimated incidence of 0.03% (new dermatology cases in hospital).[10,12] The incidence of PG increases with age with peak incidence at 20-50 yrs of age.[12] However an Indian study reported a possibility of lower mean age of onset as they reported majority of pediatric cases of PG secondary to an infective etiology.[12] PG is more commonly seen in females with incidence of 59-76%.[11]

ETIOLOGY

Causative Organism

No pathogen is yet found to be a causative agent for PG. However it is found that after giving killed injection of *E. coli* in previous PG or IBD, patient developed bullous PG, thus suggesting that gut flora antigens when introduced in skin can cause PG lesion in a susceptible individual.

Genetics

Pyoderma gangrenosum cases are reported to have autosomal dominant genetic predisposition and are commonly associated with PG, pyogenic arthritis and acne (PAPA) and PG, acne and hidradenitis suppurativa (PASH) genetic autoinflammatory syndromes with mutation in PSTPIP1/CD2BP1 gene on chromosome 5 encoding complex proline/serine/threonine phosphatase interacting proteins and is also linked to pyrin (PSTPIP1-previously called as CD2BP1). Association of PAPA with familial Mediterranean fever is reported.

Environmental Factors

Pyoderma gangrenosum occurs at the site of penetrating skin injury in 25% cases (pathergy phenomenon). Pathergy phenomenon is defined as a state of altered tissue reactivity that occurs in response to minor trauma.

PATHOGENESIS[10-12]

Pyoderma gangrenosum primarily was considered to be secondary to bacterial infection in the immunocompromised host. Fulbright et al. speculated it to be secondary to abnormal response to unknown factor. Also it is reported that PG lesions having protein complex deposition in blood vessels might represent as Arthus-like reaction.[10]

Following factors are involved:
- Neutrophilic dysfunction
- Aberrant response of innate immunity
- Defective cell mediated immunity: Leading to abnormal trafficking of neutrophils.
- Altered production of cytokines (IL-8, IL-23, TNF-α) and chemokines (CXCL1, 2, 3 and 16)
- Impaired phagocytosis
- Over-expression of MIF by lymphocytes, RANTES

ASSOCIATIONS[10-12]

Pyoderma gangrenosum is reported to be associated with other neutrophilic dermatosis in 30-35% cases thus sharing common etiopathogenesis. Because of its varied association (Box 3), PG was classified accordingly as idiopathic, drug induced, parainflammatory (associated with IBD, arthritis),

---

Box 3: Associations of pyoderma gangrenosum.

- Idiopathic
- Drug induced: Pegfilgastrim [granulocyte colony-stimulating factor (GCSF)], Gefinib [epidermal growth factor inhibitor (EGFRI)], Isotretinoin, propylthyuracil
- Para inflammatory: Inflammatory bowel disease (IBD) (20-30%), rheumatoid arthritis, psoriatic arthritis, Spondylitis, Sarcoidosis, Takayasus disease, HIV, HCV, hidradenitis suppurativa
- Paraneoplastic: Internal malignancy
- Hematological malignancies: Myelodysplasia, myeloproliferative disease, leukemia, Polycythemia vera, monoclonal gammopathy

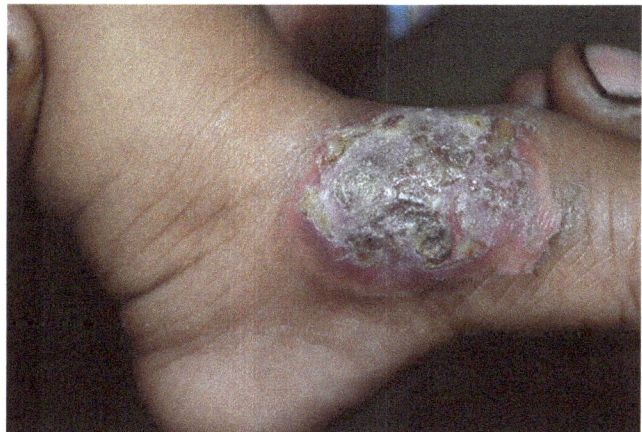

Fig. 6: Classical ulcer of Pyoderma Gangrenosum showing bluish tinge.

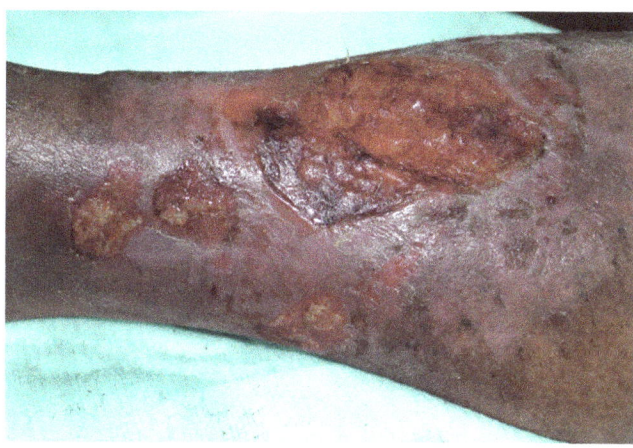

Fig. 7: Multiple ulcers of classical PG.

paraneoplastic (associated with internal malignancy) and hematological malignancies.

Other associations like chronic active hepatitis, thyroid disorders, complement deficiency, hypogammaglobinemia, hyperimmunoglobulin E syndrome, osteoarthritis, PAPA and PASH are also reported. Associated comorbidities like obesity, peripheral vascular diseases, diabetes mellitus and depression are known.

CLINICAL FEATURES[10-12]

Following is the presentation of classic PG:
- Starts as small discrete follicular pustules with surrounding halo of erythema which over few days softens with bluish tinge and forms ulceration (Figs. 6 and 7).
- The hallmark of PG is extremely painful recurrent cutaneous ulcerations with undermined bluish edematous borders having mucopurulent or hemorrhagic discharge.
- The border rapidly progresses further at rate of 1–2 cm over 24 hours with a halo of erythema around it extending into normal skin. These either regress or progress by coalescing with peripheral lesions.
- Most commonly occurs on the lower legs preferably pretibial area but can occur at other sites like breast, hand, trunk, head and neck. There are various clinical types of PG described with varied presentation (Box 4 and Table 13).

Clinical Course of Ulcerative Pyoderma Gangrenosum[12]

It can present as given in Table 13.

Table 13: Clinical course of pyoderma gangrenosum.

Explosive onset	Indolent onset
Sudden onset with rapid progression and severe necrosis	Gradual progression and spontaneous regression

Box 4: Types of pyoderma gangrenosum.

Synonyms and inclusions:
- Classical ulcerative
- Includes atypical forms
  - Parastomal
  - Pustular
  - Bullous (Fig. 8)
  - Atypical
  - Granulomatous superficial
- Variants: Neutrophilic dermatoses of dorsal hand, Pyostomatitis vegetans

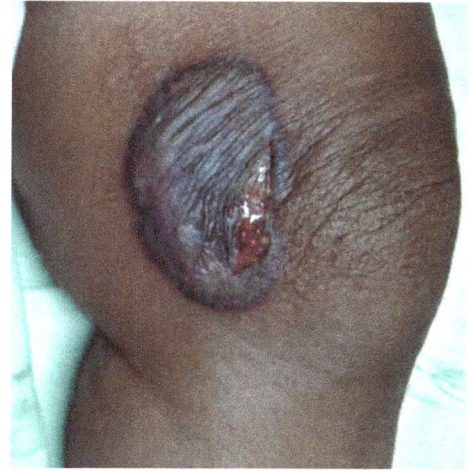

Fig. 8: Bullous Pyoderma Gangrenosum.

Extracutaneous Manifestations of Pyoderma Gangrenosum[11,12]

It can involve upper airway mucosa, eye, genital mucosa, develop sterile pulmonary or splenic neutrophilic infiltrates and myositis. It is reported that sterile cortical osteolysis can occurs at the site of PG ulcers.

DIFFERENTIAL DIAGNOSIS[12]

Pyoderma gangrenosum has to be differentiated from other diseases (Box 5).

DIAGNOSIS

Pyoderma gangrenosum is considered to be a diagnosis of exclusion of other possible diseases. The diagnosis of PG is made by its characteristic history and clinical presentation supported by histopathology and specific investigation if any associated disease exists. A diagnostic criteria has been developed for PG where it should meet 1 major criteria and 2 minor criteria (Box 6).[11]

TREATMENT

The course of PG is unpredictable; the lesions can spontaneously heal and simultaneously new lesions can occur. The mainstay of treatment is corticosteroids and immunosuppressive therapy. If PG has an associated disease, its treatment may help in remission of PG and if no underlying disease is present, then long term follow up is essential as remote chance of recurrence is present. Use of local therapy in addition to systemic therapy helps in healing and provides relief of symptoms. Aggressive surgical debridement or skin grafting is better avoided in active stage of disease because of the risk of a pathergic response. Various topical and systemic agents used in the treatment of PG are provided in Box 7.[10,12]

Box 5: Differential diagnosis of pyoderma gangrenosum.

- Vascular occlusive or venous disease
- Vasculitis (Wegener's, PAN)
- Malignancies: Lymphoma leukemia MF
- Drug induced (nicorandil, halogenoderma)
- Infections: Deep fungal infections (sporotrichosis, mucormycosis, histoplasmosis, blastomycosis and fusariosis, atypical mycobacteria and opportunistic infections
- External tissue injury: Insect bites, factitious panniculitis
- Other neutrophilic dermatoses: Atypical Sweet's syndrome, Behcets

---

Box 6: Diagnostic criteria for pyoderma gangrensoum (WP Daniel Su et al).[11]

Diagnostic criteria

Major criteria:
Rapid progression of a painful necrolytic cutaneous ulcer with an irregular; violaceous and undermined border; and the exclusion of other causes of cutaneous ulceration.

Minor criteria:
- History suggestive of pathergy or clinical finding of cribriform scarring;
- Systemic diseases known to be associated with PG;
- Histopathological findings (massive sterile dermal neutrophilia (sea of neutrophils), with or without mixed inflammation or lymphocytic vasculitis)
- Treatment response (e.g. rapid response to systemic corticosteroid which is 50% improvement within one month of therapy)

Box 7: Treatment of pyoderma gangrensoum.

First line of treatment:
- Aid healing
  - Compressions and supportive local therapy
  - Vascular disease and obesity

Second line of treatment:
- Systemic corticosteroids is the mainstay of therapy
- For more severe PG: can be combined with cyclosporine
- Still no control: Other systemic and immunosuppressives

Third line:
- Suggests effective use of TNF alpha biologicals especially those having associated IBD.

Local Therapy (Box 8)

> **Box 8:** Local measures for pyoderma gangrensoum.
>
> Local therapy[10-12]
> *Ulcers with heavy discharge*: Foam and laminate dressings preferred
> *Ulcers with purulent discharge*: Wet compresses with saline and alginate dressings
> *Peristomal pyoderma gangrensoum (PG)*: Application of betamethasone (4-puffs) are reported
> *Other topical agents*: Tacrolimus, potent corticosteroids, 20% nitrogen mustard, sodium cromoglycate 2%, 2.5% benzoyl peroxide, granulocyte macrophage colony stimulating factor, Nicotine 2% phenytoin sodium solution
> *Intralesional*: Triamcinolone acetonide and Cyclosporin
> *In nonprogressive PG*: Skin grafting or microvasular flap grafting can be successfully done
> *Under oral corticosteroid cover*: Cultured keratinocyte autografts and allografts have also been tried.
> *Hyperbaric oxygen therapy*: Helps by increasing oxygen tension in the ulcers.

Systemic Therapy

Oral corticosteroids remains mainstay of treatment with prednisolone commonly being used or with pulse therapy of methylprednisolone or dexamethasone are tried in resistant cases.[12] Oral cyclosporine is preferred drug in steroid resistant cases for its effectivity and least myelosuppression. A large RCT found no difference in mono therapy of cyclosporine (4 mg/kg day) and prednisolone (0.75 mg/kg/day).[12] A retrospective observational study of PG with IBD patients treated with infliximab or adalimumab (93.5%) showed that ulcers healed in 4–8 weeks while ulcers treated with prednisolone alone (38%) healed in 1–3 months. Thus in eastern countries biologics are now becoming the first line of treatment.[11]

Treatment of PG is described in Box 9.[10-12]

PROGNOSIS

The PG-ulcers with arthritis have a poorer prognosis and ulcers heal only in 23.4% cases as compared to others which heal up to 78.9%. PG presenting over hands commonly had association of lymphoproliferative disease rather than IBD.[11] After healing PG may recur in 16–61% of cases and a study has reported that PG has a significant mortality around 16%.[10,11]

> **Box 9:** Treatment of pyoderma gangrenosum.
>
> *Systemic steroids*
> - Prednisolone 0.5–1 g/kg.
> - Methylprednisone pulse 1 g
>
> *Immunosuppressive agents*
> - Cyclosporine 2–3 mg/kg body wt.
> - Methotrexate
> - Mycophenolate mofetil 2 g/day
> - Cyclophosphamide
> - Azathioprine 100–150 mg/day
> - Chlorambucil
> - Tacrolimus 0.1 mg/kg body wt
>
> *Biologics*
> - *Infliximab*: IV 5 mg/kg body wt 0,2,6 and every 8 wks specially PG with IBD and spondyloarthropathy
> - *Adalimumab*: Paradox PG reported
> - *Etanercept SC*: 50 mg twice weekly
> - *Anakinra*: effective in PASH with PG
> - Canakinumab
> - *Ustekinumab*: Effective in PAPA with PG
>
> *Others*
> - *Dapsone*: 200 mg/day
> - Intravenous immunoglobulin (IVIG)
> - Rifampicin
> - *Clofazimine*: 300–400 mg/day
> - Vancomycin
> - Mezlocillin
> - Minocycline
> - Sulfasalazine
> - Sulfapyridine
> - Suflamethyoxy pyridazine
> - Colchicine
> - Tetracyclines
> - Thalidomide
> - Potassium iodide
> - Mesalazine
> - Heparin
> - Tripterygium wilfordii
> - Multiglycoside (TWG) (Chinese herb)
> - *Isotretinoin*: PG paradox reported

VASCULITIC ULCER

INTRODUCTION

Vasculitis is a spectrum of clinicopathological processes leading to inflammation and damage of blood vessels. There is usually compromised vessel lumen that causes ischemia of the tissues supplied by the involved vessel leading to a heterogenous group of syndromes.[13,14]

Vasculitis and its consequences can be the primary or isolated manifestation of a disease or a secondary component of other primary disease.[13,14] Vasculitis may be restricted to a single organ, such as the skin, or it may simultaneously involve multiple organ systems.[13]

Vasculitis and autoimmune diseases are known causes for chronic wounds and non healing ulcers. Studies show that while 79.7% of leg ulcers have a vascular etiology,[13,14] 20–23% of patients have wounds because of other etiologies including vasculitis, PG and other autoimmune diseases.[13]

CLINICAL FEATURES AND MANAGEMENT

Clinical features and management of the three common causes of vasculitic ulcers namely rheumatoid associated, ANCA associated and scleroderma associated leg ulcers are provided in Tables 14 to 16 respectively.

Approach to management of vasculitic ulcers is provided in Flowchart 2.

Table 14: Leg ulcers in rheumatoid arthritis (RA).

Leg ulcers associated with rheumatoid arthritis[13]

Prevalence	• *Mayo Clinic study*: Mean disease duration for ulcer development—25.9 years.
	• *Olmsted County, Minnesota*:
	  Incidence at 5 years after RA diagnosis—4.8%
	  At 25 years after the RA diagnosis—26.2%	

Risk factors	Age, rheumatoid factor positivity, Presence of rheumatoid nodules and Venous thromboembolism.	

Role of the biopsy	• Confirmation of vasculitis on tissue biopsy is challenging.
	• In approximately 50–55% of patients with RA-associated leg ulcer there is histological evidence of vasculitis.
	• There are also non-specific findings like scar tissue, fibrosis and changes of a chronic ulcer.
	• The main role of biopsy in RA-associated leg ulcers is to exclude:
	  – atypical infections such as chronic mycobacterial infections
	  – malignancies which can develop in longstanding chronic wounds.	

Treatment	• No randomized controlled trials have been done to find out specific therapeutic interventions for RA-associated leg ulcers. Data is drawn from review of case-series reports only.	
	With CLI	Surgical revascularization: Endovascular treatment (EVT) for critical limb ischemia (CLI) has been investigated in a case series study and was found to be successful in all cases.
	Without CLI	Managed medically: While clinicians are often concerned about escalating *immunotherapy* in patients with RA-associated leg ulcers due to risks of infection and delayed wound healing, this concern is not supported by evidence. Steroids: Steroids induces skin fragility can predispose the patient to ulceration hence not used as primary therapy. However, studies have shown that use of steroids in the 100 days prior to the index surgery was not a risk factor for post-operative wound dehiscence[14] indicating that steroid therapy may not be a direct risk factor for wound development rather it is likely that the association between 'steroid use and ulceration in RA patients' may rather be a manifestation of the known relationship between 'RA severity and leg ulceration'.[15] Disease modifying antirheumatic drugs (DMARD): Mainstay of treatment. Biologic agents (TNF-α inhibtors and rituximab): Advance therapy

Table 15: Leg Ulcers due to anti-neutrophil cytoplasmic antibody (ANCA)-associated vasculitis.

Leg ulcers due to ANCA-associated vasculitis[13]

Introduction and Epidemiology	The ANCA associated vasculitides include following: • Granulomatosis with polyangiitis (GPA, formerly known as Wegener's granulomatosis) • Microscopic polyangiitis (MPA) • Churg-Strauss syndrome (CSS) All forms of systemic vasculitis, have been associated with vasculitic leg ulcers. However there is no data available on prevalence.
Pathology	• Indication of biopsy: In cases of systemic vasculitis with negative ANCA-serology, tissue biopsy has a role to confirm the diagnosis. • Ideal biopsy: should include the subcuticular tissue and biopsy of early lesions is often most informative. • Typical findings: leukocytoclastic vasculitis is seen with infiltration of arterioles and postcapillary venules by neutrophils undergoing degranulation and fragmentation. Fibrinoid necrosis of the inflamed vessels is often seen. Occasional presence of vasculitis in medium and small arteries of the reticular dermis and fat. • Direct immunofluorescence can be helpful to confirm immunoglobulin and complement deposits.
Management	• Appropriate and aggressive treatment of the underlying autoimmune disease hastens the process of wound healing. • B-cell depletion therapy—successful treatment of vasculitic leg ulcers with rituximab has been reported in many studies.

Table 16: Scleroderma and mixed connective tissue disease (MCTD) associated ulcers.

Scleroderma and MCTD associated ulcers[13]

Introduction		• Scleroderma (SSc): Autoimmune disease characterized by immune activation, vasculopathy, fibroblast stimulation and connective tissue fibrosis. • MCTD: Heterogeneous group of disorders which may have overlapping features of several autoimmune disease [often scleroderma with features of systemic lupus erythematosus (SLE) or Rheumatoid arthritis (RA). Characterized by the presence of anti- ribonucleoprotein (RNP) antibodies.
Prevalence		• Approximately 4% of patients of scleroderma have lower extremity ulcers especially common in longstanding disease.

Pathology		• Progressive tissue fibrosis and vasculopathy—End-organ damage.
		• Etiology of lower extremity ulcers in scleroderma is often - multifactorial.
		• Scleroderma ulcers are bilateral in 70% of cases.
		• Most common histologic finding—Fibrin occlusive vasculopathy with intimal thickening and some inflammation.
		• Associated conditions
		  – Coexistent prothrombotic states like antiphospholipid antibodies and genetic prothrombotic state- leads to refractory ulcers in scleroderma.
		  – Arterial and venous disease also contribute to delay in healing in cleroderma and can be associated in as many as 50% of patients.[23]

Management		Multidisciplinary approach is required for management of these patients.
	Medical management	• *Aim*: To address the pathophysiologic etiology of scleroderma associated ulcers. • Vasodilators - calcium channel blockers, prostanoids (e.g. iloprost) and endothelin receptor antagonists (e.g. Bosentan). • Topical and systemic opioids-to address the severe pain associated with these vasculopathic ulcers. Post-operative wound dehiscence data and data from the Wound Healing and Etiology (WE-HEAL) Study has revealed that higher opioid exposure is associated with relatively slower wound healing.
	Endovascular treatment	In a study with patients having CLI associated ulcers with scleroderma and connective tissue disorder, endovascular treatment gave satisfactory results.
	Bypass surgery	The data on long-term effectiveness of bypass surgery is limited due to the associated distal vasculopathy. Despite having early pain relief and wound healing, incidences of graft failure and limb loss in on longer follow up is seen.

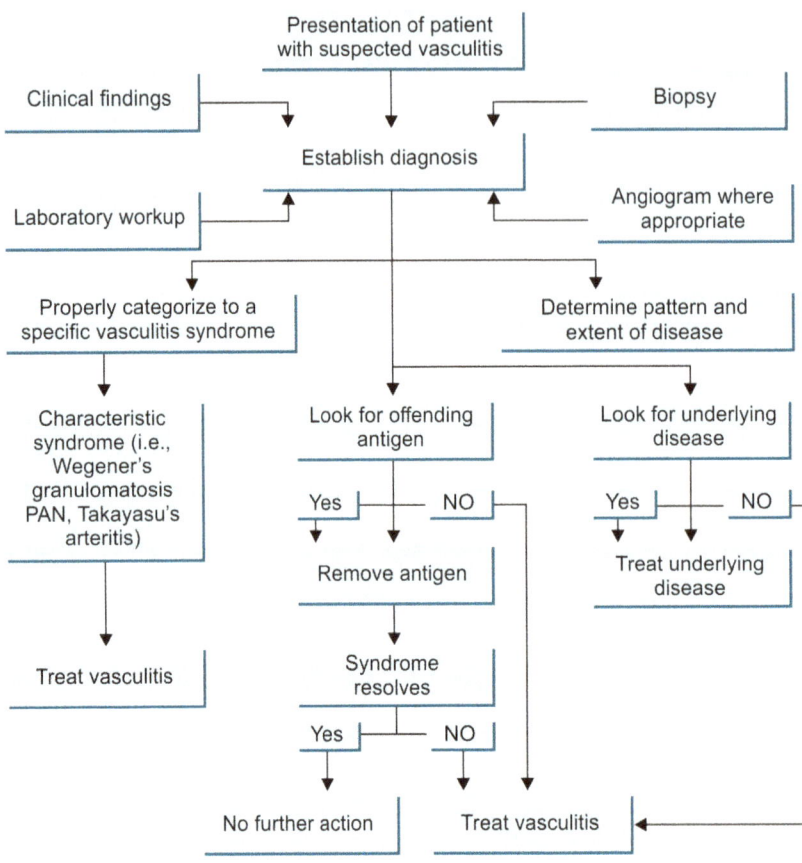

Flowchart 2: Management of vasculitic ulcer.

CONCLUSION

Ischemic, arterial ulcers and PG form a major population of leg ulcers. These ulcers have distinctive features which help their early recognition. Management of these ulcers are challenging with most of them having recurrences. Underlying ischemia, vasculitis and associated conditions have to be managed for complete recovery.

REFERENCES

1. Rahman GA, Adigun IA, Fadeyi A. Epidemiology, etiology, and treatment of chronic leg ulcer: Experience with sixty patients. Ann Afr Med. 2010;9:1-4.
2. Kahle B, Hermanns HJ, Gallenkemper G. Evidence based treatment of chronic leg ulcers. Dtsch Arztebl Int. 2011;108: 231-7.
3. Shrinivas AG, Amol W. Study of the pathogenesis and diagnosis of ulcer of lower extremity under various conditions. Int J Res Med Sci. 2016;4:621-7.
4. Grey JE, Harding KG, Enoch S. Venous and arterial leg ulcers. BMJ. 2006;332:347-50.
5. Abdulhannan P, Russell DA, Homer-Vanniasinkam S. Peripheral arterial disease: a literature review. Br Med Bull. 2012;104:21-39.
6. Olin JW, Sealove BA. Peripheral artery disease: Current insight into the disease and its diagnosis and management. Mayo Clin Proc. 2010:678-92.
7. Fu X. Skin ulcers in lower extremities: the epidemiology and management in China. Int J Low Extrem Wounds. 2005;4:4-6.
8. Sontheimer DL. Peripheral vascular disease: Diagnosis and treatment. Am Fam Physician. 2006:1971-6.
9. Alavi A, Mayer D, Hafner J, et al. Martorell hypertensive ischemic leg ulcer: an underdiagnosed entity. Adv Skin Wound Care. 2012:563-72.
10. Wollina U. Pyoderma gangrenosum – a review. Orphanet J Rare Dis. 2007;2:19.
11. Omerod AD, Hampton PJ. Neutrophilic Dermatoses. In: Griffiths C, Barker J, Bleiker T, Chalmers R, Creamer D (Eds). Rooks Textbook of Dermatology, 9th edition. Oxford, UK: Blackwell Publications; 2016. pp.49.1-49.6.
12. Bhat RM. Pyoderma gangrenosum: An update. Indian Dermatol Online J. 2012;3(1):7-13.
13. Shanmugam VK, Angra D, Rahimi H, et al. Vasculitic and autoimmune wounds. J Vasc Surg Venous Lymphat Disord. 2017;5(2):280-92.
14. Levell NJ, Mukhtyar C. Cutaneous vasculitis. In: Griffiths C, Barker J, Bleiker T, Chalmers R, Creamer D (Eds). Rooks Textbook of Dermatology, 9th edition. Oxford, UK: Blackwell Publications; 2016. pp.102.1-.102.35.

CHAPTER 11

Principles of Leg Ulcer Management

Anju George

INTRODUCTION

Leg ulcers may be classified as either acute or chronic on the basis of their duration at presentation. *Chronic leg ulcers* are defined as those that lack a healing tendency even after 3 months of adequate treatment or have still not fully healed at 12 months.[1] Acute ulcers heal in less than 4 weeks after going through the normal phases of wound healing. Clinicians commonly encounter chronic lower limb ulceration which presents a serious therapeutic challenge. Delineating the etiology tends to be cumbersome in these scenarios. The disease is associated with significant morbidity and poses a huge threat to the quality of life due to the financial burden and loss of productivity. No definite guidelines have been outlined in the management of leg ulcers as the treatment strategy varies depending on the pathophysiology and duration of ulceration. An interdisciplinary approach is therefore highly essential to derive the exact etiology and diagnosis, so as to ensure an appropriate and timely systematic management.[2,3]

Approach to a Case of Leg Ulcer

The most common cause for leg ulceration is chronic venous insufficiency (70%). Arterial disease constitutes 5% to 10% of leg ulcers while other causes include neuropathy (usually diabetic), vasculitis or a combination of these diseases. The different etiological factors in complex leg ulcers need to be reasonably and objectively compiled so as to tabulate a comprehensive approach for the management. In the previous chapters the historical details, clinical examination and relevant investigations have been clearly detailed.

Table 1 summarizes the essential points while eliciting the history:[1,2]

Table 1: History taking in evaluation of leg ulcers.

1. *Onset and duration of ulcer*: Preceding trauma; neuropathic/ factitious causes; first episode/ recurrent nature
2. *Progress of ulcer*: Whether rapid or slow; arterial ulcers tend to develop slowly, compared to venous ulcers which may progress rapidly.
3. *Pain*: Ulcers due to arterial disease, vasculitis and hypertension are more painful whereas venous ulcers are less symptomatic in the absence of secondary infection. Neuropathic ulcers on the other hand may or may not be associated with paresthesia.
4. *Associated features*: Intermittent claudication (pain on walking relieved with rest) is a feature of arterial disease whereas lower limb edema, pain on long standing associated with hyperpigmentation or dermatitis of lower legs favors a venous disease.
5. *Medical history*: History of diabetes, hypertension, previous surgeries, recurrent cellulitis of lower limbs, deep vein thrombosis, connective tissue disorders, rheumatoid arthritis, varicose veins, should be excluded as these can predispose to ulceration.
6. *Systemic involvement*: History of other organ involvement as in connective tissue diseases, certain vasculitides.
7. *Drug history*: Numerous topical and systemic medications can delay wound healing. A variety of topical medications may cause contact dermatitis. The common sensitizers include neomycin, parabens, lanolin, ethylene diamine, nitrofurazone. Systemic medications such as corticosteroids may also impair wound healing.
8. *Family history*: Sickle cell anemia, thalassemia, and hereditary spherocytosis are hematologic disorders which predispose the patient to leg ulceration.
9. *Addictions*: Cigarette smoking predisposes to arterial disease and severely impairs wound healing. Alcohol consumption is another risk factor which delays healing of the wound.
10. *General health and nutrition*.

Table 2: Differentiating features of arterial, venous and neuropathic ulcers.			
Ulcer	**Common characteristics**	**Pathomechanism**	**Clinical features**
Venous	Most common cause in 70%[4]	Venous hypertension preceding cellular events	Well defined superficial painful ulcer located mostly over the gaiter area (medial malleolus). Other features include dilated veins, edema, dermatitis, lipodermatosclerosis
Arterial	Accounts for 25% leg ulcers. Claudication pain is the most common symptom. May be associated with venous disease as well.	Tissue ischemia	Deep punched out painful ulcers with well demarcated borders, located over bony prominences. Other findings include cold shiny extremities, absent peripheral pulses, prolonged venous filling time and femoral bruit
Neuropathic	Commonly associated with diabetes mellitus	Decreased sensation in the background of trauma and uneven pressure	Mostly seen on pressure points on soles in diabetics, leprosy and other conditions with peripheral neuropathy.

The differentiating features between venous, arterial and neuropathic leg ulcers have been depicted in the Table 2.

The initial clues to a definitive diagnosis can be derived from a reliable history. Table 3 summarizes the salient points in clinical assessment of lower extremity ulceration.[2,5-12]

General Principles in Leg Ulcer Management

There are various factors which can delay or impede the normal healing process in chronic wounds.[13,14] The local factors which need to be considered include:

a. Moisture: Is essential for rapid healing of wounds which promotes epidermal cell migration and a quicker re epithelialization.
b. Pressure: Excessive pressure impedes the capillary flow and delays wound healing.
c. Necrosis: Both slough and eschar formation delay the healing process and should be removed or debrided.
d. Infection: Presence of yellowish slough, purulent foul-smelling discharge, induration, erythema, or fever is a sign of infection which can worsen the ulcer. Culture of the pus can guide in treatment with appropriate antibiotic.
e. Oxygenation: Besides excessive oxygen consumption, the metabolically active cells in chronic wounds damage the smaller vessels and deplete oxygen from the wound microenvironment, which impairs the healing process. Hypoxia is a common accompaniment of chronic wounds with oxygen tensions ranging from 5 to 20 mm Hg compared to control values of 30 to 50 mm Hg.

Systemic factors which influence proper healing of wounds are age, obesity, and nutritional status, presence of comorbidities such as diabetes mellitus, hypertension, coronary artery disease or any immunosuppression.

After defining the etiology with a definite history taking and clinical examination, the major principals in the management of chronic leg ulcers include:
- Wound cleansing
- Wound debridement
- Appropriate wound dressings
- Topical and systemic therapeutics
- Compression therapy
- Pressure off loading
- General measures and life style changes
- Role of surgery
- Tackling the psychosocial aspects

Wound Cleansing

The first and foremost step in the management of any long-standing ulcer includes cleaning and debridement. Irrigation can be done using ordinary tap water or normal saline solution.(Evidence Level E).[7,15,16]

Distilled water, boiled water and normal saline have similar effects and no significant variation have been found in studies comparing their efficacies. Studies have compared the effects of distilled water, boiled water and normal saline for wound cleansing and no significant difference in infection or healing rates have been found.[15] Dilute Potassium permanganate compresses are effective in exudative wounds.

Table 3: Salient features in clinical evaluation in leg ulcers.

1. *Location*:
   - Medial
   - Lateral

   Gaiter area is the most common location for a venous ulcer (medial malleolar region) whereas in arterial origin, ulcers tend to occur more at pressure sites.

   Hypertensive ulcer or Martorell's ulcer occurs on the lateral malleolus.

2. *Ulcer characteristics*:
   - Initial size
   - Site
   - Wound base
   - Surrounding skin changes

   These features will help in reassessment at the next visit.

3. *Photographic record*: helps in serial measurement of ulcer size at each visit.

4. *Vascular assessment*:
   - Palpate lower limb pulses to rule out significant ischemic arterial causes
   - Measure ankle brachial index

5. *Sensations*:
   - Test for diminished or impaired sensations with 10 g monofilament to rule out neuropathic causes.

6. *Associated physical findings*:
   Venous disease may show
   - Hyperpigmentation due to hemosiderin staining
   - Lipodermatosclerosis (inverted champagne bottle shaped leg)
   - Atrophie blanche
   - Stasis eczema

   Arterial disease may show
   - Shiny, hairless, pale and cool skin
   - Changes in foot structure.

   Vasculitis/panniculitis may show
   - Retiform purpura
   - Palpable purpura
   - Nodules

7. *Mobility*: Limited joint mobility and anatomical abnormalities can worsen a preexisting ulcer irrespective of the etiology.

8. *Microbiology*: Always swab the ulcer and send for culture and sensitivity studies.

9. *Biopsy*: A non-healing ulcer requires histopathological examination along with samples for cultures (bacterial, fungal, mycobacterial, atypical mycobacterial) to differentiate vasculitides, microvascular occlusion disorders, panniculitis, infections and malignancies. A wedge biopsy from the ulcer edge is recommended.

10. *Lab investigations*: to rule out underlying systemic diseases.
    - Antinuclear antibody
    - Anticardiolipin antibody
    - RPR (rapid plasma reagin)

Contd...

Contd...

- Lupus anticoagulant
- Complements
- ANCAs
- Protein C
- Cryoglobulins and cryofibrinogens
- Rheumatoid factor
- Factor V Leiden mutations

11. *Radiography*: Imaging of the affected area is essential to rule out osteomyelitis or other bony deformities

12. *Patch test*: Indicated in a background of possible allergic contact dermatitis

Wound Debridement

In infected and undermined chronic wounds debridement is obligatory to redeem wound healing. This consists of eliminating or detaching the superficial non-viable tissue which transforms wound to an acute one, which helps it to traverse through the normal wound healing processes. This can be achieved through autolytic, osmotic, mechanical enzymatic, biological or surgical debridement. Debridement is contraindicated in ulcers in a background of severe arterial insufficiency. [7,17-19]

Surgical debridement and sharp debridement are done using a sharp surgical instrument such as a scalpel with or without anesthesia. This is advocated for unhealthy necrotic wounds with slough. *In autolytic debridement,* the body's own cells and enzymes help in denudation of dead tissue and is recommended for wounds with minimal slough. The wounds are then secured with moist dressings or natural agents to promote the wound healing.

Other methods include *mechanical debridement* which utilizes wet-to-dry dressings on the wound, which can be occasionally painful. Pulsed lavage and whirlpool therapy also aid in removal of the unhealthy tissue. *Enzymatic debridement* uses enzymes that break down the affected tissue such as collagenases, papain, and urea. *Bio surgical debridement* uses maggots to debride necrotic tissue.[20]

Wound Dressings

The 'TIME' approach to wound healing emphasizes the following factors[19]:

- **T**issue: Necrotic tissue and fibrin slough should be thoroughly excised for faster wound healing.
- **I**nfection: Reduction in bacterial load.
- **M**oisture: Wound dressings which furnish an optimal "moist" environment are essential in managing chronic wounds.
- **E**dge: Ulcer edge advancement plays a pivotal role in the healing process.

A dressing should be chosen based on wound properties such as site, extend, depth, presence or absence of slough and changes in the surrounding skin.

Both SIGN (Scottish Intercollegiate Guidelines Network) and NICE (National Institute for Health and Care Excellence) guidelines recommend simple, low cost dressings, low or nonadherent, which are acceptable to the patient (Evidence Level A). Care should be taken to prevent cross infection. (Evidence level E).[7,17,21,22,23]

The frequency of change of dressings should be tailored so that the dressing is neither oversaturated nor dry and adherent to the wound when it is removed. This is continued till the wound heals.

The different types of wound dressings used are absorbent dressings, occlusive plastic films, hydrocolloids, hydrogels, calcium alginate, semipermeable films and biological dressings.

Low adherent absorbent dressings which are ideal are made of either cotton or viscose fibers and impregnated with white or yellow soft paraffin. They are apt for shallow wounds with minimal to low exudate with minimal trauma occurring at each dressing change.

Recent studies have measured the effects of wound dressings on epithelial cells, their viability and proliferative capacity. Silver-based dressings are deferred in healthy wounds as these are cytotoxic.[7,23] Alginate dressings have a high calcium content and hamper cell proliferation. Hence, these should be used with caution in cases where keratinocyte proliferation is an essential requisite. They are suitable for highly exudative wounds and when hemostasis is essential. Semipermeable films are polyurethane sheets coated with an adhesive useful in shallow to flat wounds with minimal exudate. Hydrogel sheets and hydrocolloid dressings promote autolytic debridement of dry slough and are used in dry wounds with minimal exudate.[7,23]

Topical and Systemic Therapies

Topical antimicrobials are either antiseptics or antibiotics. Silver compounds, chlorhexidine and iodides are antiseptics whereas the commonly used topical antibiotics include mupirocin, fucidic acid, metronidazole, retapamulin. Antibiotics are indicated when there are clinical signs suggesting active infection (Evidence Level C).

Chlorhexidine-impregnated dressings

The advantages of chlorhexidine-impregnated dressings include reduced bacterial colonization, fewer adverse effects on healing and lack of toxicity, though there are reports of allergic reactions to chlorhexidine.

Iodine

Iodine is available as either povidone-iodine or cadexomer iodine. It promotes healing by its antiseptic and action which reduces the bacterial count. An advantage of iodine is that it lacks cytotoxicity as compared to other antimicrobials. Cadexomer iodine has significant activity against methicillin resistant Staphylococcus aureus (MRSA) and Pseudomonas aeruginosa.

Silver (Evidence Level C)

Nano crystalline silver dressings help in decreasing the surface flora which contributes more towards the wound healing process than the deeper flora.[7]

GM-CSF (Granulocyte macrophage colony stimulating factor)

In a study on topical GM-CSF for venous ulcers, 90% of ulcers healed, with an average healing time of 19 weeks. Injections of G-CSF are avoided as they are extremely painful.

Topical Protein C

Activated protein C has a potential role in chronic non-healing ulcers as it stimulates angiogenesis and epithelialization while inhibiting inflammatory processes.

Role of growth factors

Growth factors such as, epidermal growth factor, platelet-derived growth factor, transforming growth factors, fibroblast growth factors and insulin-like growth factors enhance wound healing with minimal effects on epithelialization. Platelet rich fibrin (PRF) and platelet rich plasma (PRP) are other recent therapeutic options with varying efficacies. Homs et al. (2007) in a study on autologous platelet gel (APG) and its effects on acute human skin wounds concluded that APG not only enhanced wound closure but also increased the wound healing velocity.[24]

Systemics

Inadvertent use of systemic antibiotics can result in resistance and is administered only in cases of evident infection such as fever, localized warmth, tenderness, erythema and lymphangitis (Evidence level C).

Oral pentoxyfylline (400 mg thrice daily) helps in faster healing of venous leg ulcers. (Evidence level A).[7,23,25]

Zinc, calcium dobesilate, aspirin, stanozolol, calcium channel blockers, prostaglandin derivatives, serotonin antagonists such as ketanserin are other systemics which are used with varying efficacies in venous and arterial leg ulcers.

Iloprost, a synthetic analogue of prostacyclin is a potent vasodilator that inhibits platelet aggregation and adhesion, increases capillary permeability, alters neutrophil function, and may help repair the damaged endothelium.

Immunosuppressants such as systemic steroids, IV immunoglobulins, methotrexate, dapsone, cyclosporine, minocycline, clofazimine, thalidomide are used in vasculitic leg ulcers.

Pain is a common accompaniment of chronic leg ulcers and might require analgesics during periods of exacerbation. Neuropathic pain can be treated with amitriptyline and anticonvulsants such as gabapentin. Opioids like morphine are advocated only in extremely painful ulcers.[4,7,23,25]

Other adjuncts to wound care with controversial efficacies include hyperbaric oxygen therapy, therapeutic ultrasound and electromagnetic therapy.[26,27,28]

Vacuum assisted closure (VAC) is a non-invasive therapy which makes use of a negative pressure device which evacuates wound exudate, increases the vascularity stimulates granulation tissue formation and reduces the bacterial content in the wound. Adhesive foam is placed into the wound and sealed followed by application of sub atmospheric pressure of 125 mm Hg which is transmitted to the wound in a controlled gradient.[4]

Compression Therapy

Compression systems include stockings, short-stretch bandages and long-stretch bandages. In an edematous extremity, short stretch bandages are usually recommended (Evidence Level C). Multi-layer high compression is more effective than low compression in simple venous ulcers after ruling out a peripheral arterial disease. Compression therapy helps in preventing recurrence of ulcer. The ideal compression pressure to overcome venous hypertension around the ankle is around 40 mm Hg. The proper application of compression hosiery aids in preventing ulcers at pressure points. All compression bandages should create a uniform gradient from ankle to the knee. Intermittent pneumatic compression given rapidly can be tried along with bandages or hosiery. This improves the leg edema in venous ulcers and lymphedema.[4,29]

Pressure Off-Loading

Peripheral sensorimotor neuropathy is a known risk factor for development of leg ulcers. Pressure modulation or "off loading," is mandatory in the treatment of diabetic ulcers on the plantar aspect. The common off-loading methods include bed rest, wheel chair, use of modified footwear with felted foam, contact casts and removable cast walkers.[30]

General Measures and Lifestyle Changes

a. Chronic dermatitis surrounding the ulcer can impede the healing process especially in venous ulcers. Other common complications of chronic venous insufficiency include lipodermatosclerosis, atrophie blanche and recurrent cellulitis. Regular use of emollients breaks the itch scratch cycle and prevents erosions, fissures and eczematous damage to the surrounding skin. Topical steroid impregnated antibiotics can be used in short courses to tide over the active dermatitis.

b. Allergic contact dermatitis can result from contact sensitization and should be considered in the scenario of non-responsiveness or worsening of ulcer with topical medication. The common allergens reported include fragrance mix, colophony, neomycin, and gentamicin.

c. Patients should be advised to carefully inspect their feet and legs for blisters or erosions, especially diabetic individuals. Use of proper fitting shoes and soft footwear should be frequently stressed.

d. Correction of nutritional deficiencies especially anemia ensures faster healing.

e. Control of blood sugars and hypertension is essential in all chronic open wounds with decreased healing tendency.

f. Regular calf muscle exercise increases the venous return and enhances healing in venous leg ulcers. Isotonic exercises improve the ejection function of calf muscle pump in limbs with venous ulceration and controls recurrence of ulceration.[4,7,31]

g. Limb elevation improves cutaneous microcirculation and reduces edema in chronic venous insufficiency. Avoid prolonged standing for long duration or sitting with the feet dependent.

h. Avoid sheering forces and friction at the site.

i. Lifestyle modifications include reduction of weight as wound healing is delayed in obese individuals. Avoid smoking and alcoholism which delays the healing process.

Role of Surgery

In arterial ulcers, arterial reconstruction surgery might be required to salvage the limb. Endarterectomy or reconstruction to bypass the occluded artery is indicated in presence of a clot or atheroma. Interventions such as balloon angioplasty, femoropopliteal bypass are tried after angiographic studies in patients with ischemic rest pain, ulceration or gangrene.

Cultured epidermal cells can be used in venous ulcers as a skin graft. Cultured allografts are expensive and are reserved for the management of chronic non-healing ulcers. Apligraf is cultured from human dermal fibroblasts and keratinocytes by tissue engineering and has histological resemblance to normal skin. This is being tried in clean non-infected wounds. It acts as a biological dressing and provides temporary wound closure.[4]

Ulcers due to chronic venous insufficiency are candidates for surgery so as to hasten healing and reduce recurrences (Evidence Level B). The incompetent superficial veins can be surgically ablated if there are no signs of healing after 3 months of adequate treatment measures. For superficial varicosities and perforator incompetence, sclerotherapy can be considered. (Evidence Level D). Endovascular laser therapy (EVLT) enhances healing in chronic venous ulcers.[7]

Psychosocial Aspects

Chronic leg ulcers are often accompanied by symptoms such as pain, pruritus, joint deformity, swelling, discharge, and malodor. These symptoms can diminish the quality of life by restricting routine physical activities and such individuals are often socially stigmatized culminating in mood changes and sleep deprivation.[32]

Physicians should therefore be aware of the patient's emotional stressors and consider health counseling especially in non-compliant patients.

CONCLUSION

Though the mortality associated with leg ulcers is very minimal they carry a huge burden on the individual's well-being and health standards. A comprehensive treatment plan should be derived after examining the ulcer and the limb along with a thorough physical examination. A combined multidisciplinary approach remains the mainstay of management along with careful patient education as adherence to a specific treatment plan is highly essential for proper healing of the wound, its maintenance, as well as to prevent recurrences in the future.

REFERENCES

1. Kahle B, Hermanns H-J, Gallenkemper G. Evidence-based treatment of chronic leg ulcers. Dtsch Arztebl Int. 2011;108:231-37.
2. Miller OF, Phillips TJ. Leg ulcers. J Am Acad Dermatol. 2000;43:91-95.[online] Available from https://www.jaad.org/article/S0190-9622(00)50401-0/abstract [Accessed December 2018].
3. Ghauri AS, Nyamekye IK. Leg ulceration: the importance of treating the underlying pathophysiology. Phlebology. 2010;25:42-51.
4. Sarkar P, Ballantyne S. Management of leg ulcers. Postgrad Med J. 2000;76:674-82.
5. Ouhes N, Phillips TJ. Leg ulcers. An in-depth review of differential diagnosis and management of leg ulcers. Curr Probl Dermatol. 1995;7:109-42.
6. Mekkes JR, Loots MAM, Van der Wal AC, et al. Causes, investigation and treatment of leg ulceration. Br J Dermatol. 2003;148:388-401.
7. Dogra S, Sarangal R. Summary of recommendations for leg ulcers. Indian Dermatol Online J. 2014;5:400-7.
8. Singer AJ, Tassiopoulos A, Kirsner RS. Evaluation and management of lower-extremity ulcers. N Engl J Med. 2017;377:1559-67.
9. Dean S. Leg ulcers - causes and management. Aust Fam Physician. 2006;35:480-4.
10. Marston W, Tang J, Kirsner RS, et al. Wound Healing Society 2015 update on guidelines for venous ulcers. Wound Repair Regen. 2016;24:136-144.
11. Alavi A, Sibbald RG, Phillips TJ, et al. What's new: Management of venous leg ulcers: Treating venous leg ulcers. J Am Acad Dermatol. 2016;74:643-64.
12. McMullin GM. Improving the treatment of leg ulcers. Med J Aust. 2001;175:375-8.
13. Hess CT. Clinical Guide to Skin and Wound Care. 6th ed. Philadelphia, PA: Lippincott Williams & Wilkins; 2008.p.192.
14. Guo S, Dipietro LA. Factors affecting wound healing. J Dent Res. 2010;89:219-29.
15. Fernandez R, Griffiths R, Ussia C. Water for wound cleansing. The Cochrane Library. No. 4. Chichester: John Wiley and Sons Ltd.; 2003.
16. Rai R. Standard guidelines for management of venous leg ulcer. Indian Dermatol Online J. 2014;5:408-11.
17. Kunimoto BT. Management and prevention of venous leg ulcers: A literature-guided approach. Ostomy Wound Manage. 2001;47:36-42.
18. Fowler E, van Rijswijk L. Using wound debridement to help achieve the goals of care. Ostomy Wound Manage. 1995;41:23S-35S.
19. Mosti G, Mattaliano V. The Debridement of chronic leg ulcers by means of a new, fluidjet-based device. Wounds 2006;18:227-37.[online] Available from https://www.woundsresearch.com/article/6069 [Accessed December 2018].
20. Falabella AF. Debridement and management of exudative wounds. Dermatol Ther. 1999;9:36-43.
21. Paddle-Ledinek JE, Nasa Z, Cleland HJ. Effect of different wound dressings on cell viability and proliferation. Plast Reconstr Surg. 2006;117:110S-118S.
22. Falanga V, Margolis D, Alvarez O, et al. Rapid healing of venous ulcers and lack of clinical rejection with an allogeneic cultured human skin equivalent. Human Skin Equivalent Investigators Group. Arch Dermatol. 1998;134:293-300.
23. Tate S, Price A, Harding K. Dressings for venous leg ulcers. BMJ. 2018;361:k1604.

24. Hom DB, Linzie BM, Huang TC. The healing effects of autologous platelet gel on acute human skin wounds. Arch Facial Plast Surg. 2007;9:174-83.
25. Whitmont K, Reid I, Tritton S, et al. Treatment of chronic leg ulcers with topical activated protein C. Arch Dermatol. 2008;144:1479-83.
26. Kranke P, Bennett MH, Martyn-St James M, et al. Hyperbaric oxygen therapy for chronic wounds. Cochrane Database Syst Rev. 2012; CD004123.
27. Aziz Z, Cullum N. Electromagnetic therapy for treating venous leg ulcers. Cochrane Database Syst Rev. 2015;CD002933. [online] Available from https://www.cochranelibrary.com/es/cdsr/doi/10.1002/14651858.CD002933.pub6/media/CDSR/CD002933/CD002933.pdf/es [Accessed December 2018].
28. Flemming K, Cullum N. Therapeutic ultrasound for venous leg ulcers. Cochrane Database Syst Rev. 2000;CD001180.
29. Simon DA, Dix. FP, McCollum CN. Management of venous leg ulcers. BMJ. 2004;328:1358-62.
30. Wu SC, Jensen JL, Weber AK, et al. Use of pressure offloading devices in diabetic foot ulcers: Do we practice what we preach? Diabetes Care. 2008;31:2118-19.
31. Shenoy MM. Prevention of venous leg ulcer recurrence. Indian Dermatol Online J. 2014;5:386-9.
32. Platsidaki E, Kouris A, Christodoulou C. Psychosocial aspects in patients with chronic leg ulcers. Wounds.2017;29:306-10. [online] Available from https://www.woundsresearch.com/article/psychosocial-aspects-patients-chronic-leg-ulcers [Accessed December 2018].

CHAPTER 12

Investigations and Radiological Diagnosis of Leg Ulcers

Shwetha S, Deepak HS

INTRODUCTION

Leg ulcers are an increasing problem worldwide and represent a major healthcare burden. Patients with leg ulcers are managed by clinicians in multiple specialties, including primary care, vascular surgery, plastic surgery, podiatry, wound care, and dermatology.

A leg ulcer is a physical finding that can result from multiple etiologies, rather than a diagnosis. Thus, determination of the cause is essential for selecting appropriate treatment and determining the need for further evaluation. Hence, properly investigating leg ulcers will not only aid in diagnosis, but also useful therapeutically and to assess the prognosis as well. The most common causes of leg ulcers are venous insufficiency, arterial insufficiency, and neuropathic disease.

INVESTIGATIONS FOR LEG ULCERS DUE TO VENOUS INSUFFICIENCY AND DEPENDENCY

Post-thrombotic Syndrome

Duplex Ultrasonography

Duplex scanning is noninvasive, widely available, and portable with minimal potential for complications. Evaluation of the lower extremities includes an assessment of venous compressibility, intraluminal echoes, venous flow characteristics, and luminal color filling (Figs. 1 to 3). Among these, venous incompressibility is the most widely used and objective criterion for the diagnosis of deep vein thrombosis (DVT).[1] Despite its utility, duplex ultrasonography does have some well-recognized limitations. Among studies limited to the proximal veins, the results are indeterminate or nondiagnostic in 1–6% of patients.[2,3] Adequate evaluation of the tibial and peroneal veins may be impeded by large calf size, edema, or operator experience but is aided by the use of color-flow Doppler ultrasonography.[4,5]

Computed Tomography Venography

Peterson and colleagues,[6] however, found that computed tomography venography (CTV) is specific but not sensitive for DVT, with a sensitivity of 71% and a specificity of 93% (Fig. 4).

Magnetic Resonance Imaging

It has also been used for imaging the venous system. Conventional magnetic resonance imaging (MRI), using

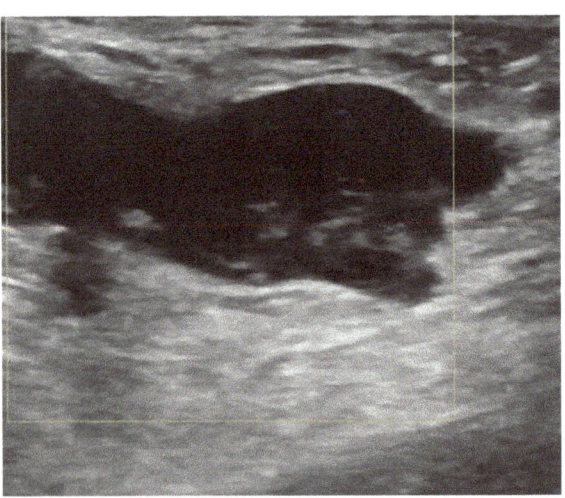

Fig. 1: A 55-year-old female with left lower extremity pain and swelling since 3 days. Ultrasound color Doppler image shows absence of flow in the left common femoral vein (CFV). The left CFV is distended by echogenic thrombus filling its lumen.

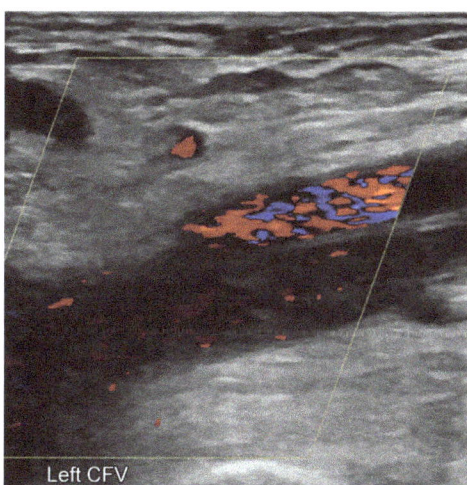

Fig. 2: Color Doppler image of common femoral vein (CFV) showing thrombus.

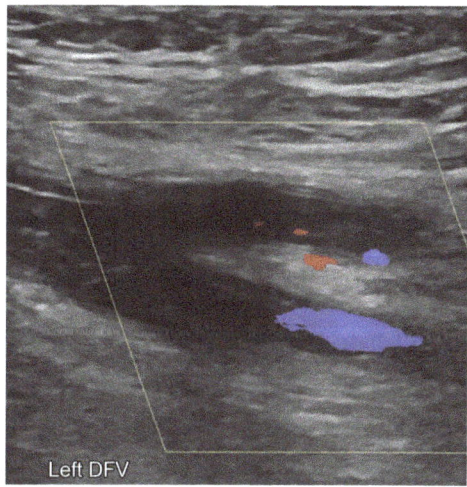

Fig. 3: Color Doppler image of left deep femoral vein showing thrombus.

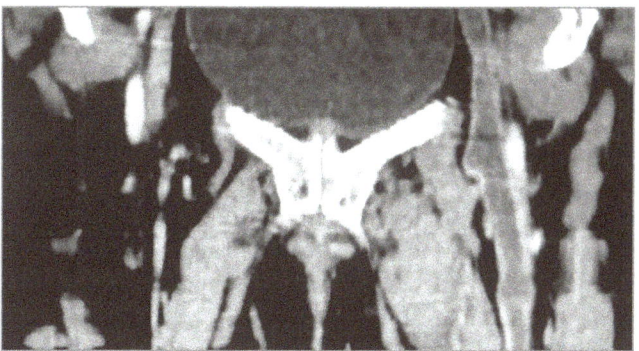

Fig. 4: Computed tomography venography of common iliac vein thrombus.
Courtesy: Dr Naveen KG, Assistant professor, Department of Radiodiagnosis, Bangalore Medical College and Research Institute.

spin-echo imaging, can detect central venous thrombi and, through its ability to identify acute perivascular edema, can provide information about the age of a thrombus.[7]

Flow-sensitive MRI Techniques

Flow-sensitive MRI techniques, or magnetic resonance venography (MRV), have been developed specifically for imaging the venous circulation. MRV takes advantage of the ability of magnetic resonance to distinguish stationary from moving signals. Various protocols have been employed, including noncontrast MRV techniques such as time-of-flight (TOF) and phase-contrast techniques as well as contrast-enhanced MRV (CE-MRV). TOF has been used as the primary noncontrast MRV modality for DVT.[7]

Newer Radiopharmaceuticals

Newer radiopharmaceuticals have also been approved for the imaging of DVT. ^{99m}Tc-apcitide is a complex of the radionuclide technetium Tc 99m and apcitide, a small synthetic peptide that binds the glycoprotein IIb/IIIa receptor on activated platelets and is specific for acute thrombus.[8,9] Imaging with ^{99m}Tc-apcitide has the advantage of being functional rather than relying on anatomic structural changes in the vein. Hence, it may avoid some of the pitfalls associated with venography and ultrasonography. Imaging is typically performed 10-60 minutes after peripheral venous administration of the radionuclide and venous segments both above and below the knee may be targeted.[10]

D-dimer Assays

D-dimers are products of the degradation of cross-linked fibrin by plasmin. Diagnostic assays for D-dimer have been based on the development of monoclonal antibodies capable of differentiating degradation products of fibrin and fibrinogen. D-dimer blood levels reflect the presence of intravascular fibrin and are sensitive for the diagnosis of venous thromboembolism. When measured by enzyme-linked immunosorbent assay (ELISA), the reference standard, sensitivity for the diagnosis of DVT is as high as 96.8%.[11] Unfortunately, these measurements are also quite nonspecific, with specificities as low as 35.2%.[12] Elevated D-dimer values are also associated with disseminated intravascular coagulation, malignancy, postoperative states, preeclampsia, infection, and recent trauma.[13]

Venous Ulcer

Various investigations can be performed to know the condition of the deep vein, position of the incompetent perforators.

List of routine investigations and special investigations mentioned in Boxes 1 and 2.

Specific Investigations

Standard Doppler Examination

In standard Doppler examination, a sound is emitted from the probe when blood flows past the transmitting and receiving crystals. If the blood flows in one direction in the absence of incompetence a uniphasic signal is received and a biphasic signal indicates bidirectional flow indicating blood refluxing down through incompetent valves. To know the saphenofemoral incompetence, Doppler probe is placed over the saphenofemoral junction and a calf squeeze is carried out. If the saphenofemoral junction is incompetent a biphasic signal is obtained. This diagnosis is further supported if all of the varices are controlled by a thigh tourniquet. The Doppler probe can be placed over distal varices when the tourniquet is released; retrograde flow is indicated by a rumbling noise as the blood refluxes down the long saphenous vein to fill the varices. This is not an accurate method of establishing incompetence of the lesser saphenous vein as its termination is variable and it is difficult to separate lesser saphenous incompetence from popliteal valvular incompetence. In all cases of short saphenous incompetence, a further investigation is desirable; this is usually carried out by duplex scanning.[14]

Box 1: Routine investigations.
- Hemoglobin estimation
- Total count and differential count
- Blood sugar estimation
- Blood urea, serum creatinine
- Urine for albumin and sugar

Box 2: Special investigations for venous insufficiency.

Noninvasive:
- Plethysmographic techniques
- Continuous wave Doppler ultrasonography
- Duplex Doppler and color flow Doppler ultrasound

Invasive imaging methods:
- Ambulatory venous pressure
- Venography
- Arm-foot venous pressure
- Radionuclide scintigraphy

Duplex Doppler Ultrasonography

The advent of color flow duplex scanning has revolutionized the assessment of venous disease. It is valuable noninvasive tool and simple in application. This technique combines B-mode real time ultrasonography with pulsed Doppler ultrasonography (Fig. 5). The B-mode image allows visualization of the underlying vessels so that a pulsed Doppler signal can then be specifically targeted to assess flow in a particular vessel.

Duplex color flow imaging can color red or blue depending on whether flow is in a forward or reverse direction thus providing additional data for analyzing the venous incompetence (Fig. 6).

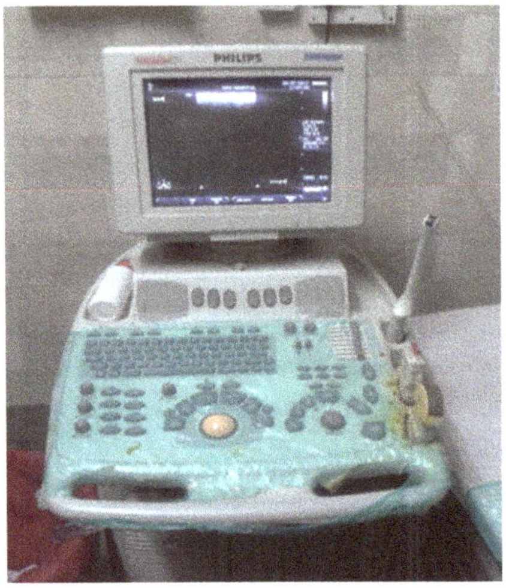

Fig. 5: Ultrasound machine.

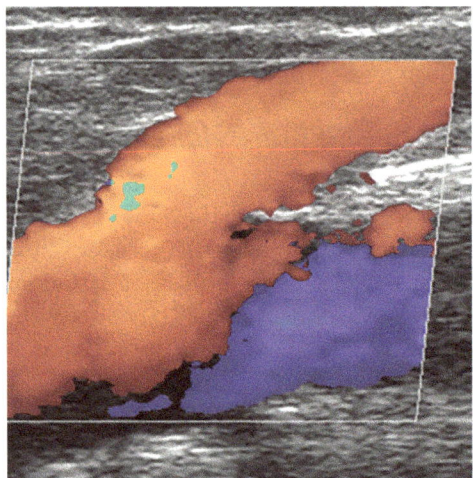

Fig. 6: Color Doppler image of the incompetent saphenofemoral (SF) junction on valsalva.

Duration and velocity of venous reflux in normal limbs, reflux during closure of competent valves does not exceed 0.45 seconds. When the color flow scanner is used, reflux is evident as persistent flow. Reflux studies have shown that if the sum of the refluxes in all vein is more than 10 mL/second there is 66% chances of skin changes and ulceration.

The duplex scan provides the following information, which will have an effect on the decision to intervene and the nature of the procedure.

- *Patency and competence of the deep veins (obstruction and incompetence)*: If the deep veins are occluded, removal or interruption of the superficial veins is likely to cause deterioration and is usually contraindicated.
- *Site and level of major incompetence*
- *Evaluation of perforator incompetence*
- *Anatomical variation and abnormalities identified*
- *Duration and velocity of venous reflux*
- *US criteria*: Great saphenous vein (GSV) insufficiency (Figs. 7 and 8):
  - Diameter more than 3 mm
  - Expansion in upright position
  - *Reflux*: Duplex and color flow reversal traceable to visible varicose vein (Table 1; Figs. 9 and 10).

Also, clinical, etiological, anatomical, and pathophysiological (CEAP) classification of chronic venous disease utilizes duplex ultrasonography mentioned in Table 2.

Varicography

Varicograpgy involves injecting a contrast directly into surface varices. The contrast is nonthrombogenic, as it is nonionic, and iso osmolar with blood. As the contrast flows through the veins, a detailed mapping of the varices to their termination is obtained. This is an extremely useful investigation in patients with recurrent varicose veins or those with complex anatomy.[14]

Venography

In this investigation, tourniquets are used to direct contrast injected into the superficial veins of the foot into the deep veins of the calf, thigh, and pelvis. It is not used as a standard investigation in patients with varicose veins but is useful if the duplex scan indicates, but cannot confirm, the presence of post-thrombotic change.[14]

Phlebography

In general, phlebography is unnecessary in the diagnosis and treatment of primary venous stasis disease and varicose

Table 1: Reflux grading by ultrasound (Fig. 9 and 10).

Type I	Perijunctional, originating from the SFJ or SPJ tributaries into the GSV or SSV
Type II	Proximal, from the SF or SP to tributary or perforating vein
Type III	Distal, from a tributary or perforating vein to the paramalleolar GSV or SSV
Type IV	Segmental, from a tributary or perorating vein to another tributary or perorating vein above the malleoli
Type V	Multisegmental, two or more distinct refluxing segments were detected
Type VI	Diffuse, entire GSV or SSV from the SFJ or SPJ to the malleoli

(GSV: great saphenous vein; SFJ: saphenofemoral junction; SPJ: saphenopopliteal junction; SSV: short saphenous vein)

Table 2: Clinical, etiological, anatomical, and pathophysiological (CEAP) classification of chronic venous disease.

Classification	Description/definition
C: clinical (subdivided into A for asymptomatic, S for symptomatic)	
0	No venous disease
1	Telangiectasias
2	Varicose veins
3	Edema
4	Lipodermatosclerosis or hyperpigmentation
5	Healed ulcer
6	Active ulcer
E: etiologic	
Congenital	Present since birth
Primary	Undetermined etiology
Secondary	Associated with post-thrombotic, traumatic
A: anatomic distribution (alone or in combination)	
Superficial	Great and short saphenous veins
Deep	Vena cava, iliac, gonadal, femoral, profunda, popliteal, tibial, and muscular veins
Perforator	Thigh and leg perforating veins
P: pathophysiological	
Reflux	Axial and perforating veins
Obstruction	Acute and chronic
Combination of both	Valvular dysfunction and thrombus

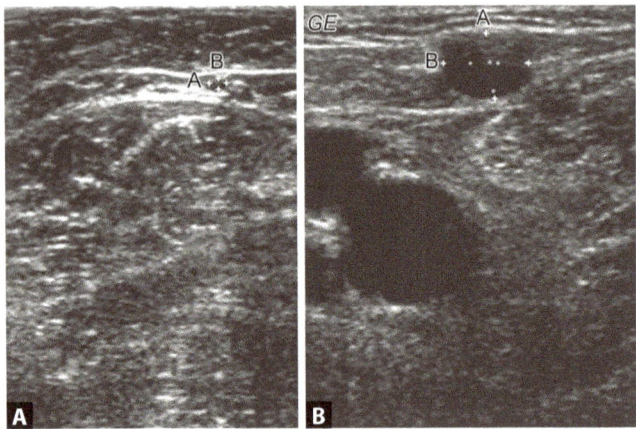

Figs. 7A and B: (A) Great saphenous vein (GSV) undilated and (B) GSV vein dilated.

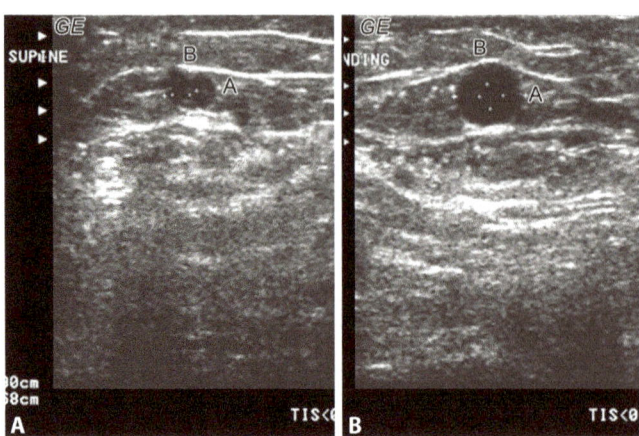

Figs. 8A and B: Positional change in the great saphenous vein (GSV) luminal dimension: (A) shows supine position and (B) GSV dilated in standing position.

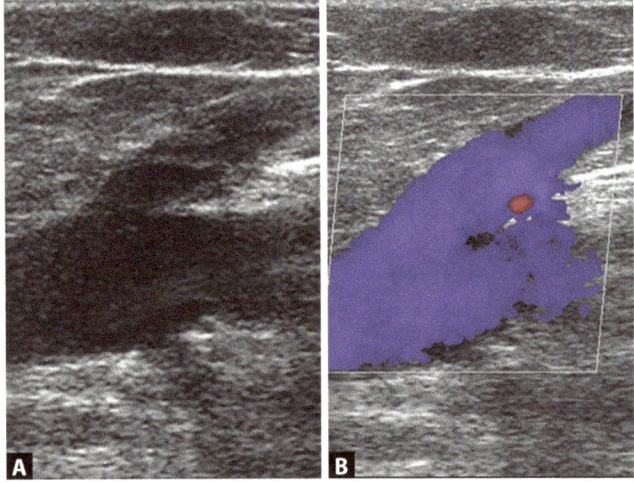

Figs. 9A and B: Demonstration of reflux: (A) saphenofemoral junction (SFJ) on gray scale; (B) color Doppler in neutral position.

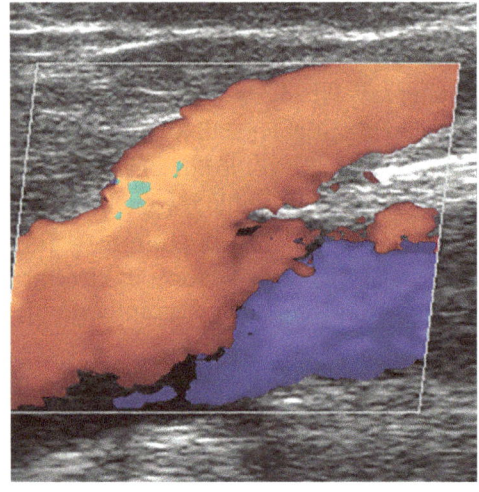

Fig. 10: Color Doppler image of the incompetent saphenofemoral (SF) junction on valsalva.

veins. In cases of severe chronic venous insufficiency (CVI), phlebography has specific utility. Ascending phlebography defines obstruction. Descending phlebography identifies specific valvular incompetence suspected on B-mode scanning and clinical examination.[15]

Ambulatory Venous Pressure

Ambulatory venous pressure (AVP) monitoring is the gold standard in assessing CVI.[16] In this technique, a needle is inserted into the pedal vein with connection to a pressure transducer. The pressure at rest and after exercise is performed is noted, usually in the form of toe raises. The pressure also is determined before and after the placement of an ankle cuff to help distinguish deep from superficial reflux. AVP has been shown to be useful in assessing the severity and clinical outcomes in CVI.[17] The mean ambulatory venous pressure (normal range of 20–30 mm Hg) and refill time (normal range of 18–20 seconds) are the most useful measurements. AVP provides information on the global competence of the venous system; however, there is concern about the failure of pressure to accurately reflect the pressure within the deep system.[18] AVP seldom is done in clinical practice because of the invasive nature and alternative diagnostic modalities.

Histopathological Examination

Histopathological examination of lipodermatosclerosis shows thickening and infiltration of the subcutaneous septa with lymphocytes and histiocytes. Fat cells are replaced by hyalinized masses of collagen. Dermal changes include a superficial and deep perivascular mixed cell infiltrate. Direct immunofluorescence shows deposition of fibrin around the blood vessels in the dermal papillae.[19] However, biopsy is not usually indicated in lipodermatosclerosis, as the biopsy site may fail to heal. A bone scan, computed tomographic scan or bone biopsies should be considered, if there is suspicion of osteomyelitis.[20]

INVESTIGATIONS FOR ARTERIAL CAUSE OF LEG ULCERS

Routine blood tests may be indicated in the evaluation of patients with suspected serious compromise of vascular flow to an extremity. Complete blood count (CBC), blood urea nitrogen (BUN), creatinine, and electrolyte studies help evaluate for signs of end-organ injury and for factors that might lead to worsening of peripheral perfusion. The hemoglobin A1c (HbA1c) level indicates the patient's level of glycemic control over the previous 120 days. Risk factors for the development of vascular disease (lipid profile, coagulation tests) can also be evaluated, though not necessarily in the emergency department (ED) setting. Elevated levels of inflammatory blood markers such as D-dimer, C-reactive protein, interleukin-6, and homocysteine have been linked to decreased lower extremity tolerance of exercise. A baseline electrocardiogram should be obtained. Any previous cardiac testing, including echocardiography, stress echocardiography, dobutamine-adenosine sestamibi scan, and coronary catheterization, should be reviewed and documented. In such circumstances, radioisotope ventriculography or echocardiography may be attractive as a noninvasive method of assessing left ventricular function. Patients must also be assessed for lung disease by chest radiograph and, if necessary, pulmonary function tests.[21]

Investigations for Acute Ischemia of Leg/Peripheral Arterial Disease

Pressure Measurement

Measurement of pressure has distinct advantages over measurement of flow for identifying the presence of arterial disease and for assessing its severity. Even though resting flow levels may remain in the normal range, there is almost always a pressure drop across a stenotic lesion that increases resistance to arterial flow.[22,23,24,25] Pressure measurements can be made more sensitive by augmentation of blood flow through a stenotic segment. This can be accomplished by exercise, the induction of reactive hyperemia, or the intra-arterial administration of vasodilating drugs. With increased blood flow, pressure drops are greater, and even those that were not noticeable under baseline conditions become evident.[26]

- *Ankle pressure*: Of all the noninvasive tests available for evaluating the functional severity of peripheral arterial disease, none is more useful than measurement of systolic blood pressure at the ankle. This test not only provides a simple, reliable means of diagnosing obstructive arterial disease but is also readily applicable to follow-up studies.[22]

Systolic ankle pressure is measured as follows:[22]

- A pneumatic cuff is placed around ankle just above the malleolus. A Doppler ultrasound probe is placed over the posterior tibial artery, and the pressure is measured at this site. The Doppler probe is placed over the dorsalis pedis artery, and the pressure is measured at this site.
- In normal individuals, the pressure measured at these two sites should differ by no more than 10 mm Hg. A pressure difference greater than 15 mm Hg suggests that there is a proximal occlusion or stenosis in the artery with the lower pressure.[25] The pressure at the site giving the higher value is taken as the ankle pressure.
- Occasionally, no audible Doppler flow signal can be obtained over either the posterior tibial or the dorsalis pedis artery. In these cases, a careful search often reveals a peroneal collateral signal anteriorly, near the lateral malleolus. When no Doppler signal can be found, the ankle pressure can often be measured with a plethysmograph placed around the foot or applied to one of the toes.
- *Ankle-brachial index*: Because the ankle systolic blood pressure varies with the central aortic pressure, it is convenient to normalize these values by dividing the ankle pressure by the brachial blood pressure.[25,27] Doppler instrument is advantageous to document flow within the smaller arteries and, most important, to provide an objective and quantitative assessment of the extent of arterial insufficiency through the calculation of a Doppler-derived ankle-brachial index (ABI). Normally, the ABI is greater than 1.0. The index is decreased to 0.40–0.80 in patients with claudication and to lower levels in patients with pain at rest or tissue loss. The ABI may be normal in some patients with mild-arterial narrowing; treadmill exercise has been used in these cases to increase the sensitivity of the test.[28] Falsely elevated ABI may be seen in patients with diabetes mellitus or renal failure as they may have calcific lower leg arteries, making them incompressible. In these cases, a toe-brachial pressure index gives more predictive value about significant arterial disease (Table 3).[22,29]

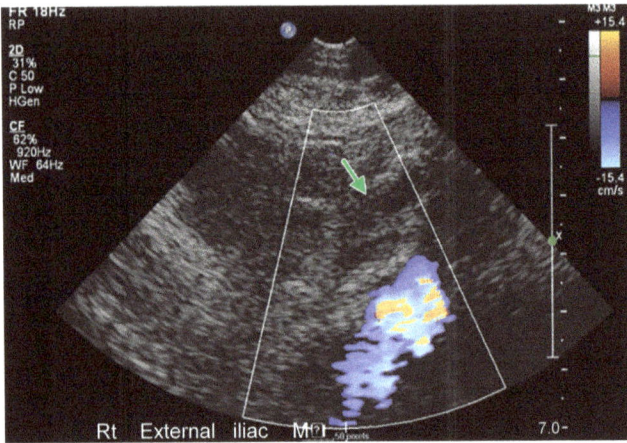

Fig. 11: Color Doppler image showing no flow in the right common iliac artery (green arrow).

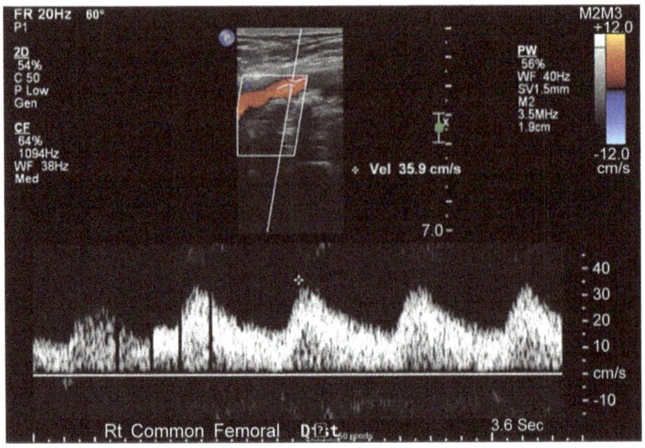

Fig. 12: Color Doppler of right common femoral artery shows low resistance spectral pattern suggesting proximal obstruction.

Table 3: Clinical category ankle-brachial pressure.	
Normal	>0.97
Claudication	0.40–0.80
Rest pain	0.20–0.40
Ulceration, gangrene	0.10–0.40
Acute ischemia	<0.10

The Transcutaneous Pressure of Oxygen

Measure of transcutaneous pressure of oxygen ($TcPO_2$) gives an idea about the degree of microvascular perfusion, which in turn reflects the metabolic state of the limb. It is measured with an oxygen electrode coupled directly to the skin of the foot or leg. The limb is adequately perfused when $TcPO_2$ more than 30 mm Hg. Improvement after hyperbaric oxygen therapy can also be measured by performing $TcPO_2$.[30]

Duplex Ultrasonography

It is a safe, inexpensive, and can provide functional information about vessel stenosis. It uses the combination of gray scale (B-mode) for vessel morphology and color pulsed-wave Doppler techniques.[31] The primary criteria of intra-arterial peak systolic velocity (PSV) and ratio of PSV between the site of stenosis and adjacent normal vessel are used to gauge the degree of stenosis. A PSV ratio of more than 2.5 suggests a stenosis of 50–74% and if the end-diastolic velocity is more than 60 cm/s, this suggests a tighter stenosis, in the range of 75–99%.[32] However, the most commonly used criteria is PSV ratio more than 2.0, along with peak systolic velocity more than 200 cm/s and aliasing and/or spectral broadening seen with color Doppler to diagnosis a stenosis more than 50%.[33] The addition of color flow imaging improves the diagnostic performance of duplex ultrasonography for aortoiliac and femoropopliteal arteries.[34] If no color Doppler signal is visible in the vessel, arterial occlusion is suggested (Figs. 11 and 12). The evaluation of infrapopliteal vessels while feasible by ultrasonography is time consuming and may be technically challenging. Thus, a complete evaluation of the native lower extremity arterial system may not be feasible in many patients.[35]

Plethysmography

Plethysmography performed in a vascular laboratory with measurements taken at the thigh, calf, ankle, metatarsal, and digital levels will assess disease progression through volume recordings, which are quantified through the pulse volume recorder. This procedure measures the small volume changes that occur in tissues during systole.[36,37]

Angiography (Synonym: Arteriography)

In lower limb disease, symptoms and their severity determine whether intervention is needed. Angiography is only appropriate, if intervention is being contemplated. Even then, it is often advisable to have a duplex scan first. Classical angiography involves the injection of a radiopaque solution into the arterial tree, generally by a retrograde percutaneous catheter method (Seldinger technique) usually involving the femoral artery. Hazards include thrombosis, arterial dissection, hematoma, renal dysfunction, and allergic reaction. Rather than taking simple films, nowadays a computer system digitizes the images, allowing the image before injection of contrast agent to be subtracted from the contrast image, thereby removing

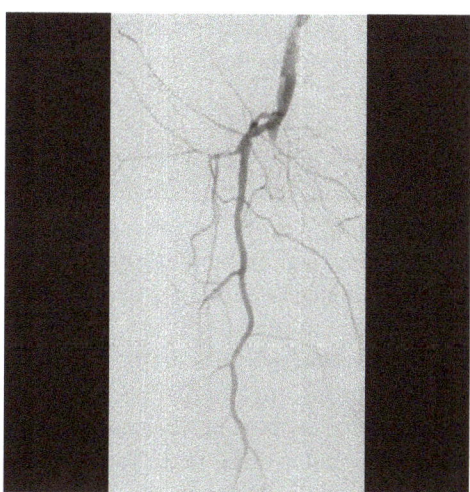

Fig. 13: Digital subtraction angiography (DSA) of right saphenous femoral artery occlusion.

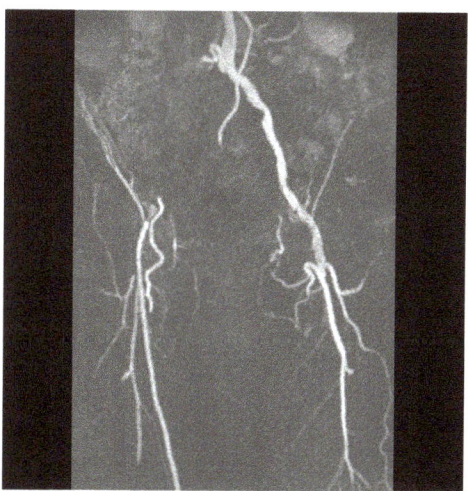

Fig. 14: A 62-year-old male with history of right extremity claudication. Magnetic resonance angiography (MRA) showing complete occlusion right common iliac artery (CIA) and right external iliac artery (EIA) with distal reconstitution of common femoral artery via circumflex artery.

extraneous background and providing great clarity. Such digital subtraction angiography (DSA) may be carried out by arterial or venous injection of contrast agent (Fig. 13). The former allows the use of fine catheters and relatively small amounts of contrast agent; although the latter avoids the need for arterial puncture completely, a high volume of contrast agent must be used.[38]

MR Angiography

The new millennium has seen the introduction of MR angiography, which offers the prospect of multiplanar imaging without the need for ionizing radiation or direct arterial puncture. MR angiography is being used with greater frequency in patients with peripheral arterial disease.[39] Using gadolinium as an MR contrast agent, the specificity and sensitivity of the test exceed that of duplex ultrasonography and approach the accuracy of standard arteriography (Fig. 14). MR angiography has been effective in demonstrating patent tibial arteries undetected with less sensitive conventional arteriography, identifying potential target vessels for an otherwise unfeasible lower extremity reconstructive bypass procedure. Today, MR angiography is widely employed in patients with chronic renal insufficiency to limit the dye load.

Computed Tomography Angiography

Another noninvasive imaging modality, computed tomographic (CT) angiography, is gaining appeal as a means of delineating anatomy to provide a means of localizing the extent and severity of occlusive disease.[40] The widespread

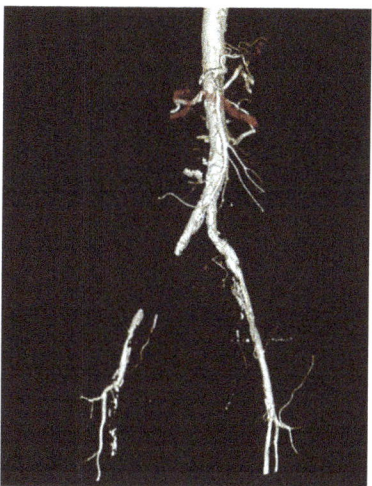

Fig. 15: Volume rendered reconstruction of computed tomographic angiography (CTA) showing right distal common iliac artery (CIA) and proximal external iliac artery (EIA) occlusion.

use of multidetector row CT scanners has improved the speed, volume coverage, and slice thickness of images so that a single contrast bolus can be imaged as it passes through the arterial system. One advantage of CTA is the depiction of the entire vessel, with the ability to appreciate thrombus and calcification; arteriography typically characterizes only the lumen of the artery. Thin slices of 0.625 mm allows for three-dimensional reconstructions and multiplanar reformatting that is not routinely achieved with conventional arteriography (Figs. 15 and 16). CTA disadvantages are similar to those of arteriography, with

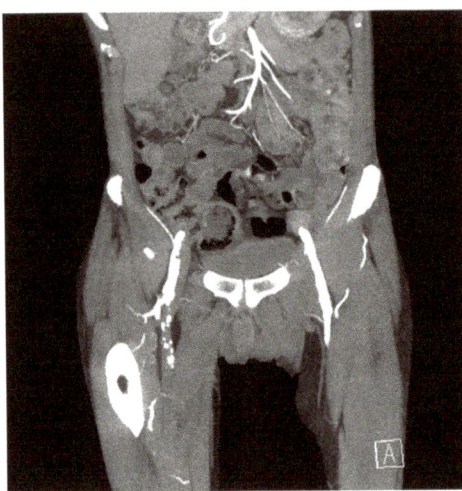

Fig. 16: Coronal (maximum intensity projection) MIP reconstruction of computed tomographic angiography (CTA) showing right superficial femoral artery (SFA) occlusion.

the potential for complications from the use of iodinated contrast agents and significant accumulation of radiation exposure.[21]

Carbon Dioxide Angiography

Angiography using CO_2 as a contrast medium can be helpful in patients with severe chronic renal insufficiency. CO_2 temporarily displaces the blood in the artery being imaged. CO_2 rapidly dissolves, but 3–5 minutes must be allowed to pass between injections. The limitations to use of this contrast agent include poor detail, especially for distal vessels. The bolus may cause significant patient discomfort. Sequelae of CO_2 embolus, with gas trapping leading to mesenteric ischemia, have been described. CO_2 is not used for arch or cerebral arteriography.[21]

Intravascular Ultrasound

With improvements in high-frequency smaller transducers, the use of catheter-based intravascular ultrasound (IVUS) has increased. IVUS provides a transverse, 360° image of the lumen of the vessel to be imaged throughout its length and provides qualitative data about the wall anatomy. It has been used in peripheral interventions for opening chronic total occlusions (CTOs) and has been instrumental in the endovascular treatment of aortic dissection.[21] As a diagnostic tool, adjuncts such as color flow Doppler enable the delineation between flow and thrombus, whereas virtual histology, in which color is assigned to plaque components of fibrous, fibrofatty, calcified, and necrotic lipid core densities, has been shown to correlate well with actual histology in assessment of coronary[41] and carotid arteries disease.[42] The use of IVUS, however, increases the length of procedures and its expense limits its applicability.

Investigations for Embolism

Angiography can be helpful in differentiating emboli from thrombosis. Typically, emboli are associated with a sharp cutoff, sometimes with a convex filling defect, or "reversed meniscus", in an otherwise fairly normal vessel. Owing to the acute nature of embolic occlusion, scant and poorly developed collateral vessels are another hallmark of an embolic event. The absence of disease elsewhere in the arterial tree implies embolism. Furthermore, multiple filling defects within several arterial beds are pathognomonic for embolization. Finally, the location of the occlusion is more frequently at a bifurcation in embolic disease. In contrast, patients with acute thrombosis have more obvious and diffuse atheromatous changes and better developed collaterals. The point of obstruction is generally associated with an irregular tapering and occurs in regions commonly afflicted with atherosclerotic disease, such as Hunter's canal. Unfortunately, many of these findings may become obscured with the propagation of clot.[43]

Investigations for Atheromatous Embolism

The diagnosis of cholesterol embolization syndrome remains a significant challenge for physicians. The symptoms and signs are nonspecific and diverse explaining why this disease is sometimes referred to as the "great masquerader."[44,45] For this reason, a high index of suspicion and a thorough understanding of the various clinical manifestations are needed in order to correctly make the diagnosis antemortem. The diagnosis can often be made on clinical grounds alone, without histological evaluation, in a patient who has a precipitating event, acute or subacute renal failure, hypertension that is difficult to control, and evidence of peripheral embolization.[46]

No specific laboratory test is diagnostic. Eosinophilia can be found in up to 80% of cases and is probably related to the generation of complement component C5, which has chemotactic properties for eosinophils. The eosinophilia, however, tends to be transient and short-lived.[47,48] Laboratory markers of inflammation, including levels of C-reactive protein, fibrinogen, and erythrocyte sedimentation rate, have also been found to be elevated in many patients. Other reported laboratory findings are leukocytosis, anemia, thrombocytopenia, and decreased complement levels.[49] Laboratory data may also

> **Box 3:** List of investigations for atheromatous embolism.
>
> *Complete hemogram*: Eosinophilia, thrombocytopenia, leukocytosis can be noted
> *Laboratory markers of inflammation*: C-reactive protein, fibrinogen, ESR
> Serum amylase
> RFT
> LFT
> Creatine phosphokinase
> Urinalysis for proteinuria, microhematuria, hyaline, and granular casts
> CT angiography, magnetic resonance angiography
> Transesophageal echocardiography

(CT: computed tomography; ESR: erythrocyte sedimentation rate; LFT: liver function test; RFT: renal function test).

reflect specific organ involvement. Elevations in serum concentrations of amylase, hepatic transaminases, blood urea nitrogen, creatinine, and creatine phosphokinase may be seen with involvement of the pancreas, liver, kidney, and muscle, respectively. Mild proteinuria, microhematuria, and hyaline or granular casts are the most common urinary findings in patients with confirmed cholesterol embolism.[50] Proteinuria in the nephrotic range and eosinophiluria has also been reported, although less commonly.[51]

Invasive vascular procedures requiring aortic instrumentation should be avoided as diagnostic modalities because of the potential risk of producing recurrent atheroembolism. Noninvasive imaging studies, such as multidetector CT angiography, magnetic resonance angiography, and transesophageal echocardiography, can assist in confirming the diagnosis, if any of these modalities demonstrates a markedly irregular and shaggy aorta (Box 3).[52]

Diagnosis of Thromboangiitis Obliterans

There are no specific laboratory tests to aid the diagnosis of thromboangiitis obliterans (TAO). Arteriography of all four limbs should be done in patients with TAO, even though they present with clinical involvement of only one limb. It shows segmental occlusion with the presence of collaterals around the areas of occlusion (corkscrew collaterals). Arteriography is suggestive but not diagnostic. Histopathology shows there will be panvasculitis of arteries and veins in the acute stage, characterized by the presence of a highly cellular inflammatory thrombus, with less inflammation in the wall of the blood vessels. The normal structure of the vessel wall, including the internal elastic lamina, is generally intact, in contrast to systemic vasculitis.[15]

INVESTIGATIONS FOR ULCER SECONDARY TO VASCULITIS

Exclusion of Vasculitis Mimics[53]

- Hepatitis B and C screen
- HIV test
- Electrocardiogram
- Complete antiphospholipid antibodies (APLA) workup
- Blood culture
- Antiglomerular basement membrane
- Antinuclear antibody.

Routine Blood Tests and to Rule Out Systemic Involvement

- Complete blood count (CBC) with erythrocyte sedimentation rate (ESR)
- Absolute eosinophil count (AEC)
- Renal function test, liver function test
- Urine dipstick and microscopy
- Chest X-ray
- Nerve conduction studies/electromyography
- Ultrasonography (USG) abdomen and pelvis
- Antistreptolysin O (ASLO) titers
- RA factor
- Mantoux test, Quantiferon Gold test to rule out tuberculosis.

Confirmation

Biopsy

Clinical evaluation should be focused toward identifying a suitable site for biopsy, as tissue diagnosis is vital to confirming the diagnosis of vasculitis. The site to be biopsied depends on clinical presentation. Common favored sites include skin, kidney, temporal artery, muscle, nasal mucosa, lung, sural nerve, and testis. If clinical evidence of multisystem involvement was present, choice of biopsy site would depend on its likelihood of affecting treatment decisions. In patients with skin and renal involvement, renal biopsy is preferred, as detection of necrotizing glomerulonephritis not only helps to confirm the diagnosis of vasculitis but also to decide how aggressive treatment should be. Blind biopsies to "exclude vasculitis" in patients with nonspecific generalized systemic symptoms are usually unhelpful. Biopsy findings might sometimes not be helpful even in patients with definite vasculitis. Histological examination could be normal (yield with sural nerve biopsies in patients with definite vasculitis is only around 45%[54]) or show only nonspecific findings. For example, necrotizing granulomas are not always seen in nasal mucosal or lung biopsy specimens from patients with suspected Wegener's granulomatosis.[55]

Angiogram

If tissue diagnosis is impractical (patients with large or medium vessel vasculitis with no accessible tissue for obtaining histological proof), angiogram should be considered. For example, mesenteric and celiac axis angiograms are useful in patients with suspected gastrointestinal tract vasculitis, while renal angiogram is useful in those with suspected renal artery involvement (not glomerulonephritis, which is best diagnosed with renal biopsy). Recently, computed tomographic angiography has been used to permit rapid diagnosis in patients with suspected polyarteritis nodosa.[56] Characteristic angiographic findings in patients with medium vessel vasculitis (polyarteritis nodosa) include multiple microaneurysms (attributable to necrotizing inflammation through vessel wall with consequent weakening).[57] Magnetic resonance angiogram of the thoracic aorta is the investigation of choice in patients with suspected large vessel vasculitis such as Takayasu's arteritis.[58] This would show stenosis, occlusion, or aneurysm formation.

Identify Specific Type of Vasculitis

- *Antineutrophilic cytoplasmic autoantibody (ANCA)*: Two types of ANCA staining patterns are seen on immunofluorescence (IF), namely cytoplasmic (c-ANCA), and perinuclear (p-ANCA).[59] ELISA should then always be performed in patients with positive results on immunofluorescence (IF) to identify the specific antigen targeted by ANCA. Presence of c-ANCA with antiproteinase-3 (anti-PR3) is highly suggestive of Wegener's granulomatosis, while p-ANCA with antimyeloperoxidase (anti-MPO) is more often encountered in those Churg-Strauss syndrome and microscopic polyangiitis.
- Cryoglobulins
- Complement levels
- Eosinophil counts/IgE levels
- Specific findings on biopsy (necrotizing granulomatous inflammation, presence of IgA deposits, evidence of immune complex formation or its absence)

NEUROPATHIC ULCERS

Diabetes Mellitus

Diabetes is readily detected by routine laboratory investigations, which in the case of ulcer patients should include:
- Serum glucose (and, if elevated, HbA1c)
- Cholesterol and triglycerides
- Prealbumin levels and urinary albuminuria levels
- Liver function test (LFT), renal function test (RFT)
- Iron profile, hemoglobin, erythrocyte sedimentation rate, and differential leukocyte counts.
- In case of diabetes, neuropathy may be assessed by measuring the thresholds for perception of vibration (using a biothesiometer) and light touch (using 10 g Semmes–Weinstein monofilaments).
- Plain radiographs to rule out osteomyelitis are suggested when there is sinus tracking or when probing to bone is possible.[60]
- It is important to evaluate underlying blood flow characteristics and determine the need for surgical consultation. Low ABI and $TcPO_2$ significantly increase the odds ratio of amputation in diabetics.[61]

Leprosy

Leprosy is a chronic infectious condition caused by *Mycobacterium leprae* (*M. leprae*) and affects mainly skin and peripheral nerves. It presents a wide spectrum of clinical manifestations dependent on the interaction of *M. leprae* with host and related to the degree of immunity to the bacillus. The diagnosis of this disease is a clinical one. However, in some situations, laboratory examinations are necessary to confirm the diagnosis of leprosy or classify its clinical form (Box 4).

Box 4: List of laboratory tests.

- *Intradermal reaction*
- *Inoculation on the foot pad of mice*
- *Slit skin smear: Bacterial index and morphological index*
- *Histopathology of skin and peripheral nerve*
- *Serological testing: Anti-PGL-1 antibodies and antigen assay*
- *Immunohistochemical reaction*
- *Molecular identification of M. leprae bacillus*
- *Imaging tests to asses bone, joint involvement, and peripheral nerve lesions*
- *Electroneuromyography*

Intradermal Reaction

Intradermal reaction consists of performing an intradermal injection of the lepromin antigen (synthesized from *M. leprae*) on the flexor surface of the forearm. There are two types of response: an early response, Fernandez reaction, which is assessed from 48 hours to 72 hours after injection and is considered positive, if the onset of an erythema measuring between 10 mm and 20 mm is observed; and a delayed response, Mitsuda reaction, which is assessed 4 weeks after injection and is considered positive, if the onset of a papule measuring 5 mm or more is observed. Mitsuda is positive in tuberculoid pole, which shows good cellular immunity and negative in lepromatous pole.[62]

Inoculation

M. leprae can be isolated from infected tissues after bacillus inoculation on the foot pad of mice, nine-banded armadillos (Dasypus novemcinctus), athymic mice, and monkeys.[5-8] It is a cumbersome and time-consuming technique that is employed only in referral centers.[62]

Skin Smear Microscopy

Skin smear examination for *M. leprae* is one of the simplest and most valuable laboratory tests available for diagnosis, and for monitoring the progress of patients under treatment. The skin is cleaned with methylated spirit and allowed to dry. The site to be examined is tightly pinched between the thumb and index finger to make it as avascular as possible, as detection of *M. leprae* becomes difficult, if the smear is full of blood. With a sterile scalpel, a 5-mm long and 2-mm deep cut is made at the edge of the skin lesion. The sides and bottom of the cut are quickly scraped to collect material for examination. The material on the blade is smeared on a clean slide with a circular motion to make a smear about 8 mm in diameter. The usual sites skin smear taken is from earlobes, forehead, chin, and active lesional skin. The slide is stained with ZN stain and observed under oil immersion microscope. At least, a hundred fields across the smear should be examined before declaring a smear as negative. For the sake of documenting the bacillary load and for following up progress on treatment, the Bacterial Index (BI) of Ridley is widely used.[63]

Ridley's logarithmic scale:
- 0: No bacilli in 100 oil immersion fields
- 1+: 1–10 bacilli in 100 oil immersion fields
- 2+: 1–10 bacilli in 10 oil immersion fields
- 3+: 1–10 bacilli in an average oil immersion field
- 4+: 10–100 bacilli in an average oil immersion field
- 5+: 100–1,000 bacilli in an average oil immersion field
- 6+: More than 1,000 bacilli in an average oil immersion field

The Morphological Index (MI) is calculated as the percentage of solidly staining bacilli in a smear after examining 200 bacilli. It was introduced as a measure of viability.

Histopathology

Histopathological examination is usually performed in fragments of skin lesions or nerves (Fig. 17). Hematoxylin-eosin staining should be complemented with Faraco-Fite staining or one of its variations for the investigation of acid fast bacilli. Depending on Ridley and Jopling criteria, histopathology is discussed here.

- *Indeterminate group*: The histopathological changes in indeterminate leprosy are minimal. Periadnexal and perivascular infiltrate of lymphocytes and histiocytes can be seen. The deep dermal nerves are usually thickened and show intraneural infiltration of lymphocytes.
- *Polar tuberculoid leprosy*: Well-defined tuberculoid granulomas constituted by macrophages with epithelioid differentiation and Langhans multinucleated giant cells, as well as by lymphocytes in the center and surrounded by a dense lymphocytic halo. The granuloma extends from the deeper dermis into the papillary layer of the dermis and causes erosion of the epidermis and atrophy. There are no bacilli or they are scarce.[62]
- *Borderline tuberculoid (BT) leprosy*: Epithelioid granulomas with many giant cells and fewer lymphocytes than polar tuberculoid lesions. Occasional bacilli may

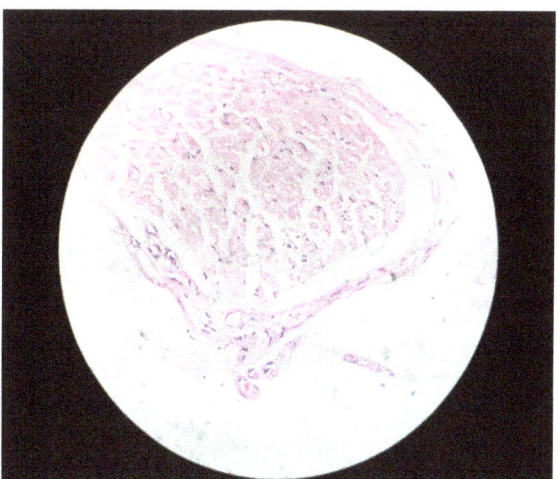

Fig. 17: Cross-section of nerve showing lymphocytic and epithelioid cell infiltrate.

be demonstrated in nerves on careful microscopic examination.
- *Mid borderline leprosy*: Diffuse collections of epithelioid cells, not focalized by a rim of lymphocytes and often associated edema. This group is unstable and very prone to reactions, and may upgrade to BT or downgrade to borderline lepromatous pole.
- *Lepromatous leprosy*: Sheets of macrophages extensively infiltrating the dermis except for a narrow subepidermal zone (Grenz zone), which is free of infiltration. In acid-fast stain preparations, the macrophages are found to be full of *M. leprae* (Figs.18A and B). Foamy macrophages are found around dermal blood vessels, sweat glands, hair follicles, and nerves. Proliferation of perineurial cells produces a characteristic "cut onion" or "onion peel" appearance and these cells also contain bacilli.
- *Borderline lepromatous leprosy*: Lepromatous leprosy except for a larger number of lymphocytes in BL lesions, suggesting a better host immune response to *M. leprae*. The dermal nerves also show lymphocytic infiltration, in addition to the presence of *M. leprae* in Schwann cells and macrophages. The subepidermal clear zone is preserved.[62]

Serological Testing

The presence of anti-PGL-1 antibodies reflects bacillary load and helps to classify clinical forms, since multibacillary (MB) patients show high antibody titers and paucibacillary (PB) patients show scarce or absent titers, with a percentage of PGL-1 seropositive patients ranging from 80% to 100% in cases of lepromatous leprosy and 30–60% in those of tuberculoid leprosy.[64,65] More recently, studies on the genomic sequences of *M. leprae* identified proteins and peptides specific for this bacillus and tested its immunoreactivity in leprosy patients and their contacts, through the detection of antigen-specific G immunoglobulins (IgG) of several recombinant proteins of *M. leprae*.[66,67]

Immunohistochemical Reaction

Immunohistochemical reaction using monoclonal or polyclonal antibodies to detect *M. leprae* antigens may provide higher sensitivity and specificity than conventional methods, representing an important auxiliary tool in the diagnosis of leprosy, especially at the initial phases or in PB cases.[68,69]

Molecular Identification of M. Leprae Bacillus

Polymerase chain reaction (PCR) allows detecting slow growth or uncultivable microorganisms, and, based on the available genetic data, has been used to detect *M. leprae*, since 1989.[70,71] PCR made it possible to detect, quantify, and determine *M. leprae* viability, showing significantly better results compared to common microscopic examinations. It is based on the amplification of specific sequences of *M. leprae* genome and in the identification of the fragment of amplified deoxyribonucleic acid (DNA) or ribonucleic acid (RNA).[72]

Imaging Tests

- Evaluation of bone and joint involvement:
  - X-ray may show signs of osteomyelitis, resorption of the extremities
  - Scintigraphy may help to differentiate between active and inactive disease, because it allows performing a

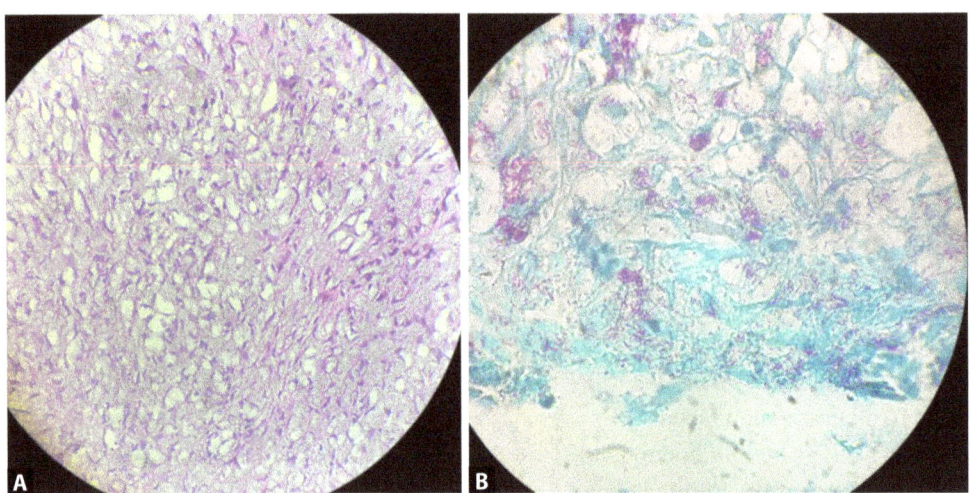

Figs. 18A and B: (A) Sheets of foamy macrophages on histopathology of lepromatous leprosy; (B) Multiple acid-fast bacilli on Fite–Faraco staining.

functional assessment of organs and systems, making it possible to analyze infection activity and evaluate therapeutic results.[62]
- CT scan accurate to analyze bone and joint lesions, especially those secondary to neurological involvement.
- Magnetic resonance imaging (MRI) may more accurately reveal soft tissue changes, such as subcutaneous fat infiltration, cellulitis, and abscess, in addition to osteomyelitis and neuropathic osteoarthropathy.[62]
- *Evaluation of peripheral nerve involvement*:
  - *Ultrasound (US)*: US may evaluate thickening, structural anomalies, edema, and neural vascularization, in addition to identifying nerve abscess and compression. The cross-sectional area of the nerve may be measured in order to assess thickening. High-resolution color Doppler US shows an increase in neural vascularization at the acute phase of neuritis in type 1 and 2 reactions, with greater signs of blood flow in perineural plexus or in intrafascicular vessels in type 1 reactions.[62]
  - MRI is a supplementary tool in the differential diagnosis between leprosy neuropathy and other peripheral nerve diseases.

Electroneuromyography

Electroneuromyography is indicated at the time of diagnostic evaluation in cases of suspected primary neural leprosy in order to help to choose the site of nerve biopsy. Electroneuromyographic changes include peripheral neurogenic involvement, with no evidence of disease in cells from the ventral horn of the spinal cord, usually leading to multiple mononeuropathy or, less commonly, to isolated mononeuropathy or distal polyneuropathy. In general, no changes are observed in the muscles not affected by leprosy.[73] Paralyzed muscles showed good response to stimulation, which suggests evidence of axonal interruption without actual degeneration, a finding that was consistent with the involvement of Schwann cells or interstitial tissue.[74] The most common and early finding is the decrease in the amplitude of motor and sensitive responses, which is usually more common than the decrease in the velocity of nerve conduction. The most frequently altered nerve seems to be the ulnar nerve, with the possible presence of cubital and carpal tunnel syndromes; however, a study demonstrated the involvement of the following nerves, in descending order of frequency: sural, median, ulnar, fibular, posterior tibial, and frontal branch of the facial nerve.[75]

Tabes Dorsalis

Tabes dorsalis is a late manifestation of untreated syphilis that is characterized by ataxia, lancinating pains, and urinary incontinence. A form of tertiary syphilis or neurosyphilis, it is the result of slow, progressive degeneration of the nerve cells in the spinal cord.
- Venereal disease research laboratory test (VDRL) of serum and cerebrospinal fluid (CSF)
- CSF treponemal hemagglutination assay
- CSF examination for glucose, proteins, and inflammatory cells
- X-ray suggests Charcot joint usually involving hip, knee, or spine
- *MRI of spine*: Multiple hyperintensities on T2-weighted images are seen in gray as well as white matter structures of dorsal columns of spinal cord. Secondary signs of vasculitis may be seen such as small infarctions.

HEREDITARY SENSORY NEUROPATHY TYPE 1C: CHARCOT–MARIE–TOOTH DISEASE

In a single patient, the clinical diagnosis of hereditary sensory neuropathy type 1 (HSN I) is based on the observation of signs and symptoms described above, and is supported by a family history suggesting autosomal-dominant inheritance.
- In HSN I, there is broad variability of electrophysiological abnormalities within and between families. Primarily axonal nerve damage of both motor and sensory nerves has been shown. Sensory potentials are usually absent in the lower limbs but are often recordable or even normal in the upper limbs, particularly in females.[76,77]
- The study of Whitaker *et al.* in the family later shown to carry a *SPTLC1* mutation and the study by Dubourg *et al.* also show motor conduction slowing, possibly implying a demyelinating process.[78,79]
- Neurophysiological studies in CMT2B patients with a *RAB7* mutation showed a mixed motor and sensory neuropathy with axonal and sometimes also demyelinating nerve damage.[80,81]
- Sural nerve biopsy findings were well studied in six English patients with a *SPTLC1* mutation. In severely affected nerves, only a very few myelinated fibers remained but electron microscopy showed a reasonable number of unmyelinated axons although the presence of stacks of flattened Schwann cell processes suggested

Table 4: Other causes of neuropathic ulcer.	
Syringomyelia	• MRI and CT of spine
Spina bifida	• X-ray of spine
	• MRI and CT of spine
Paraplegia	• CT and MRI of spine
	• Myelography
	• Evoke potential nerve test
	• Lumbar puncture
	• CBC
Poliomyelitis	• Stool sample or pharynx swab for polio virus
	• Antibodies to polio virus
	• CSF analysis
	• Oligonucleotide mapping
	• PCR amplification
Multiple sclerosis	• MRI of brain
	• CNS evoked electric potentials
	• Oligoclonal bands by agarose gel electrophoresis in CSF

(CSF: cerebrospinal fluid; CT: computed tomography; CBC: complete blood count; CNS: central nervous system; MRI: magnetic resonance imaging; PCR: polymerase chain reaction)

unmyelinated axon loss. There was also some evidence for primary demyelination (Table 4).[77,82]

LABORATORY SCREENING TESTS FOR CLOTTING DISORDERS[83]

- Activated partial thromboplastin time
- Prothrombin time
- Thrombin time
- Factor V (Leiden) mutation (506R fi 506Q)
- Factor II (prothrombin) mutation (20210G fi 20210A)
- Antithrombin III
- Protein C and protein S
- Lupus anticoagulant
- Anticardiolipin.

METABOLIC CAUSES OF LEG ULCERS

List of investigations is given in Table 5.

INFECTIOUS CAUSES OF LEG ULCER

Wound cultures are often routinely performed, but give only information about the bacterial flora in the superficial layers. The decision to prescribe systemic antibiotics should be based on the combination of culture results and clinical criteria, such as signs of infection (fever, erythema, color). The diagnosis has become easier after the introduction of labeled leukocyte scanning and especially, magnetic resonance imaging.

Apart from infectious causes of leg ulcers, all chronic leg ulcers are secondarily contaminated, a quantitative bacterial culture is more specific, and should be performed once wound infection is suspected.[84] This is performed by curetting or biopsying the bed of the ulcer. The quantitative biopsy is the current gold standard for assessing the quality and quantity of microbial pathogens within a wound. Quantitative biopsies containing greater than 10^5 organisms per gram of tissue are considered significant, and systemic antibiotherapy should be considered.[85] Ulcers that probe to bone should be considered osteomyelitic until proven otherwise. Radiographs will usually show characteristic changes such as translucency corresponding to areas of osteolysis. The sensitivity, specificity, and likelihood ratios of probing to bone are better than those of plain radiograph and bone scan but are worse than those of 111-indium scanning and magnetic resonance imaging.[86] More specific tests such as white blood cell scans are more sensitive than bone or gallium scan. In a comparative study of 107 patients, Sommezoghi et al.[87] found that 99mTc-labeled ciprofloxacin (Infecton) has a better specificity for bacterial infections than WBC scans in detecting infectious foci in bones and joints. One should keep in mind that even in the presence of osteomyelitis, constitutional symptoms, and leukocytosis may be lacking in immunocompromised and some diabetic patients.[30]

HEMATOLOGICAL CAUSES OF LEG ULCERS (TABLE 6)

The hematological causes of leg ulcers are discussed in Table 6.

INVESTIGATING ATYPICAL LEG ULCERS[30]

- Guided by the medical history and physical examination, some specific laboratory investigations and procedures may be performed. Significantly elevated antinuclear antibodies, rheumatoid factors, or other more specific immunologic tests may tend to support the diagnosis of vasculitic process.
- Serologic tests for syphilis, or polymerase chain reaction for mycobacterium DNA may be performed on specimens

Table 5: List of investigation for metabolic causes of leg ulcer.

Diabetes	• HbA1C • Lipid profile • RFT • Threshold of perception of vibration using biothesiometer • Plain radiograph to rule out osteomyelitis
Necrobiosis lipoidica	• Blood tests to rule out diabetes • *Skin biopsy*: Variable degree of granulomatous inflammation around degenerated collagen in the dermis with the involvement of subcutaneous fat. The degenerated collagen appears paler with gray hue and more haphazardly arranged on H- and E-stained sections. This alteration in the collagen is known as necrobiosis. Few scattered multinucleated or Langhans giant cells and histiocytes with extensive sclerosis.
Porphyria cutanea tarda	• *Urine*: Increased uroporphyrin III, heptacarboxyporphyrin • *Feces*: Increased isocoproporphyrin, heptacarboxyporphyrin • *Plasma spectrofluorimetry*: Peak is seen at 615–620 nm • *Liver biopsy*: To rule out—hemochromatosis, hepatitis C, alcoholic cirrhosis • Ultrasound and alpha fetoprotein—to rule out liver carcinoma, as porphyrins are carcinogenic • Periodic acid-Schiff (PAS) stain reveals a mild degree of thickening of the papillary vessel wall on histopathology
Gout	• Raised uric acid • Leukocytosis, raised ESR • Polarized microscopy shows intracellular, negatively birefringent, needle-shaped crystals • Histopathology; granulomatous fluffy infiltrate surrounding radially arranged needle-like spaces. Special stain-like deGalantha used to stain urate
Calciphylaxis	• RFT • Parathyroid hormone levels • Thyroid profile • Serum calcium and phosphorous levels • Serum albumin levels • Protein C and S levels • *Histopathology*: von Kossa stain used to detect calcium deposits
Homocystinuria	• CBC with peripheral smear • ESR • Vitamin B_{12} levels • Sodium nitroprusside test of urine • Serum homocysteine levels (normal range 4.60–12.44 µmol/L)
Prolidase deficiency	• CBC • USG abdomen • Complement levels • Iminopeptiduria greater than 5 mmol/24 hours • Detection of either biallelic PEPD pathogenic variants or reduced prolidase enzyme activity in a proband
Hyperoxaluria	• Urinary oxalate excretion • Testing of AGXT, GRHPR, HOGA1 genes • Skin biopsy • Radiological imaging for multiorgan involvement (USG, CT, etc.) • ECG and echo, if heart is involved

(RFT: renal function test; CBC: complete blood count; CT: computed tomography; USG: ultrasonography; ECG: electrocardiography; ESR: erythrocyte sedimentation rate)

from an ulcer suspected of being of mycobacterial origin (e.g. erythema induratum of Bazin: Mycobacterial panniculitis with subsequent ulceration usually involving the calves).[30]

• Cryoglobulins may be associated with hepatitis C and leg ulceration. Therefore, hepatitis C serologies and serum level of cryoglobulins may be helpful tests.[88] Like cryoglobulins, cryofibrinogens may be associated with

Table 6: Hematological causes of leg ulcers relevant investigations.

Sickle cell anemia	• Hemoglobin electrophoresis • Mass spectroscopy • Sickling test
Thalassemia	• Hemoglobin electrophoresis • Peripheral smear
Hereditary spherocytosis	• Peripheral smear • Osmotic fragility • Acid glycerol lysis test • Eosin-5'-maleimide binding test • SDS gel electrophoresis
Glucose-6-phosphate dehydrogenase	• Peripheral smear • DNA testing
Waldenstrom disease	• Serum electrophoresis • Bone marrow biopsy • Positive Coombs test
Leukemia	• Peripheral smear • Bone marrow sampling

(SDA: sodium dodecyl sulfate).

Table 7: Investigations for ulcerating skin diseases.

Bullous pemphigoid	• Skin biopsy • Direct and indirect immunofluorescence • Tests to rule out associated diseases
Panniculitis	• *Skin biopsy*: Septal or lobular panniculitis with or without vasculitis features
Erythema elevatum diutinum	• *Skin biopsy*: Leukocytoclastic vasculitis • Direct immunofluorescence • Immunoelectrophoresis • Tests to rule out associated autoimmune conditions, malignancies and infections
Malignant atrophic papulosis	• Skin biopsy • ANA, lupus anticoagulant and anticardiolipin antibodies • Imaging studies, if neurological and gastrointestinal involvement present
Sarcoidosis	• *Skin biopsy*: Naked granulomas, asteroid bodies, Schaumann bodies, reticulin stain • ACE levels • Serum calcium levels • Chest X-ray, ECG • Peripheral blood counts • LFT, RFT
Behcet's disease	• *Skin biopsy*: Leukocytoclastic vasculitis • MRI of brain • Angiography, if vascular lesions • Pathergy test
SLE and scleroderma	• ANA titer • ANA profile • Skin biopsy • Routine blood tests

(ACE: angiotensin-converting enzyme; ANA: antinuclear antibody; ECG: electrocardiography; LFT: liver function test; RFT: renal function test; MRI: magnetic resonance imaging; SLE: systemic lupus erythematosus)

recurrent leg ulcers, especially if there is a history of worsening of symptoms with exposure to cold.

- Leg ulcers of atypical presentation or those that fail to heal should alert the clinician to consider uncommon etiologies. (1) When a wound fails to heal after 3–4 months of conventional treatment, biopsy of the ulcer edge (either excisional or multiple punch biopsy techniques) should be performed to rule out malignancy. The most common type of cancer developing in chronic wounds is squamous cell carcinoma.
- Patients with leg ulcers are prone to developing contact dermatitis to dressings. When necessary a patch testing should help to determine specific allergens.
- *Ulcerating skin diseases*: Pyoderma gangrenosum is a noninfective ulcer, which usually presents with undermined borders. It may be associated with inflammatory bowel disease, inflammatory arthropathies, or myeloproliferative disorders. Appropriate workup for associated disease should be considered in patients with pyoderma gangrenosum. Other causes of ulcerating skin diseases mentioned in Table 7.

REFERENCES

1. Lensing AW, Prandoni P, Brandjes D, et al. Detection of deep-vein thrombosis by real-time B-mode ultrasonography. N Engl J Med. 1989;320:342-5.
2. Lewis BD, James EM, Welch TJ, et al. Diagnosis of acute deep venous thrombosis of the lower extremities: Prospective evaluation of color Doppler flow imaging versus venography. Radiology. 1994;192:651-5.
3. Vaccaro JP, Cronan JJ, Dorfman GS. Outcome analysis of patients with normal compression US exams. Radiology. 1990;175:645-9.
4. Mattos MA, Melendres G, Sumner DS, et al. Prevalence and distribution of calf vein thrombosis in patients with symptomatic deep venous thrombosis: A color-flow duplex study. J Vasc Surg. 1996;24:738-44.
5. Messina LM, Sarpa MS, Smith MA, et al. Clinical significance of routine imaging of iliac and calf veins by color flow duplex scanning in patients suspected of having acute lower extremity deep venous thrombosis. Surgery. 1993;114:921-7.

6. Peterson DA, Kaverooni EA, Wakefield TW, et al. Computed tomographic venography is specific but not sensitive for diagnosis of acute lower extremity deep venous thrombosis in patients with suspected pulmonary embolus. J Vasc Surg. 2001;34:798-804.
7. Cook J, Meissner MH. Clinical and diagnostic evaluation of the patient with deep vein thrombosis. In: Cronenwett JL, Gloviczki P, Johnston KW, Krupski WC, Ouriel K, Sidawy AN (Eds). Rutherford vascular surgery, 6th edition. Philadelphia: Elsevier Saunders; 2005.
8. Muto P, Lastoria S, Varella P, et al. Detecting deep venous thrombosis with technetium-99m-labeled synthetic peptide P280. J Nucl Med. 1995;36:1384-91.
9. Pearson DA, Lister-James J, McBride WJ, et al. Thrombus imaging using technetium-99m-labeled high potency GPIIb/IIIa receptor agonists: Chemistry and initial biological studies. J Med Chem. 1996;39:1372-82.
10. Carretta RF. Scintigraphic imaging of lower-extremity acute venous thrombosis. Adv Ther. 1998;15:315-22.
11. Horellou MH, Conard J, Samama MM. Venous thromboembolism: An Evidence-Based Atlas. Armonk, NY: Futura; 1996.
12. Kelly J, Hunt BJ. Role of D-dimers in diagnosis of venous thromboembolism. Lancet. 2002;359:456-8.
13. Gaffney PJ, Creighton LJ, Callus MJ, et al. Monoclonal antibodies to cross-linked fibrin degradation products (XL-FDP). II: Evolution in a variety of clinical conditions. Br J Haematol. 1988;68:91-6.
14. Burnard K. Venous disorders. In: Williams NS, Bustrode CJK, O'Connell PR (Eds). Bailey and Love's short practice of Surgery, 25th edition. London: Edward and Arnold Ltd; 2008. pp. 925-43.
15. Sacchidanand S, Shwetha S, Rajendran SC. Diseases of arteries, veins and lymphatics. In: Sacchidanand S, Oberoi C, Inamadar AC, (Eds). IADVL textbook of dermatology, 4th edition. Mumbai: Bhalani Publishing House; 2015: pp.1117-50.
16. Freischlag JA, Heller JA. Venous disease. In: Townsend CM, Beauchamp RD, Evers BM, Mattox KL, (Eds). Sabiston textbook of surgery: the biological Basis of modern surgical practice, 19th edition. Philadelphia: Elsevier Saunders; 2012. pp. 1807-24.
17. Singh S, Lees TA, Donlon M, et al. Improving the preoperative assessment of varicose veins. Br J Surg. 1997;84:801-2.
18. Masuda EM, Arfvidsson B, Eklof B, et al. Direct venous pressure: role in the assessment of venous disease. In: Gloviczki P, Yao JS (Eds). Handbook of venous disorders, 2nd edition. New York, NY: Arnold; 2001: pp. 140-5.
19. Nicolaides AN, Hussein MK, Szendro G, et al. The relation of venous ulceration with ambulatory venous pressure measurements. J Vasc Surg. 1993;17:414-9.
20. Neglen P, Raju S. Ambulatory venous pressure revisited. J Vasc Surg. 2000;31:1206-13.
21. Silva MB, Vhoi L, Cheng CC. Peripheral arterial disease. In: Townsend CM, Beauchamp RD, Evers BM, Mattox KL (Eds). Sabiston textbook of surgery: the biological Basis of modern surgical practice, 19th edition. Philadelphia: Elsevier Saunders; 2012. pp. 1731-90.
22. Zierler RG, Sumner DS. Physiologic assessment of peripheral arterial disease. In: Cronenwett JL, Gloviczki P, Johnston KW, Krupski WC, Ouriel K, SidawyAN (Eds). Rutherford vascular surgery, 6th edition. Philadelphia: Elsevier Saunders; 2005.
23. Sumner DS, Strandness Jr DE. The relationship between calf blood flow and ankle blood pressure in patients with intermittent claudication. Surgery. 1969;65:763.
24. Tønneson KH, Noer I, Paaske W, et al. Classification of peripheral occlusive arterial diseases based on symptoms, signs, and distal blood pressure measurements. Acta Chir Scand. 1980;146:101.
25. Wyss CR, Matsen III FA, Simmons CW, et al. Transcutaneous oxygen tension measurements on limbs of diabetic and nondiabetic patients with peripheral vascular disease. Surgery. 1984;95:339.
26. Tønnesen KH, Noer I, Paaske W, et al. Classification of peripheral occlusive arterial diseases based on symptoms, signs, and distal blood pressure measurements. Acta Chir Scand. 1980;146:101.
27. Carter SA. Indirect systolic pressures and pulse waves in arterial occlusive disease of the lower extremities. Circulation. 1968;37:624.
28. Barnes RW, Hafermann MD, Petersen J, et al. Noninvasive assessment of altered limb hemodynamics and complications of arterial catheterization. Radiology. 1973;107:505.
29. Barnes RW, Shanik GD, Slaymaker EF. An index of healing in below-knee amputation: Leg blood pressure by Doppler ultrasound. Surgery. 1976;79:13.
30. Khachemoune A, Kauffman C. Diagnosis of Leg Ulcers. Int J Dermatol. 2001;1(2):1-8.
31. Norgren L, Hiatt WR, Dormandy JA, et al. Intersociety consensus for the management of peripheral arterial disease. J Vasc surg. 2007;45:S5-S67.
32. De Smet AEA, Ermers EJM, Kitslaar PJEH. Duplex velocity characteristics of aortoiliac stenoses. J Vasc Surg. 1996;23:628-36.
33. Rooke TW, Hirsch AT, Misra S, et al. 2011 ACCF/AHA Focused Update of the Guideline for the Management of Patients With Peripheral Artery Disease (Updating the 2005 Guideline): A Report of the American College of Cardiology Foundation/American Heart Association Task Force on Practice Guidelines. J Am Coll Cardiol. 2011;58:2020-45.
34. De vries SO, Hinik MG, Polak JF. Summary receiver operating characteristics curves as a technique for metanalysis of the diagnostic performance of duplex ultrasonography in peripheral arterial disease. Acad Radiol. 1996;3:361-9.
35. Pollak AW, Patrik N, Kramer CM. Multimodal imaging of lower extremity peripheral arterial disease: Current role and future directions. Circ Cardiovasc Imaging. 2012;5(6):797-807.
36. Goldstein DR, Vogel KM, Mureebe L, et al. Differential diagnosis: assessment of the lower-extremity ulcer—is it arterial, venous, neuropathic? Wounds. 1998;10(4):125-31.
37. London NJ, Donnelly R. Ulcerated lower limb. BMJ. 2000; 320(7249):1589-91.
38. Murie JA. Arterial disorders. In: Williams NS, Bustrode CJK, O'Connell PR, (Eds). Bailey and Love's short practice of Surgery, 25th edition. London: Edward and Arnold Ltd: 2008. pp. 899-924.

39. Schoenberg SO, Londy FJ, Licato P, et al. Multiphase-multistep gadolinium-enhanced MR angiography of the abdominal aorta and runoff vessels. Invest Radiol. 2001;36:283-91.
40. Rubin GD, Dake MD, Semba CP. Current status of three-dimensional spiral CT scanning for imaging the vasculature. Radiol Clin North Am. 1995;33:51-70.
41. Nair A, Kuban BD, Tuzcu EM, et al. Coronary plaque classification with intravascular ultrasound radiofrequency data analysis. Circulation. 2002;106:2200-6.
42. Diethrich EB, Pauliina Margolis M, Reid DB, et al. Virtual histology intravascular ultrasound assessment of carotid artery disease: The Carotid Artery Plaque Virtual Histology Evaluation (CAPITAL) study. J Endovasc Ther. 2007;14:676-86.
43. Fecteau SR, Darling III RC, Roddy SP. Arterial Thromboembolism. In: Cronenwett JL, Gloviczki P, Johnston KW, Krupski WC, Ouriel K, SidawyAN (Eds). Rutherford vascular surgery, 6th edition. Philadelphia: Elsevier Saunders; 2005.
44. Lie JT. Cholesterol atheromatous embolism: The great masquerader revisited. Pathol Annu. 1992;27:17-50.
45. Olin JW. Syndromes that mimic vasculitis. Curr Opin Cardiol. 1991;6:768-774.
46. Belenfant X, Meyrier A, Jacquot C. Supportive treatment improves survival in multivisceral cholesterol crystal embolism. Am J Kidney Dis. 1999;33:840-50.
47. Fabbian F, Catalano C, Lambertini D, et al. A possible role of corticosteroids in cholesterol crystal embolization. Nephron. 1999;83:189-90.
48. Moolenaar W, Lamers CB. Cholesterol crystal embolization in the Netherlands. Arch Intern Med. 1996;156:653-7.
49. Fine MJ, Kapoor W, Falanga V. Cholesterol crystal embolization: A review of 221 cases in the English literature. Angiology. 1987;38:769-84.
50. Haqqie SS, Urizar RE, Singh J. Nephrotic-range proteinuria in renal atheroembolic disease: Report of four cases. Am J Kidney Dis. 1996;28:493-501.
51. Greenberg A, Bastacky SI, Iqbal A, et al. Focal segmental glomerulosclerosis associated with nephrotic syndrome in cholesterol atheroembolism: Clinicopathological correlations. Am J Kidney Dis. 1997;29:334-44.
52. Rose R, Bartholomew J, Olin JW. Atheromatous embolization. In: Cronenwett JL, Gloviczki P, Johnston KW, Krupski WC, Ouriel K, SidawyAN (Eds). Rutherford vascular surgery, 6th edition. Philadelphia: Elsevier Saunders; 2005.
53. Suresh E. Diagnostic approach to patients with suspected vasculitis. Postgrad Med J. 2006;82(970):483-8.
54. Oh SJ. Diagnostic usefulness and limitations of sural nerve biopsy. Yonsei Med J. 1990;31:1-26.
55. Devaney Ko, Travis WD, Hoffman G, et al. Interpretation of head and neck biopsies in Wegener's granulomatosis. A pathologic study of 126 biopsies in 70 patients. Am J Surg Pathol. 1990;14:555-64.
56. Ozcakar ZB, Yalcinkaya F, Fitoz S, et al. Polyarteritis nodosa: successful diagnostic imaging utilizing pulsed and color Doppler ultrasonography and computed tomography angiography. Eur J Pediatr. 2006;165:120-3.
57. Stanson AW, Friese JL, Johnson CM, et al. Polyarteritis nodosa: spectrum of angiographic findings. Radiographics. 2001;21: 151-9.
58. Schmidt WA, Gromnica-Ihle E. What is the best approach to diagnosing large-vessel vasculitis? Best Pract Res Clin Rheumatol. 2005;19:223-42.
59. Seo P, Stone JH. The antineutrophil cytoplasmic antibody-associated vasculitides. Am J Med. 2004;11:739-50.
60. Caputo GM, Cavanaugh PR, Ulbrecht JS, et al. Assessment and management of foot disease in patients with diabetes. N Engl J Med. 1995;332:854-60.
61. Reiber GE. The epidemiology of diabetic foot problems. Diabic Med. 1996;13:S6-11.
62. Lastória JC, Morgado de Abreu MAM. Leprosy: a review of laboratory and therapeutic aspects—Part 2. An Bras Dermatol. 2014;89(3):389-403.
63. Ridley DS. Therapeutic trials in leprosy using serial biopsies. Lepr Rev. 1958;29:45-52.
64. Ananias MTP, Araújo MG, Gontijo ED, et al. Estudo do antiPGL-1 em pacientes hansenianos utilizando técnica de ultramicroelisa. An Bras Dermatol. 2002;77:425-33.
65. Barro RPC, Oliveira MLW. Detecção de anticorpos específicos para antigen glicolipíde fenólico-1 do M. Leprae (anti PGL-1IgM): aplicações e limitações. An Bras Dermatol. 2000;75: 745-53.
66. Aráoz R, Honoré N, Cho S, et al. Antigen discovery: a postgenomic approach to leprosy diagnosis. Infect Immun. 2006;74:175-82.
67. Duthie MS, Goto W, Ireton GC, et al. Use of protein antigens for early serological diagnosis of leprosy. Clin Vaccine Immunol. 2007;14:1400-8.
68. Mshana RN, Belehu A, Stoner GL, et al. Demonstration of mycobacterial antigens in leprosy tissues. Int J Lepr Other Mycobact Dis. 1982;50:1-10.
69. Natrajan M, Katoch K, Katoch VM. Histology and immunohistology of lesions clinically suspicious of leprosy. Acta Leprol. 1999;11:93-8.
70. Hartskeerl RA, de Wit MY, Klatser PR. Polymerase chain reaction for the detection of Mycobacterium leprae. J Gen Microbiol. 1989;135:2357-64.
71. Woods SA, Cole ST. A rapid method for the detection of potentially viable Mycobacterium leprae in human biopsies: a novel application of PCR. FEMS Microbiol Lett. 1989;53:305-9.
72. Roselino AM. Biologia molecular aplicadaàs dermatoses tropicais. An Bras Dermatol. 2008;83:187-203.
73. DeFaria CR, Silva IM. Electromyographic diagnosis of leprosy. Arq Neuropsiquiatr. 1990;48:403-13.
74. Brasil-Neto JP. Electrophysiologic studies in leprosy. Arq Neuropsiquiatr. 1992;50:313-8.
75. Morgulis RF, Nóbrega JAM, Lima JGC. Comparative study of evidence of neurological and electromyographic alterations in leprosy. Neurobiologia. 1988;51:31-42.
76. Dyck PJ. Neuronal atrophy and degeneration predominantly affecting peripheral sensory and autonomic neurons. In: Dyck PJTP, Griffin JW, Low PA (Eds). Peripheral Neuropathy, 3rd edition. Philadelphia: WB Saunders; 1993. pp. 1065-93.

77. Houlden H, King R, Blake J, et al. Clinical, pathological and genetic characterization of hereditary sensory and autonomic neuropathy type 1 (HSAN I). Brain. 2006;129:411-25.
78. Dubourg O, Barhoumi C, Azzedine H, et al. Phenotypic and genetic study of a family with hereditary sensory neuropathy and prominent weakness. Muscle Nerve. 2000;23:1508-14.
79. Whitaker JN, Falchuck ZM, Engel WK, et al. Hereditary sensory neuropathy. Association with increased synthesis of immunoglobulin A. Arch Neurol. 1974;30:359-71.
80. Auer-Grumbach M, De Jonghe P, Wagner K, et al. Phenotype-genotype correlations in a CMT2B family with refined 3q13–q22 locus. Neurology. 2000;55:1552-7.
81. Auer-Grumbach M, De Jonghe P, Verhoeven K, et al. Autosomal dominant inherited neuropathies with prominent sensory loss and mutilations: a review. Arch Neurol. 2003;60:329-34.
82. Grumbach MA. Hereditary sensory neuropathy type 1. Orphanet J Rare Dis. 2008;3:7.
83. Mekkes JR, Loots MAM. Causes, investigations and treatment of leg ulceration. Br J Dermatol. 2003;148:388-401.
84. Sibbald RG, Williamson D, Falanga V, et al. Venous leg ulcers. In: Krasner DL, Rodeheaver GT, Sibbald RG (eds). Chronic Wound Care: A clinical Source Book for Healthcare Professionals, 3rd edition. Wayne, PA: HMP Communications; 2001. pp. 483-94.
85. O'Meara SM, Cullum NA, Majid M, et al. Systematic review of antimicrobial agents used for chronic wounds. Br J Surg. 2001;88(1):4-21.
86. Eckman ME, Greenfield S, Mackey WC, et al. Foot infections in diabetic patients. Decision and cost-effectiveness analyses. JAMA. 1995;273:712-20.
87. Sonmezoglu K, Sonmezoglu M, Halac M, et al. Usefulness of (99m)Tc-Ciprofloxacin (Infecton) scan in diagnosis of chronic orthopedic infections: comparative study with (99m)Tc-HMPAO leukocyte scintigraphy. J Nucl Med. 2001;42(4):567-74.
88. Mahabir RC, Taylor CD, Benny WB, et al. Necrotizing Cutaneous Cryoglobulinemic Vasculopathy. Plast Reconstr Surg. 2001;107(5):1221-4.

CHAPTER 13

Topical Therapy for Leg Ulcers

Nagesh TS, Sneha M

INTRODUCTION

Chronic leg ulcers can occur due to various causes. The most common cause for leg ulcer are due to venous disease, arterial insufficiency (peripheral arterial disease), or a combination of both. Other less common causes include lymphedema, infection, trauma, vasculitis, calciphylaxis, drug induced, malignancy, autoimmune disease, and pyoderma gangrenosum. In general, leg ulcers are slow to heal as they are on the most distal aspects of the circulatory, lymphatic, and nervous system. Because of weight bearing and gravity, the lower extremities are prone to edema, which prolongs the healing process.[1] The treatment of leg ulcers needs a multimodal approach with topical therapy, dressings, debridement, and surgical treatment. Also, the treatment of leg ulcer depends on the etiology of the ulcer. In this chapter, we discuss the different topical treatment options available for various types of leg ulcers.

HISTORY AND PHYSICAL EXAMINATION

A detailed history and physical examination are important to establish the etiology of the leg ulcer. The onset and chronicity of the ulcer including previous treatment taken has to be assessed. A comprehensive medical and surgical history including diabetes, hypertension, cardiovascular disease, peripheral arterial disease, venous insufficiency, autoimmune disorders, venous thromboembolism, inflammatory bowel disease, and connective tissue disease should be taken.

MANAGEMENT OF LEG ULCER

Preparation of the ulcer bed is the most important step in the management of chronic leg ulcers. TIME acronym was coined by Schultz GS et al. to describe the steps in the management of leg ulcer and also to help in taking appropriate decisions to prepare the wound bed.[2]

The acronym stands for T: tissue removal, I: infection control, M: moisture balance, E: edge of wound.[2]

Tissue removal: Removal of the necrotic tissue will help in reducing the risk of infection, to eliminate senescent cells, damaged extracellular matrix, and proteolytic enzymes. This can be done by gently rinsing with normal saline initially. If the necrotic tissue is more, other debridement methods can be used.

Infection control: Most of the ulcers are contaminated by bacteria. However, only the presence of bacteria might not interfere with healing of the ulcer.

When the bacteria replicate and influence the healing process without invading the adjacent tissue or inducing signs of infection, it is termed as colonization. It is referred to as critical colonization when the bacteria replicate to an extent to impact the healing process of an ulcer. The signs of critical colonization include friable, grayish granulation tissue, absence of granulation tissue, increased exudates, discharge with an abnormal smell, increased pain, and failure to improve despite proper treatment.[3]

The ulcer is considered as infected when the number of bacteria exceeds 100,000 per gram of tissue. Also, other signs of infection like fever, enlarged lymph nodes, cellulitis, and pus discharge will be present.

Culture is considered when there are signs of critical colonization or infection.

Moisture balance: Various types of dressings are used to maintain the moisture balance of the ulcer bed.

Edge of the wound: Optimal condition for the edge of the wound is necessary for healing of the ulcer. Debridement of the edges can be done, if necessary. If there is any eczematous change in the surrounding skin, it can be treated with topical corticosteroids, which accelerate the healing process.

Topical Antimicrobials/Antiseptics[3]

Regular use of topical antimicrobials and antiseptics for leg ulcers is still debatable. Traditional antiseptics such as chlorhexidine, hydrogen peroxide, or povidone–iodine are not routinely recommended as they are considered toxic to keratinocytes and fibroblasts.

When necessary, less toxic antibacterial agents like silver impregnated dressings, cadexomer iodine, or polyhexanide are used.

Cadexomer iodine causes slow release of iodine and can be painful in few patients and precaution to be taken in children and patients with thyroid disease. It is available in gel and powder form.

Polyhexanide is available in gel and solution forms.

Cochrane review about the use of antibiotics and antiseptics in venous leg ulcers and pressure ulcers states that cadexomer iodine might improve healing of ulcer. It does not give any definitive conclusion about the use of other agents like chlorhexidine, povidone–iodine, framycetin, mupirocin, and peroxide-based solutions.[4-6]

A study by Salavastru et al. has used topical agents like Castellani's paint, methylene blue, and gentian violet. Also, they have used other topical antimicrobials like metronidazole, fusidic acid, colistin, and neomycin depending on the culture reports. They conclude that use of topical antimicrobials is beneficial in accelerating the healing of the ulcer. Also, use of topical antimicrobials is recommended when there is infection rather than colonization of the ulcer.[7]

The following are the advantages of topical application over systemic antibiotic therapy:[8]
- Concentration of the antimicrobial agent at the site of infection is high and sustained
- Only a limited quantified of the antimicrobial needs to be applied
- Systemic toxicity is avoided
- Ability to use agents not approved for systemic use
- Easy application
- Better patient adherence.

Other Topical Agents used in Leg Ulcers

Phenytoin

Topical phenytoin has been used in various studies for the management of different types of leg ulcers. There has been a moderate evidence to support the use of phenytoin for leg ulcers, leprosy wounds, and diabetic foot ulcers.[9] The use of topical phenytoin powder has shown to effectively relieve pain, clear discharge, and enhance formation of granulation tissue and hence promote healing of ulcer.[10]

Honey

Topical honey has been used for the treatment of wounds since long time. It acts mainly because of the antibacterial properties. Manuka honey is known to inhibit bacterial growth, reduce virulence, motility, and biofilm formation.[11] A systematic review by Kateel R et al. on the topical treatment of diabetic leg ulcers with honey has shown that honey dressing is safer for treatment of diabetic foot ulcer, however, the efficacy could not be realistically concluded.[12] A study by Gethin G et al. has shown a positive wound healing outcome but arterial wounds showed minimal improvement.[13] Topical honey can be used as an adjunctive therapy as dressings in the treatment of leg ulcers.

Topical Granulocyte–Macrophage Colony-stimulating Factor

Granulocyte–macrophage colony-stimulating factor (GM–CSF) has been used locally in a study for the treatment of diabetic leg ulcers. Receptors for GM–CSF are expressed on various cells of granular and monocytes line, on Langerhans, dendritic and endothelial cells, and on muscle fibroblasts. T-lymphocytes, macrophages, endothelial cells, fibroblasts, and keratinocytes produce GM–CSF. The growth factor GM–CSF is produced by the keratinocytes immediately after the ulcer formation and contributes to the multiplication of the epidermis cells. This results in the multiplication of the keratinocytes on the ulcer edges, increased formation of granular tissue and increase of neovascularization. Consequently, the growth factor GM–CSF contributes to the healing of the full skin thickness in the ulcerated area. Furthermore, it probably contributes to increased neovascularization, through the de-novo production of vascular endothelial growth factor (VEGF) by the inflammatory cells. The correct use of growth factor in ulcer healing can prevent amputations.[14]

Topical Hemoglobin Spray

A study by Norris R has evaluated the role of topical hemoglobin spray in the treatment of leg ulcers, which are not responding to standard lines of therapy.[15]

Topical oxygen is a potential treatment for the chronic wound, as the wound:
- Is originally caused by depletion of oxygen to the tissues
- Worsens due to resultant chronicity, causing a further reduction in oxygen levels.

The mechanism of action is based on the premise that hemoglobin, the natural oxygen carrier, will carry oxygen from the normal atmosphere and deliver it directly into the wound bed. It is proposed, this will improve the oxygen supply to a chronic wound through facilitated diffusion, in turn promoting and accelerating healing.[15,16]

It should not be used along with other topical agents like antibiotics and also in infected wounds or during pregnancy as sufficient data is not available in evaluating these cases.

This pilot study has shown a good response in healing of chronic leg ulcers. With further studies, it can be a cost-effective alternative in treating unresponsive chronic wounds.[15]

Topical Steroids[17,18]

Chronic wounds are commonly characterized by an excessive inflammatory response, essentially getting "stuck" in the inflammatory phase. They are therefore associated with a greater number of inflammatory cells such as neutrophils, lymphocytes, and macrophages.

The resultant inflammatory milieu contains high levels of inflammatory cytokines, proteases [especially matrix metalloproteases (MMPs) and elastase] and reactive oxygen species, and low levels of protease inhibitors such as the tissue inhibitors of metalloproteases. This milieu results in excessive degradation of the extracellular matrix and failure of progression of wound healing. This factor has been identified as one of the four key components of wound bed preparation. From the above evidence, it would appear that aberrations in inflammation retard healing.

The use of topical steroids on a wound bed displaying evidence of excessive inflammation would therefore be a logical approach for treating such wounds. Case series exist of the successful use of topical corticosteroids for excessive granulation tissue, but they are few in number.

A study by Bosanquet et al. has shown good healing rates in chronic ulcers having abnormal inflammation. Also a study by Hofman D et al. concludes that suppression of inflammation plays an important role in healing and pain relief in chronic ulcers.[17]

However, topical steroids should be used with caution as there can be risk of sensitization with prolonged use and also a potential risk of infection.

Topical steroids can be used around the ulcer area in cases of venous ulcers where there can be a stasis eczema coexisting with ulcers.

Bioengineered Skin Substitutes

Newer skin substitutes are products of tissue engineering. These promote healing similar to native tissues, with an added advantage of not getting rejected.[19] Bioengineered skin substitutes are defined as, "the use of methods that promote biological repair or regeneration of tissues or organs by providing signaling, structural, or cellular elements with or without systems that contain living tissue or cells".[20] These substitutes not only limit bacterial colonization and fluid loss by acting as a layer of protective dressing, but also stimulate healing.

The design of the bioengineered skin substitutes is varied, and is dependent on the layer of skin they are suppose to replace.[19] In the laboratory, patient-derived keratinocytes are expanded and are used as epidermal replacements.[21]

An attachment to a certain carrier material before being transferred back to the patient for application on the wound may or may not be necessary. However, dermal substitutes based upon three-dimensional matrix behave like extracellular matrix (ECM). Bioactive molecules and cells may be incorporated to dermal substitutes.[19]

The structure and cellular constituents of skin substitutes may vary. The induction of the influx of endogenous cells including fibroblasts, keratinocytes, endothelial cells, macrophages, and neutrophils into the wound bed is brought about by both cellular and acellular substitutes.

The secretion of a various cytokines and growth factors, which stimulate angiogenesis, ECM deposition, and reepithelialization, takes place via the process of dynamic reciprocity.[1] The native tissue eventually replaces the skin substitute resulting in a healed wound.

Neutrophils release nitric oxide (NO), matrix metalloproteinases (MMP), and serine protease. Platelet-derived growth factor (PDGF), transforming growth factor-α (TGF-α), interleukins-1 (IL-1) and IL-6 are released by macrophages.[19] The complex interplay of cytokines, growth factors, and cells is given in Table 1.

Table 1: Regulation of various cytokines, growth factors, and cells in substitutes.[19]		
Cytokine, growth factor, or cell	Upregulation	Downregulation
Keratinocyte growth factor-2 (KGF-2)	Keratinocytes	
Nitric oxide	Keratinocytes	Bacteria
Transforming growth factor-β (TGF-β)	VEGF (vascular endothelial growth factor)	
VEGF	Endothelial cells	
IL-6	Keratinocytes, endothelial cells, and fibroblasts	
Keratinocytes	VEGF, IL-6, and nitric oxide	
Serine protease	VEGF and fibroblast	

(IL: interleukin)

The above factors in the wound bed may act as a stimulus to favor the wound microenvironment to promote healing, this has been described in the dynamic reciprocity model of wound healing.[22] Bilayer substitutes have features of both epidermal and dermal substitutes.

Epidermal Substitutes

In the laboratory, patient cell samples are expanded to form most of the epidermal grafts.[22,23] Wound healing can be initiated and barrier function restored by transferring suitable cell mass once it has grown in the laboratory.[1] First reliable culture of autologous keratinocytes was done 35 years ago.[24] Further, this leads to production of small sheets of cells with two to three layers thickness known as cultured epithelial autografts (CEA), which was used to treat burns victims.[25,26] Autograft derived from split thickness skin grafting or cell line bioreactor expansion is the gold standard epidermal substitute. Although they may take about 2–3 weeks to generate enough tissue to cover the defect, these are not subject to rejection.[24] Preparations of both autologous keratinocytes and allogeneic keratinocytes are available in the markets. Keratinocytes can be delivered to the wound by application as CEAs, delivery on carrier dressings such as bovine collagen or chemically defined polymers, and as suspensions which can be sprayed onto wound sites.[27] A well-vascularized dermal bed is essential for CEAs, else they are fragile.[28]

Primary cells derived from human donors possess low expansion capability. The phenotypes of these cells are known to adapt to in vitro conditions, which restrict their ability to form new tissues. Allografts, xenografts, inert membranes such as silicone and epidermal or bilayer substitutes give temporary wound coverage as they are not composed of autologous keratinocytes. The expected healing time is faster and they are easily available, which makes the best option for beginning the treatment.[22]

Dermal Substitutes

If the dermis has been destroyed, use of epidermal substitute is not enough to ensure optimal wound healing, dermis is essential for skin elasticity and mechanical resistance.[21] Blistering, contractures, scarring, and poor cosmesis may develop in increased frequency on the new skin surface and it is very fragile.[19] Ex-vivo functions of epidermal cells are facilitated by epithelial–mesenchymal communications, the absence of which can lead to fibrotic conditions.[27] Keratinocytes initiate growth factors in fibroblasts, which stimulate keratinocyte proliferation, this concept is called double paracrine signaling.[21] The differentiation of fibroblasts to myofibroblasts is controlled by keratinocytes. Dermal reconstruction is very essential in cases where none of the dermis is left on the wound bed. Debridement through proper preparation of chronic granulomatous tissue results in good uptake of grafts, if not, only 15% get incorporated successfully.[19]

Dermal replacements can have a synthetic or biological origin and consist of a three-dimensional biomaterial matrix material, which must behave like ECM forming a template to infiltrate the host and act as a physical support guiding the differentiation and proliferation of cells, which take part in cutaneous wound healing. There is evidence to support that the process of cellular differentiation and positioning of specific cell types is influenced by matrix elasticity.[19]

Excellent biocompatibility, biodegradability, and suitable mechanical properties on the macro-, micro-, and nanoscale are necessary properties of an ideal scaffold.[1] Cell intrusion, proliferation, and function are influenced by micropore size, shape, distribution, and porosity.[1] Cellular infiltration does not take place via nanopores as they are very small, but nanopores play a vital role in promoting diffusion of gas and nutrient through the matrix to support cell survival. A matrix with mechanical properties similar to injured tissue is essential to promote healing. The scaffold mediates beneficial cellular activity, such as adhesion, cytoskeletal organization, and differentiation.[19]

Dermal tissue substitutes are rendered acellular to minimize immunogenic responses.[23] The acellular products provide scaffold that eventually gets repopulated with patient's own fibroblast and endothelial cells.[27] These have come to be known as "acellular dermis", not only are they nonimmunogenic, but also mechanically robust, used off the shelf, and possess favorable handling characteristics.[1] Some products incorporate neonatal cells from neonatal human foreskin fibroblasts (NHFFs) and/or keratinocytes as they are less prone to elicit an immune response than adult cells.[27]

The important growth factors are secreted in reasonable concentration via the cells impregnated onto the matrix, which replaces those that have been downregulated in order to support wound healing. The tissue-engineered dermal matrices with seeded cells lead to dermal regeneration, which was noted in vivo regeneration of organized skin at 35 days using a biodegradable collagen glycosaminoglycan matrix impregnated with a dilute suspension of freshly isolated autologous keratinocytes. Living dermal fibroblast in dermal substitutes resulted in better wound healing with less myofibroblastic activity.[19]

Autologous cells were preferred to allogeneic ones, fibroblast from dermis showed better results than those from adipose tissue. Cellular infiltration, angiogenesis, and epithelialization are stimulated by dermal graft. Cellular dermal substitutes promote more rapid revascularization than acellular counterparts.[19]

Bilayer Substitutes

Bilayer substitutes structurally mimic natural skin and can be divided into cellular and acellular, however, they are expensive. The first bilayer product developed in 1981, composed of a silicone membrane, which composed of a silicone membrane that functions as a temporary barrier to prevent dehydration and also provide a flexible coverage of the wound. Bovine collagen type I and shark chondroitin-6-sulfate are components of the dermal layer.[19] The matrix is degraded and replaced by the newly synthesized native tissue primarily composed of collagen, this process takes place by the host cells that migrate into the scaffold. The grafting is done onto the wound bed, once vascularization takes place, the silicone epidermis is removed and a split-thickness skin grafting is done or tissue-engineered epidermal substitutes are placed.[22] The products that contain living keratinocytes and fibroblasts have an advantage of angiogenesis and inflammatory mediators these cells produce.

For chronic skin ulcers, a bilayer cellular substitute is which has upper layer of neonatal human foreskin keratinocytes and a lower layer of bovine-derived collagen matrix seeded with NHFFs is preferred. The graft releases cytokines (interferon-alpha, interferon-beta, IL-1, IL-6, and IL-8), growth factors (e.g. PDGF), and ECM components to the wound bed which ensures healing.[19]

To summarize various types of bioengineered skin substitutes have been tried in treatment of chronic leg ulcers not responding to conventional therapy. They have been shown to accelerate healing of ulcer. However, the type of skin substitute to be used depends on the morphology of the ulcer.

Frequency-rhythmic Electrical Modulation System

Electric current has been recommended for use on chronic wounds. Frequency-rhythmic electrical modulation system (FREMS) is an innovative type of transcutaneous electrotherapy used in a rehabilitation setting for the treatment of pain, especially in diabetic patients. The ability of this modality to improve healing of various types of chronic ulcers has been shown in few studies. They have established that FREMS system accelerated ulcer healing and also reduced pain in chronic leg ulcers. However, larger studies are needed for confirmation.[29,30]

CONCLUSION

Topical therapy plays an important role in the management of chronic leg ulcers. Various topical therapies include topical antimicrobials, phenytoin, honey, zinc, skin substitutes, and other modalities like FREMS. Topical antimicrobials are used mainly when there are any signs of infection. Topical phenytoin has shown to accelerate the healing process by formation of granulation tissue. Honey dressings act mainly by antimicrobial action and helps when there is antimicrobial resistance and biofilm formation. Topical steroids are shown to be of benefit when there is evidence of abnormal inflammation. Bioengineered skin substitutes are helpful in long-standing ulcers not responding to conventional methods of treatment. Other physical modalities like FREMS help in accelerating healing and reducing pain particularly in diabetic foot ulcers. Overall, the topical therapy used depends on the type of ulcer.

REFERENCES

1. Fukaya E, Margolis DJ. Approach to diagnosing lower extremity ulcers. Dermatol Ther. 2013;26(3):181-6.
2. Schultz GS, Sibbald RG, Falanga V, et al. Wound bed preparation: a systematic approach to wound management. Wound Repair Regen. 2003;11:S1-28.
3. Velasco M. Diagnostic and treatment of leg ulcers. Actas Dermo Sifiliográficas (English Edition). 2011;102(10):780-90.
4. O'Meara S, Al-Kurdi D, Ologun Y, et al. Antibiotics and antiseptics for venous leg ulcers. Cochrane Database System Rev. 2014;(1):CD003557.
5. Norman G, Dumville JC, Moore ZE, et al. Antibiotics and antiseptics for pressure ulcers. Cochrane Database System Rev. 2016;4:CD011586.
6. O'meara S, Richardson R, Lipsky BA. Topical and systemic antimicrobial therapy for venous leg ulcers. JAMA. 2014;311(24):2534-5.
7. Salavastru CM, Nedelcu LE, Țiplica GS. Management of leg ulcers in patients with chronic venous insufficiency: the experience of a Dermatology Clinic in Bucharest, Romania. Dermatol Ther. 2012;25(4):304-13.
8. Dumville JC, Lipsky BA, Hoey C, et al. Topical antimicrobial agents for treating foot ulcers in people with diabetes. Cochrane Database System Rev. 2017 ;6:CD011038.
9. Shaw J, Hughes CM, Lagan KM, et al. The clinical effect of topical phenytoin on wound healing: a systematic review. Br J Dermatol. 2007;157(5):997-1004.
10. Carneiro PM, Nyawawa ET. Topical phenytoin versus EUSOL in the treatment of non-malignant chronic leg ulcers. East Afr Med J. 2003;80(3):124-9.
11. Carter DA, Blair SE, Cokcetin NN, et al. Therapeutic manuka honey: no longer so alternative. Front Microbiol. 2016;7:569.
12. Kateel R, Adhikari P, Augustine AJ, et al. Topical honey for the treatment of diabetic foot ulcer: a systematic review. Complementary therapies in clinical practice. 2016;24:130-3.
13. Gethin G, Cowman S. Case series of use of Manuka honey in leg ulceration. Int Wound J. 2005;2(1):10-5.
14. Karlafti E, Savopoulos C, Hatzitolios A, et al. Local use of granulocyte-macrophages colony stimulating factor in treatment of chronic diabetic neuropathic ulcer (case review). Georgian Med News. 2018;(277):21-7.
15. Norris R. A topical haemoglobin spray for oxygenating chronic venous leg ulcers: a pilot study. Br J Nurs. 2014;23(Sup20):S48-53.
16. Arenbergerova M, Engels P, Gkalpakiotis S, et al. Topical hemoglobin promotes wound healing of patients with venous leg ulcers. Hautarzt. 2013;64(3):180-6.
17. Bosanquet DC, Rangaraj A, Richards AJ, et al. Topical steroids for chronic wounds displaying abnormal inflammation. Ann Royal Coll Surg Engl. 2013;95(4):291-6.
18. Hofman D, Moore K, Cooper R, et al. Use of topical corticosteroids on chronic leg ulcers. J Wound Care. 2007;16(5):227-30.
19. Greaves NS, Iqbal SA, Baquneid M, et al. The role of skin substitutes in the management of chronic cutaneous wounds. Wound Rep Reg. 2013;21:194-210.
20. Hashimoto K. Regulation of keratinocyte function by growth factors. J Dermatol Sci. 2000;24:546-50.
21. Lazic T, Falanga V. Bioengineered skin constructs and their use in wound healing. Plast Reconstr Surg. 2011;127:75S-90S.
22. Mac Neil S. Progress and opportunities for tissue-engineered skin. Nature. 2007;445:874-8.
23. Clark RAF, Ghosh K, Tomesen MG. Tissue engineering for cutaneous wounds. J Invest Dermatol. 2007;127:1018-29.
24. Rheinwald JG, Green H. Epidermal growth factor and the multiplication of cultured human epidermal keratinocytes. Nature. 1977;265(5593):421-4.
25. Fuchs E. Epidermal differentiation: the bare essentials. J Cell Biol. 1990;111:2807-14.
26. Gambardella L, Barrandon Y. The multifaceted adult epidermal stem cell. Curr Opin Cell Biol. 2003;15:771-7.
27. Germain FAADLL. Skin substitutes and wound healing. Skin Pharmacol Physiol. 2009;22:94-102.
28. Rovee DT, Maibach HI. The epidermis in wound healing. Boca Raton, FL: CRC Press; 2004.
29. Janković A, Binić I. Frequency rhythmic electrical modulation system in the treatment of chronic painful leg ulcers. Arch Dermatol Res. 2008;300(7):377.
30. Santamato A, Panza F, Fortunato F, et al. Effectiveness of the frequency rhythmic electrical modulation system for the treatment of chronic and painful venous leg ulcers in older adults. Rejuvenation Res. 2012;15(3):281-7.

CHAPTER 14

Systemic Therapy of Leg Ulcers

Brijesh Nair

INTRODUCTION

Leg ulcers are debilitating and painful, greatly reducing patient's quality of life. These ulcers are often difficult to treat and the successful treatment of leg ulcers depends upon the accurate diagnosis and treatment of the underlying cause. According to most of the Western and European studies, the most common type of leg ulcer is venous ulcer the others being neuropathic ulcer and arterial ulcers. These three kinds of ulcers account for almost 90% of cases of lower leg ulceration.[1]

In tropical countries like India, there is a paucity of epidemiological studies regarding prevalence and etiology of leg ulcers. A study from one center in India suggests leprosy (40%), diabetes (23%), venous disease (11%), and trauma (13%) causes of lower extremity wounds.[2]

The most common type of chronic wound in the extremities is venous leg ulcer or varicose ulcer resulting from chronic venous insufficiency. Venous Leg Ulcers is a disorder which requires judicial, multimodal, multispecialist therapy. The value of systemic therapy is to act as an adjuvant to compression therapy, when compression alone fails to heal Venous Leg Ulcers (VLUs). Systemic therapy can be a valuable alternative in those cases who fail compression and refuse surgery as an option.[3] Besides, the compliance with compression therapy is poor among patients with VLU, particularly among older patients.[3] Oral therapy is a viable alternative in these non-compliant patients. The classification of systemic therapeutic options for treatment of Venous Leg Ulcers are mentioned in Table 1.

PENTOXIFYLLINE

Pentoxifylline increases microcirculatory blood flow, oxygenation of ischemic tissues, increase red and white cell filterability, and decrease whole blood viscosity,

Table 1: Systemic therapeutic options for VLUs.

Alpha-Benzopyrones	Coumarine
Gamma-Benzopyrones $	Micronized Purified Flavonoid Fraction
	Oxerutin, Rutin, Rutosides
	Diosmine
Saponins	Ruscus extract, Escin (Horse chestnut extract)
Other plant extract	Maritime Pine tree extract
Synthetic Phlebotonics	Calcium Dobesilate $
Antibiotics	
Miscellaneous Drugs	Pentoxifylline$
	Aspirin $
	Stanozolol#
	Defibrotide
	Zinc
	Platelet Rich Plasma
	Prostaglandin E-1 and Prostacyclines
	Sulodexide
	Thromboxane A2 antagonist (Ifetroban)

$ Drugs which have significant evidence for efficacy
# Stanozolol is effective in lipodermatosclerosis
(VLUs: venous leg ulcers)

platelet aggregation and fibrinogen levels.[4] Falanga et al.[5] demonstrated statistically significant improvement in the pentoxyfylline group when compared to placebo group, both groups receiving compression. A Cochrane collaboration study done in 2012 reported that pentoxifylline is effective as an adjuvant to compression therapy for treating VLUs.[6] Pentoxifylline was found to be more effective than placebo in terms of complete ulcer healing or in causing a significant improvement (greater than 60% reduction in ulcer size). A well conducted review identified 11 RCTs comparing pentoxifylline with placebo or no treatment. Treatment with Pentoxifylline 400 mg three times daily improved VLU healing rates by 21% when used as adjuvant to compression or by 23% when used as solo therapy. The chief adverse effect was gastro-intestinal.[7] However pentoxifylline is contraindicated in patients with severe hemorrhages, acute myocardial infarction, angina, or marked liver and kidney disease.[8]

ASPIRIN

The mechanism of action of Aspirin in healing VLU is unknown. However it is postulated that the purported reason for beneficial effects of Aspirin could be inhibition of platelet activation and reduction of pain and inflammation.[9] An RCT with methodological deficiencies in randomization, blinding and lack of mention of other treatments simultaneously and low sample size (n=20) studied effect of Aspirin (300 mg daily for 4 months) in healing VLU. A significant reduction in ulcer size was seen in the control as opposed to placebo group.[10] A meta-analysis of Aspirin as intervention in VLU therapy has been conducted.[11] The evidence was deemed to be of low quality due to potential selection bias and imprecision due to the small sample size in the only two RCTs conducted. Another study using aspirin and compression also showed an improvement in time taken to heal.[12] There was little difference in complete healing rates between groups (21/28 aspirin and 17/23 compression bandages alone) but the average time to healing was shorter (12 weeks in the treated group vs 22 weeks in the compression only group) and the average time for recurrence was longer in the aspirin group (39 days: [SD 6.0] compared with 16.3 days [SD 7.5] in the compression only group).

Three on-going randomized trials investigating aspirin in subjects with venous leg ulcers are currently recruiting patients. The ASPiVLU (Aspirin in Venous Leg Ulcers) clinical trial in Australia; the AVURT (Aspirin for Venous Ulcers) in the United Kingdom and the Aspirin4VLU (Low Dose Aspirin for Venous Leg Ulcers) in New Zealand. A positive point in this study is that proinflammatory cytokines including IL-1b, IL-6, IL-10, TNF-a will be measured in patient plasma samples as well as markers of platelet activation, p-selectin and soluble CD40 ligand.[13] This will hopefully rest the doubts regarding efficacy of aspirin in VLU therapy.

ZINC

Zinc is an essential trace metal that is necessary for some enzymes and hormones to function. Its mechanism in healing VLU is not known, but purported benefits include an anti-inflammatory effect on phagocytes. It has also been noticed that zinc deficient individuals show delayed wound healing and increased risk of wound infection.[14] A Cochrane review to determine effect of zinc sulfate orally in case of arterial, venous and mixed ulcers analyzed 6 RCTs consisting of 183 participants. Four out of the 6 trials under consideration pertained to venous ulcers. Zinc did not show any significant difference in placebo in the healing of VLU.[15]

ANTIBIOTICS/ANTIMICROBIALS

Antimicrobials: A Cochrane review analyzed 5 RCTs of oral systemic antimicrobial therapy involving 232 study subjects. The conclusion was that there is no routine role of systemic antibiotics in treatment of VLU, when there is no evidence of infection.[16]

Levamisole: Levamisole, a drug used for roundworm infestation, is purported to have an antibacterial action in wounds. Usually, it is administered at a dose of 150 mg/day for 2-4 days each week.[17] A RCT analyzed effect of Levamisole in treating VLU. At 20 weeks all ulcers in treatment group had healed as opposed to 76% healing in placebo group[18], Evidence level C)

Doxycycline: Doxycycline besides its antibiotic action is known to inhibit proinflammatory cytokines like TNF-α and Matrix Metalloproteinases which are involved in pathogenesis of VLU, thereby healing them.[19] A pilot study analyzed two dosage schedules of oral Doxycycline in combination with compression in recalcitrant venous leg ulcers in 20 subjects. Doxycycline 100 mg twice a day schedule showed a median ulcer area reduction of 48% and greater suppression of ulcer fluid matrix metalloproteinase as opposed to Doxycycline 20 mg per day schedule, with compression given in both arms.[20] Further studies are required to evaluate the therapeutic utility of Doxycycline in healing of VLU.

Dapsone: Fromm and Wittman first formulated dapsone (4,4'-diaminodiphenylsulfone, DDS) in 1908, Besides its role in leprosy by inhibiting the folic acid pathway, it has a role in Neutrophilic dermatoses like Pyoderma gangrenosum and Behcets and in cases of Vasculitis, by inhibition of neutrophil myeloperoxidase, inhibition of neutrophil adhesion to endothelium. Successful use of dapsone has been described in individual cases or small series of patients with a variety of neutrophilic dermatoses, such as Sweet's syndrome and pyoderma gangrenosum, as well as in cutaneous leukocytoclastic vasculitis and erythema elevatumdiutinum.[21,22] Monitoring of complete blood count is essential while treating the patients on dapsone.

SYSTEMIC STEROIDS

Pyoderma gangrenosum (PG) is a rare inflammatory disease of unknown etiology characterized by neutrophilic infiltration of the dermis and destruction of the tissue.[23] Management of PG is often complex and will depend on comorbidities, associated diseases and the site and extent of the lesions. Systemic corticosteroids have been the most predictable and effective treatment of acute, rapidly progressive form of the disease.

High doses of prednisolone or pulse therapy with suprapharmocologic doses of methylprednisolone/dexamethasone may have to be used in resistant disease.[24,25] In general, 40–60 mg daily of prednisone, tapered over 1 month to low-dose alternate-day therapy, is successful as initial therapy. Gradual tapering of doses below 20–30 mg on alternate days is in order.

Prednisone is frequently used for a relatively brief duration in children with various subsets of PG.[26] Prednisone therapy initiated at 1 mg/kg daily is useful in rapidly attaining disease control in patients for whom dapsone will be used for long-term maintenance therapy. Both drugs are started simultaneously, with prednisone tapered after 1–3 months, depending on the rate of disease response. Intralesional CS may be a useful adjunct to the above two systemic drugs.

PHLEBOTONICS/FLAVONOIDS

Flavonoids address deficiencies in microcirculatory parameters such as decreasing leucocyte adhesion, free radical formation, decreasing venous wall permeability, increasing venous tone and protecting cells from effects of hypoxia.[27] Phlebotonics are a heterogenous group of medications both synthetic and plant origin, whose exact mechanism of action is unknown. The postulated benefits include effect on macrocirculation like improving venous tone and on microcirculation by decreasing capillary hyperpermeability.[28] A Cochrane meta-analysis selected 44 RCTs involving 4413 participants—23 of rutosides, ten of hidrosmine and diosmine, two of centellaasiatica, of maritime pine bark extract (Pycnogenol), one of aminaftone, and one of grapeseed extract. The study was to assess efficacy in relieving clinical symptoms in chronic venous insufficiency and not VLU. No evidence was obtained to recommend global use of phlebotonic drugs in cases of chronic venous insufficiency. They helped in relieving edema in some studies, but this was of uncertain clinical relevance.[29] Gastro-intestinal disorders was the most common adverse event.

Micronized Purified Flavonoid Fraction: Micronized Purified Flavonoid Fraction(MPFF) which consists of 90% Diosmine and 10% other flavonoids including Hesperidin is the most widely studied among the Phlebotonic drugs. It is free of any known major side effects.[30] Coleridge Smith et al. identified 7 RCTs in which MPFF was added to compression. No benefit was seen in VLU less than 6 months in terms of healing. Larger ulcers of 6-12 months duration were found to benefit more from MPFF treatment. These ulcers tend to heal more slowly and hence the role of an adjunctive therapy is required more in such ulcers.[31] Another meta-analysis revealed 37% increases chances of healing in VLU on treatment with MPFF.[32] MPFF also has value in reducing other clinical symptoms like pain, edema, restless legs and cramps as revealed in the largest study conducted in 5000 patients.[33] MPFF is available as Daflon in 500 mg dosage According to Konstantinos et al., Daflon 500 mg tablet taken twice in a day for 6 months has proven to shorten the duration of the venous ulcer.[34] Hence MPFF has utility in treating venous ulcers of more than 6 months duration.

Hydroxyethylrutosides: Oxerutins and hydroxyethylrutosides have also demonstrated hemodynamic and quality of life benefits in chronic venous insufficiency.[35,36] However high quality evidence is lacking in case of healing VLU for oxerutins and rutosides. The same is case with other flavonoids like catechins and epicatechins. It was reported in a review by Scallon et al. that although the overall estimated number of healed ulcers seemed to show a significant effect in favor of flavonoids [both MPFF and hydroxyethylrutosides], the results must be interpreted with caution because most of the trials were inadequately reported and thus had a risk of bias in randomization, allocation concealment, blinding and methods for addressing incomplete outcomes with a possibility of publication bias.[37] Further well-designed studies must be undertaken to reliably assess the efficacy of this group of drugs in VLU.

Calcium dobesilate: It is a synthetic venoactive drug thought to have anti-oxidant properties, reduce capillary permeability, increase venous tone and reduce inflammation. A meta-analysis identified 3 RCTs which demonstrated improvement in pain and other symptoms, more so with severe than mild disease.[38] However a later involving 509 patients failed to show any edema, symptoms and quality of life in patients consuming calcium dobesilate in comparison with placebo.[39] A trial demonstrated the increased efficacy of dobesilate with combination with oxerutins.[40] Low quality evidence supports the use of calcium dobesilate in therapy of VLU.

Escin/horse chestnut extract: A Cochrane meta-analysis demonstrated benefits of escin in reducing symptoms and edema in CVI[41], but no evidence exists to demonstrate efficacy in healing VLU.

FIBRINOLYTIC ENHANCERS

Stanozolol: Stanozolol is an anabolic steroid with fibrinolytic activity and decreases level of tissue plasminogen activator inhibitor(PAI).[42] In vitro studies have demonstrated procollagenase synthesis enhancement in fibroblasts.[43] Multiple studies have demonstrated the efficacy of clearing of fibrosis on therapy of lipodermatosclerosis by Stanozolol in combination with compression.[44,45] But multiple studies have demonstrated a lack of effect on healing venous ulcers located within the lipodermatosclerotic patches.[46,47] The reason of same is not known. Evidence does not support the use of stanozolol routinely in treatment of VLU, but it is certainly effective in the management of lipodermatosclerosis.

Defibrotide: Defibrotide is an antithrombotic and profibrinolytic drug. In a cross over trial involving 32 patients Defibrotide 400 mg tid along with compression was compared with placebo and was found to be more efficacious in healing VLU.[48]

Mesoglycans: Mesoglycans are Glycosaminoglycans extracted from porcine intestine and is composed of heparan sulfate, dermatan sulfate and chondroitin sulfate. Its exact mechanism of action is not known but it has a profibrinolytic action, microrheologic and macrorheologic benefits and has been reported to be useful in treating venous disorders.[49] It inhibits neutrophil adhesion and activation, and enhancement in process of wound healing.[50] One multicenter RCT compared mesoglycan IM / Oral and compression with placebo and compression therapy and demonstrated clinically significant benefit in time to healing. However the study was compromised by baseline differences between groups and non-standardization of compression therapy.[51]

Sulodexide: Sulodexide, a highly purified glycosaminoglycan (a naturally occurring molecule) has antithrombotic and profibrinolytic properties (it reduces the formation of blood clots) as well as anti-inflammatory effects. Meta-analysis of three RCTs suggests an increase in the proportion of ulcers completely healed with sulodexide as an adjuvant to local treatment (including wound care and compression therapy) compared with local treatment alone. Sulodexide may increase the healing of venous ulcers, when used alongside local wound care, however the evidence is presently of low quality.[52]

Cilostazol: Cilostazole is a phosphodiesterase-3 (PDE3) inhibitor and is a vasodilator and platelet inhibitor by increasing the levels of Protein Kinase A[53] and has been used in treatment of intermittent claudication. There is no good quality evidence currently for recommending Cilostazol in routine therapy of VLU.

Platelet Rich Plasma: Platelet derived growth factors are messengers/mediators of wound healing and have been found to be deficient or trapped in chronic wounds, so theoretically they could be useful in treatment of VLU.[54] Platelet releasates are supernatants of autologous platelets activated in vitro with thrombin whereas platelet lysates are platelets disrupted by sonication and centrifuged to remove platelet fragments from the solution.[55] The results in treatment of chronic venous ulcers have not been encouraging.[56-58] In an RCT, Frozen Autologous Plasma(FAP) in saline was studied for up to 12 weeks in patients of VLU in whom topical and compression therapy had already been tried. Autologous plasma was found to have no adjuvant effects on healing of CVLU.[59] The possible reasons for failure of platelets to heal VLU were presence of wound proteases leading to degradation of exogenous growth factors, decreased mitogenecity of fibroblasts to growth factors, and presence of antiangiogenic factors like TIMP -1 in the CVLU milieu. Platelet products have yet to be shown to have statistically significant results of effectiveness to recommend them as adjuvant in routine treatment of VLU.

PROSTAGLANDIN AND PROSTACYCLINE ANALOGUES

Milio et al. to know whether prostaglandin E1 (PGE-1) had beneficial effects on the treatment of venous ulcers via its anti-ischaemic properties, conducted an RCT (n = 87) of Prostaglandin E-1 versus placebo. After 120 days, period in the PGE-1 treated group, 100% of ulcers had healed in 100 days whereas in the placebo group 84% of ulcers had healed at 120 days.[60] It demonstrated that PGE-1 reduces healing time in venous ulcers with an acceptable side effect profile and good tolerability.

Iloprost, a prostacyclin analogue, has been shown to reduce the expression of leukocyte adhesion molecules, TNF and IL 6 production by monocytes which makes it a potential therapy for VLU. Iloprost in saline was compared to saline infusion only thrice a week in an RCT as an adjunct to venous ulcer treatment including compression and local therapy. In the treatment group, all of the ulcers had healed after 90 days whereas in the placebo group only 50% of ulcers had healed after 105 days and only 84.09% of ulcers had healed by the end of the study (at 150 days).[61]

CONCLUSION

Systematic therapies are an important value addition as a noninvasive option for therapy of venous leg ulcers. The efficacy as monotherapy is unproven. These drugs can be a valuable adjunct to compression in accelerating healing of venous leg ulcers. Robust evidence levels support the use of pentoxifylline and Micronized purified Flavonoid fraction (MPFF) in this condition. However, the verdict on the efficacy of Aspirin is still pending the completion of 3 large trials. Oral pharmacological adjuncts offer good alternatives to compression which is contraindicated in co-existent arterial disease and due to high rates of noncompliance by patients.

REFERENCES

1. London NJ, Donnelly R. ABC of arterial and venous disease. Ulcerated lower limb. BMJ. 2000;320:1589-91.
2. Saraf SK, Shukla VK, Kaur P, et al. A clinico-epidemiological profile of non-healing wounds in an Indian hospital. J Wound Care. 2000;9:247-50.
3. Gohel MS, Davies AH. Pharmacological treatment in patients with C4, C5 and C6 venous disease. Phlebology. 2010; 25:35-41.
4. Colgan MP, Dormandy JA, Jones PW, et al. Oxpentifylline treatment of venous ulcers of the leg. BMJ. 1990;300: 972-5.
5. Falanga V, Fujitani RM, Diaz C, et al. Systemic treatment of venous ulcer with high doses of pentoxifylline: efficacy in a randomized, placebo-controlled trial. Wound Repair Regen.1999;7:208-13.
6. Jull AB, Arroll B, Parag V, et al. Pentoxifylline for treating venous leg ulcers. Cochrane Database Syst Rev. 2012;12:CD001733.
7. Jull AB, Waters J, Arroll B. Pentoxifylline for the treatment of venous leg ulcers: a systematic review. Lancet. 2002;359: 1550-4.
8. Nair B.Venous leg ulcer: Systemic therapy.Indian Dermatol Online J. 2014 Jul-Sep; 5(3): 374–377.
9. Ibbotson SH, Layton AM, Davies JA, et al. The effect of aspirin on hemostatic activity in the treatment of chronic venous insufficiency. Br J Dermatol. 1995;132:422-6.
10. Layton AM, Ibbotson SH, Davies JA, et al. Randomized trial of oral aspirin for chronic venous leg ulcers. Lancet. 1994;344:164-6.
11. de Oliveira Carvalho PE, Magolbo NG, De Aquino RF, et al. Oral aspirin for treating venous leg ulcers. Cochrane Database Syst Rev. 2016;2:CD009432.
12. del Rio Sola ML, Antonio J, Fajardo G, et al. Influence of aspirin therapy in the ulcer associated with chronic venous insufficiency. Ann Vasc Surg. 2012;26:620-9.
13. Weller CD, Barker A, Darby I, et al. Aspirin in venous leg ulcer study (ASPiVLU): study protocol for a randomized controlled trial. Trials. 2016;17:192.
14. Seymour CS. Trace Metal Disorders. In: Warren DJ, Ledingham JG, Warrel DA (Eds). Oxford Textbook of Medicine. Oxford: Oxford University Press; 1996. pp. 1423-4.
15. Wilkinson EAJ, Hawke CC. Oral zinc for arterial and venous leg ulcers. Cochrane Database Syst Rev. 1998;4:CD001273.
16. O'Meara S, Al-Kurdi D, Ologun Y, et al. Antibiotics and antiseptics for venous leg ulcers. Cochrane Database Syst Rev. 2010;1: CD003557.
17. Scheinfeld N, Rosenberg JD, Weinberg JM. Levamisole in dermatology: A review. Am J Clin Dermatol. 2004;5:97-104.
18. Morias J, Peremans W, Campaert H, et al. Levamisole treatment in ulcus cruris. A double-blind placebo-controlled trial. Arzneimittelforschung. 1979;29:1050-2.
19. Stechmiller J, Cowan L, Schultz G. The role of doxycycline as a matrix metalloproteinase inhibitor for the treatment of chronic wounds. Biol Res Nurs. 2010;11:336-44.
20. Sadler GM, Wallace HJ, Stacey MC. Oral doxycycline for treatment of chronic leg ulceration. Arch Dermatol Res. 2012;304:487-93.
21. Aram H. Acute febrile neutrophilic dermatosis (Sweet's syndrome). Response to dapsone. Arch Dermatol. 1984;120:245-7.
22. Prystowsky JH, Kahn SN, Lazarus GS. Present status of pyoderma gangrenosum. Review of 21 cases. Arch Dermatol. 1989;125: 57-64.
23. Powell FC, Hackett BC. Pyoderma Gangrenosum. In: Wolff K, Goldsmith LA, Katz SL, Gilchrist BA, Paller AS, Leffell DJ (Eds). Fitzpatrick's Dermatology in General Medicine. 7th edition. Vol. 1. New York: McGraw Hill;2007. pp. 296-302.
24. Ruocco E, Sangiuliano S, Gravina AG, et al. Pyoderma gangrenosum: an updated review. J Eur Acad Dermatol Venereol. 2009;23:1008-17.
25. Bhat RM. Management of pyoderma gangrenosum—an update. Indian J Dermatol Venereol Leprol. 2004;70:329-35.
26. Graham JA, Hansen KK, Rabinowitz LG, et al. Pyoderma gangrenosum in infants and children. Pediatr Dermatol. 1994;11:10-7.
27. Pascarella L, Schonbein GWS, Bergan JJ. Microcirculation and venous ulcers: A review. Ann Vasc Surg. 2005;19: 921-7.
28. Tsouderos Y. Are the phlebotonic properties shown in clinical pharmacology predictive of a therapeutic benefit in chronic venous insufficiency. Our experience with Daflon 500 mg. Int Angiol. 1989;8:53-9.
29. Martinez-Zapata MJ, Bonfill CX, Moreno RM, et al. Phlebotonics for venous insufficiency. Cochrane Database Syst Rev. 2005;3: CD003229.
30. Katsenis K. Micronized Purified Flavonoid fraction (MPFF): a review of its pharmacological effects, therapeutic efficacy and benefits in the management of chronic venous insufficiency. Curr Vasc Pharmacol. 2005;3(1):1-9.
31. Coleridge Smith P, Lok C, Ramelet AA. Venous leg ulcer: A meta-analysis of adjunctive therapy with micronized purified flavonoid fraction. Eur J Vasc Endovasc Surg. 2005;30:198-208.
32. Smith PC. Daflon 500 mg and venous leg ulcer: new results from a meta-analysis. Angiology. 2005;56:S33-39.

33. Jantet G. Chronic venous insufficiency: worldwide results of the RELIEF study: Reflux assessment and quality of life improvement with micronized Flavonoids. Angiology. 2002; 53:245-56.
34. Konstantinos Katsenis. Micronized purified flavonoid fraction (MPFF): A review of its pharmacological effects, therapeutic efficacy and benefits in the management of chronic venous insufficiency. Current Vascular Pharmacology. 2005;3:1-9.
35. Petruzzellis V, Troccoli T, Candiani C, et al. Oxerutins venoruton: Efficacy in chronic venous insufficiency—A double blind, randomized, controlled study. Angiology. 2002;53:257-63.
36. Cesarone MR, Belcaro G, Pellegrini L, et al. Venoruton versus Daflon: evaluation of efects on quality of life in chronic venous insufficiency. Angiology. 2006;57:131-38.
37. Martinez MJ, Bonfill X, Moreno RM, et al. Phlebotonics for venous insufficiency. Cochrane Database Syst Rev. 2016; 4(3):CD003229.
38. Ciapponi A, Laffaire E, Roque M. Calcium dobesilate for chronic venous insufficiency: a systematic review. Angiology. 2004; 55:147-54.
39. Martinez-Zapata MJ, Moreno RM, Gich I, et al. A randomized, double-blind multicentre clinical trial comparing the efficacy of calcium dobesilate with placebo in the treatment of chronic venous disease. Eur J Vasc Endovasc Surg. 2008;35:358-65.
40. Akbulut B. Calcium dobesilate and oxerutin: effectiveness of combination therapy. Phlebology. 2010;25:66-71.
41. Pittler MH, Ernst E. Horse chestnut Seed extract for chronic venous insufficiency. Cochrane Database Syst Rev. 2006: CD003230.
42. Davidson JF, Lochhead M, McDonald GA, et al. Fibrinolytic enhancement by stanozolol: a double blind trial. Br J Haematol. 1972;22:543-49.
43. Wright JK, Smith AJ, Cawston TE, et al. The effect of the anabolic steroid, stanozolol on the production of procollagenase by human synovial and skin fibroblasts in vitro. Agents Actions. 1989;28:279-82.
44. Burnand K, Clemenson G, Morland M, et al. Venous lipodermatosclerosis: treatment by fibrinolytic enhancement and elastic compression. BMJ. 1980;280:7-11.
45. McMullin GM, Watkin GT, Coleridge Smith PD, et al. Efficacy of fibrinolytic enhancement with stanozolol in the treatment of venous insufficiency. Aust N Z J Surg. 1991;61:306-9.
46. Browse NL, Jarrett PEM, Morland M, et al. Treatment of liposclerosis of leg by fibrinolytic enhancement: a preliminary report. BMJ. 1977;2:434-5.
47. Stacey MC, Burnand KG, Layer GT, et al. Transcutaneous oxygen tensions in assessing the treatment of healed venous ulcer. Br J Surg. 1990;77:1050-4.
48. Belcaro G, Marelli C. Treatment of venous lipodermatosclerosis and ulceration in venous hypertension by elastic compression and fibrinolytic enhancement with defibrotide. Phlebology. 1989;4:91-106.
49. Andreozzi GM. Effectiveness of mesoglycan in patients with previous deep vein thrombosis and chronic venous insufficiency. Minerva Cardioangiol. 2007;55:741-53.
50. McGrath JA, Eady RA. Heparan sulphate proteoglycan and wound healing in skin. J Pathol. 1997;183:251-2.
51. Arosio E, Ferrari G, Santoro L, et al. A placebo-controlled, double-blind study of mesoglycan in the treatment of chronic venous ulcers. Eur J Vasc Endovasc Surg. 2001;22:365-72.
52. Wu B, Lu J, Yang M, et al. Sulodexide for treating venous leg ulcers. Cochrane Database Syst Rev. 2016;(6):CD010694.
53. Taniguchi K, Ohtani H, Ikemoto T, et al. Possible case of potentiation of the antiplatelet effect of cilostazol by grapefruit juice. J Clin Pharm Ther. 2007;32:457-9.
54. Knighton DR, Fiegel VD, et al. Classification and treatment of chronic nonhealing wounds: Successful treatment with autologous platelet-derived wound healing factors (PDWHF). Ann Surg. 1986;204:322-30.
55. Stacey MC, Mata SD, Trengove NJ, et al. Randomised double-blind placebo controlled trial of topical autologous platelet lysate in venous ulcer healing. Eur J Vasc Endovasc Surg. 2000; 20:296-301.
56. Coerper S, Koveker G, Flesch I, et al. Ulcus cruris venosum: surgical debridement, antibiotic therapy, and stimulation with thrombocytic growth factors. Langenbecks Arch Chir. 1995;380: 102-7.
57. Reutter H, Bort S, Jung MF et al. Questionable effectiveness of autologous platelet growth factors(PDWHF) in the treatment of venous ulcers of the leg. Hautarzt. 1999;50:859-65.
58. Senet P, Bon FX, Benbunan M, et al. Randomized trial and local biological effect of autologous platelets used as adjuvant therapy for chronic venous leg ulcers. J Vasc Surg. 2003;38:1342-8.
59. Seung JL. Cytokine delivery and tissue engineering. Yonsei Med J. 2000;41:704-19.
60. Milio G, Mina C, Cospite V, et al. Efficacy of the treatment with prostaglandin E-1 in venous ulcers of lower limbs. J Vasc Surg. 2005;42:304-8.
61. Ferrara F, Meli F, Raimondi F, et al. The treatment of venous leg ulcers: a new therapeutic use of iloprost. Ann Surg. 2007;246: 860-5.

CHAPTER 15

Compression Therapy and Dressings

Shilpa K, S Sacchidanand, Sachin S

INTRODUCTION

Compression therapy is a commonly advised conservative therapy in chronic venous and lymphatic insufficiency of the lower limbs, like varicose veins, lymphedema, venous eczema and ulceration, deep vein thrombosis and post thrombotic syndrome.[1]

MECHANISM OF COMPRESSION STOCKINGS

The stockings work by exerting the greatest degree of compression at the ankle, with the level of compression gradually decreasing up the garment. This pressure gradient ensures that blood flows in the upward direction towards the heart instead of refluxing downward to the foot or laterally into the superficial veins due to valvular or perforator insufficiency. Also the graduated compression reduces the diameter of major veins, which in turn increases the velocity and volume of blood flow.[2] These graduation compression stockings can reverse venous hypertension, enhance skeletal-muscle pump, improve venous return and facilitate lymphatic drainage.[3] The use of graduated compression stockings, especially with high compression stockings are known to increase the limb oxygenation.[4] Another study showed that levels of proinflammatory cytokines (e.g. interleukin-1α, interleukin-6 and interferon-γ) in ulcer tissue in patients with active ulcers were significantly reduced following compression therapy.[5] It also initiates complex physiologic and biochemical effects involving the venous, arterial and lymphatic systems, although the exact mechanisms remain unclear.

TYPES OF COMPRESSION STOCKINGS

Depending on the indication, compression pressure exerted different types of compression stockings are available and are tabulated in Table 1.

GRADING THE STRENGTH OF COMPRESSION STOCKINGS

Graduated compression stockings are classified according to the sub-bandage compression pressure applied by the garment at the ankle level. The pressures are determined by the manufacturer based on laboratory measurements. The degree of pressure is classified into several standards. Unfortunately, there is no single standard used worldwide, which may cause confusion. The British and European standards for classifying the strength of compression hosiery differ and are presented below in Table 2.

There are many different makes and types of graduated compression hosiery available on prescription. These include different lengths (knee or thigh length) (Figs. 2A to D) and different compression strengths.

Indications

- Primary chronic venous disease
- Uncomplicated varicose veins
- Chronic venous insufficiency
- Postsurgical or interventional treatment of varicose veins
- Prevention of venous thromboembolism
- Lymphedema and chronic leg edema
- Post-thrombotic syndrome
- Superficial thrombophlebitis
- Pregnancy.

Table 1: Types of compression stockings.

Graduated or medical compression stockings (Fig. 1)	• Graduated compression stockings exert the greatest degree of compression at the ankle, and the level of compression gradually decreases up the garment. • They are often used to treat chronic venous disease and edema. • They are designed for ambulatory patients and are manufactured under strict medical and technical specifications, including consistency and durability, to provide a specific level of ankle pressure and graduation of compression.
Antiembolism stockings	• Antiembolism stockings are used to reduce the risk of deep vein thrombosis. • Like graduation compression stockings, they provide gradient compression. • They are designed for bedridden patients and do not meet the technical specifications for use by ambulatory patients. • Although the terms "antiembolism stockings" and "graduated compression hosiery" are often used interchangeably and both types of stockings offer graduated compression, they have different levels of compression and indications.
Nonmedical support hosiery	• Nonmedical support hosiery, including flight socks and elastic support stockings, are often used to provide relief for tired, heavy and aching legs. • They usually exert considerably less compression than graduated compression stockings. • The compression is uniform and not graduated. • They do not need to meet the strict medical and technical specifications as those of graduated compression stockings. • They can often be bought over the counter without a prescription.

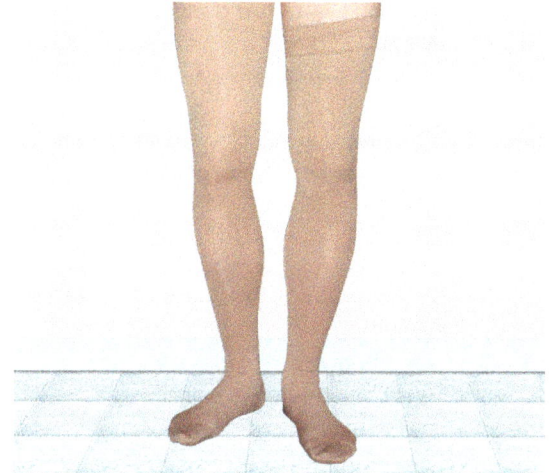

Fig. 1: Graduated compression stockings.

Table 2: The British and European standards for classifying the strength of compression hosiery. (Conservative Management Varicose Veins in the Legs: The Diagnosis and Management of Varicose Veins. NICE Clinical Guidelines, No. 168. National Clinical Guideline Centre (UK). London: National Institute for Health and Care Excellence (UK); 2013 Jul).

Class of Stocking	European/RAL standard	British Standard
Class I	18–21 (mm Hg)	14–17 (mm Hg)
Class II	23–32 (mm Hg)	18–24 (mm Hg)
Class III	34–46 (mm Hg)	25–35 (mm Hg)

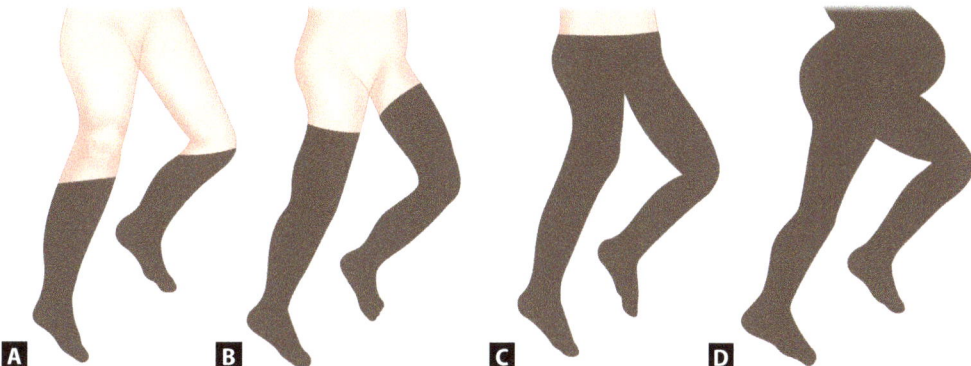

Figs. 2A to D: A. Below knee compression stockings; B. Thigh compression stockings; C. Above waist; D. During pregnancy.

Table 3: Relative contraindications and possible solution.

Relative contraindication	Possible solution
Pronounced exudating dermatoses	First reduce with decongestive treatment with bandages, then compression is usually possible
Intolerance to the material of compression stockings	Choose other materials, such as natural rubber or cotton-covered yarn
Severe sensory disturbances of the lower limbs	Compression treatment only under regular monitoring by medical or nursing staff
Minor peripheral neuropathy	Use lower compression class, monitor symptoms
Advanced peripheral neuropathy	Compression treatment only under regular monitoring by medical or nursing staff
Rheumatoid polyarthritis	Decision for compression treatment after weighing up the risk/benefit ratio by the attending physician

Contraindications

Relative contraindications are tabulated in Table 3.

Absolute Contraindications

- Advanced stage peripheral arterial occlusive disease
- Septic phlebitis
- Phlegmasia Cerulea Dolens
- Decompensated heart failure
- Extreme deformity of the leg, or unusual leg shape or size preventing correct fit.
- Allergy to stocking material.

ASSESSMENT TO BE DONE BEFORE PRESCRIBING COMPRESSION THERAPY

Before prescribing compression hosiery, the patient should be assessed for the following:
- Rule out intermittent claudication: observe for painful cramping in calf muscles after activity, such as walking or climbing stairs
- Lower limb numbness or weakness
- Signs of arterial insufficiency: Pale, cold clammy toes, feet or legs with gangrene/ulceration.
- Look for pulsations
- Poor capillary refill: should be less than 2 seconds
- Drop in pulse oximetry on leg elevation
- An arterial-brachial pressure index (ABPI) should be requested if any one or more of these is present and compression stockings chosen based on it (Table 4)
- Graduated compression hosiery is palliative rather than curative, and their use needs to continue for as long as there is evidence for venous disease. In most cases, this is lifetime
- After the clinical examination and assessment, the appropriate class of stockings can be chosen as given in Table 5.

Table 4: Choice of compression stockings based on ABPI.

ABPI	Compression stockings
Less than 0.5	Compression stockings should not be worn, as severe arterial disease is likely.
Between 0.5 and 0.8	No more than light (class 1) compression should be applied, as arterial disease is likely and compression may further compromise arterial blood supply.
Greater than 0.8	Compression stockings are safe to wear.
Greater than 1.3	Compression should be avoided, as high ABPI values may be due to calcified and incompressible arteries.

Table 5: Choosing the appropriate compression stockings.

Class	Conditions
Class 1	• Superficial or early varicose veins • Varicose veins during pregnancy
Class 2	• Varicose veins of medium severity • Treatment of and prevention of the recurrence of leg ulcers • Mild edema • Varicose veins during pregnancy
Class 3	• Gross varicose veins • Post-thrombotic venous insufficiency • Gross edema • Treatment of and prevention of the recurrence of leg ulcers

Table 6: Information to be given to patients.	
• The reason why graduated compression stockings have been prescribed	• It provides external support for the week dilated tortuous vessels while upright and prevent edema, swelling of lower limbs
• The benefits of wearing them regularly	• It reduces pain swelling and heaviness of the limb
• How to apply them correctly	• Choose the right hosiery as prescribed by the physician regarding class and length
	• It should be applied before getting off the bed and before swelling develops
	• First it should be put on the foot slowly pulled over heels and then up depending on the length
	• See to it that the stockings end 2 centimeters below the joint fold or skin crease
	• If it is too long do not roll at the edge as it may hamper blood supply
	• If open wound is there first put a dressing and stockings worn above that
• How long to wear them each day	• Throughout the day till they go to bed
• When to take them off	• During bedtime or while taking shower
• Daily hygiene	• Can be washed in washing machines
	• While drying it should be kept flat on towel on floor so that it doesn't stretch
• When to replace them	• An ideal stocking should snuggly fit and comfortable
	• It has to be replaced if it is too loose
	• If maintained properly each stocking will last for six months
• How to recognize potential problems	• Severe pain, swelling, numbness or discoloration of the digit-indicate complications
• What to do or whom to contact if problems occur	• In above situation patient should contact treating physician immediately

Information to be given to patients has been tabulated in Table 6:

DRESSINGS

A chronic wound is a wound that does not heal in an orderly set of stages and in a predictable amount of time the way most wounds do. Wounds that do not heal within three months are often considered chronic.[6] Chronic ulcers are debilitating; increasing hospital stay and morbidity. Dressings enhance wound healing capacity by providing an optimal healing environment. Various types of dressings from simple composite dressings to impregnated dressings are available in the market. The choice of dressing depends on factors like condition of wound, i.e. necrotic, infected, sloughy, presence or absence of granulation tissue, epithelialization and amount of discharge. A prescribing doctor should have a knowledge about different types of dressing suitable for any particular wound or ulcer.

Aim of Dressing

1. To facilitate healing in the shortest possible time.
2. To reduce pain.
3. To reduce foul odor.
4. To remove necrosed tissue.
5. To absorb excessive discharge.
6. To provide a moist environment for better wound healing.

Types of Dressings

Multilayer compression bandaging has been identified as the gold standard in the treatment of venous leg ulcers. Dressings are usually placed over the ulcer before compression bandages or hosiery are applied with the intention of promoting healing and preventing the bandages sticking to the wound. Large numbers of different wound dressings are available with many ways of classifying them—

> **Table 7:** Different types of dressing.
> - Simple/non-adherent dressings
> - Foams (Fig. 3A)
> - Alginate (Fig. 3B) Hydrocolloids (Fig. 3C)
> - Collagen (Fig. 3D)
> - Hydrogel (Fig. 3E)
> - Transparent (Fig. 3F)
> - Impregnated dressings (Fig. 3G)

for example, by physical composition or by describing them as passive, active, or reactive. However, the evidence for their use is equivocal. Whether any particular dressing or type of dressing affects the healing of ulcers still needs to be established. The various type of dressings is tabulated in the Table 7.

Foam Dressings

Foam dressings were one of the first advanced (modern) dressings to be used in wound management. Foam wound dressings are very absorptive, so they are a good choice for moderate to heavy exudate production. Wound exudate slows down healing and can increase bacteria which can damage the newly healed tissue. There are different variants like silicon foam dressing, polyurethane, hydrocellular foam dressings, adhesive, non-adhesive, waterproof etc. These vary in their ability to absorb exudate. Some are suitable only for lightly- to moderately-exuding wounds, whilst others have a greater fluid-handling capacity.

Advantages

- Ability in handling exudate through absorption of exudate into the fabric of the dressing and via transmission through a top sheet.
- Permeable to water vapor but blocks entry of bacteria and contaminants.
- Reducing the risk of maceration of skin around the ulcer as it keeps moisture away from the wound margin.
- Foam dressings can remain in place for longer than other dressing types, so decreased frequency of dressing changes needed thus reducing cost.
- Works well for granulating and epithelializing wounds.
- Doesn't adhere to the wound and thus leads to a non-traumatic dressing removal.[7]

Disadvantages

- Possibility of saturation leading to maceration of healthy peri-ulcer skin
- Potential reduction in fluid-handling capacity if used beneath compression devices.
- Wound bed may desiccate if there is no exudate from the wound.

A meta-analysis by Susan O'Meara et al.[8] concluded that there is no evidence to suggest that polyurethane foam dressings are significantly better or worse than hydrocellular foam dressings in venous leg ulcer healing. Similarly, they found no evidence to suggest that foam dressings are significantly better or worse than other types of dressings (paraffin-impregnated gauze dressings, hydrocapillary dressings, hydrocolloid dressings, knitted viscose dressings, or protease-modulating matrix dressings), for the healing of venous leg ulcers.

Alginate Dressings

Alginate dressings are made from natural polysaccharide fibers that are derived from processed seaweed.[9] These non-woven, non-adhesive dressings are highly absorbent, soft, and conformable. They are easy to pack, tuck or apply over wounds of irregular shapes. When the dressing comes into contact with wound exudate, the alginate fibers form a soft, moist gel-like substance, through a process of ion exchange. Alginate dressings are indicated for venous insufficiency ulcers, pressure ulcers, diabetic ulcers, surgical wounds, donor sites, first and second-degree burns. In addition, they are the ideal primary dressing for infected wounds, since infected wounds tend to have significant levels of exudate.

Advantages

- It can absorb large amounts of exudate; up to 20 times their own weight.
- The gel formed helps to provide a moist wound healing environment.
- The gel formation blocks lateral wicking of exudate, helping to reduce wound maceration.
- Its non-adherent, changing of dressing is painless and does not disturb the healing wound. The gel is easily removed from the wound site by irrigation with saline solution.
- Alginates can be used on both granulating and slough-covered wounds.

Disadvantages

- Because they have no adhesive properties, secondary dressings must be used to secure alginate dressings.
- Because of their high absorbency, they are unsuitable for a dry or minimally-draining wounds particularly full-thickness, third-degree burns, wounds with

Compression Therapy and Dressings

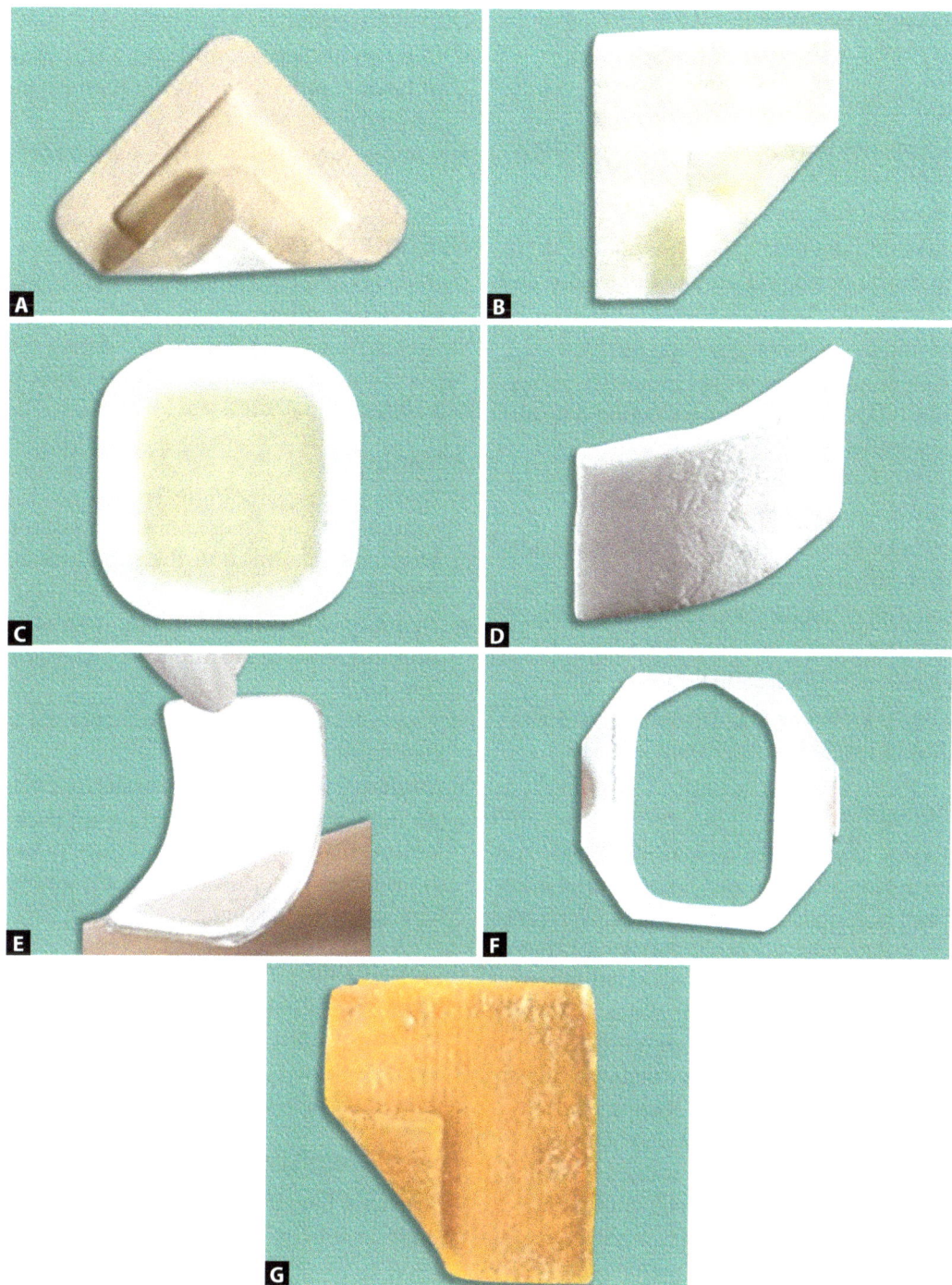

Figs. 3A to G: Different types of dressings. A. Foams; B. Alginate; C. Hydrocolloids; D. Collagen; E. Hydrogel; F. Transparent; G. Impregnated dressings.

exposed tendon, joint capsule, or bone due to the risk of desiccating tissue with high collagen content.
- Some people have a known sensitivity to alginates, and alginate dressings should naturally be avoided in these patients.

Hydrocolloid Dressings

Hydrocolloid dressings are occlusive wafer type dressings that contain gel-forming agents in an adhesive compound laminated onto a flexible, water-resistant outer layer. They are self-adhering and available with or without an adhesive border and in various thicknesses and pre-cut shapes for body areas such as the sacrum, elbows, and heels.

Advantages
- Being occlusive, they provide a moist healing environment, autolytic debridement and insulation.
- Impermeable to bacteria and other contaminants
- Dressings are self-adherent but do not adhere to the wound, only to the intact skin around the wound and mold well.
- Can be used under venous compression products.
- Can be kept for more number of days without changing- i.e. every 3 to 7 days depending upon the exudate and manufacturer guidelines.

Disadvantages
- Not recommended for wounds with heavy exudate, sinus tracts, or when infection is present.
- Must be used with caution in patients with diabetes.
- May become dislodged if the wound produces heavy exudate and may curl or roll at the edges.
- May cause hyper granulation, peri-wound maceration, trauma/injury to fragile skin upon removal.

Collagen Dressings

Collagen dressings attract cells such as fibroblasts and keratinocytes to the wound, which encourages debridement, angiogenesis, and re-epithelialization thus stimulating new tissue growth. It also stimulates deposition and organization of newly formed collagen fibers and granulation tissue in the wound bed. Matrix metalloproteinases (MMPs) found in the extracellular fluid of wounds normally attack and break down collagen. So these dressings provide an alternative collagen source to MMPs, leaving the body's natural collagen available for normal wound healing.

Topical formulations of collagen are available in various forms, such as freeze-dried sheets, pastes, pads, powder, and gels. Formulations with alginates or even antimicrobial additives are also available. Bovine, porcine, or avian are the source of these collagen.

Advantages
- They can be used in all stages of wound healing.
- They reduce inflammatory mediators in the wound.
- It is useful in granulating or necrotic wounds and chronic non-healing wounds. The frequency of dressing changes varies depending on the brand, but ranges from daily to every 7 days.

Disadvantages
- Contraindicated in third-degree burns, patient sensitivity to bovine, porcine, or avian products and in wounds covered in dry eschar.
- Some collagen products will require a secondary cover dressing.

Hydrogel Dressings

Hydrated polymer (hydrogel) dressings, contain 90% water in a gel base[10], which helps regulate fluid exchange from the wound surface. It is a clear or translucent dressing, which varies in size and thickness. There are three general forms of hydrogel wound dressings (Table 8).

Advantages
- Hydrogel dressing holds sufficient moisture in the superficial layer of the wound site, thus fastening wound healing. It is advised to change the hydrogel dressing every four days.
- Due to its high water content, it gives a comfortable soothing effect to the wound site which can lasts for six hours.
- High moisture content is also beneficial in providing a barrier for infections.
- Wounds which are very dry or necrotic wounds.
- As this hydrogel dressing does not stick or allow the necrotic tissue to slough off during the healing process, it promotes faster healing process and painless while changing the dressing.

Disadvantage
- Hydrogel is contraindicated in wounds which are extremely moist or have heavy exudate.
- When not covered, hydrogel may be dehydrated easily, so that the benefits are limited.

Transparent Wound Dressings

Transparent film dressings are waterproof dressings acting as a blister roof or "second skin" Because they're flexible,

Table 8: Different forms of hydrogel wound dressings.

Type	Descriptions
Amorphous hydrogel	It is a free-flowing gel, which is packed in tubes, foil packages, or spray bottles
Impregnated hydrogel	In this, the gel is saturated onto a gauzed pad, non-woven spongy ropes or strips
Sheet hydrogel	In this, hydrogel is held together by a thin fiber mesh. It may come with or without the adhesive borders.

these dressings can conform to wounds located in awkward locations such as the elbow.

Advantages
- They provide a moist, healing environment; enhance autolytic debridement; protect the wound from external trauma and secondary bacterial infections. The average time between transparent film dressings is 3 to 5 days, although the dressing may be left in place up to 7 days.
- The transparency makes it easy to visualize the wound bed.
- Although these dressings cannot absorb fluid, they are permeable to moisture—allowing one-way passage of carbon dioxide and excess moisture vapor away from the wound.
- They are useful in wounds with no or minimal exudate and when protection is needed for intact skin, for example, protection of bony prominences of the heel from friction.
- It promotes debridement of eschar.
- It can also be used to secure another dressing.

Disadvantages
- A transparent film dressing would not adhere to a moist surface because its adhesive properties are deactivated by moisture.
- Not suitable in wounds with moderate to heavy exudate, third-degree burns, suspected or active infection.
- These dressings can cause maceration in the surrounding skin.
- May cause epidermal stripping or skin tears in patients with fragile or thin skin like elderly patients, or in patients receiving steroids.

Impregnated Wound Dressing

Certain dressings are treated with chemicals to enhance wound healing. In these the dressing material either gauze or bandage is treated with a special chemical agent that promotes rapid wound healing and create sterile environment. They are combined with a secondary dressing as they are non-adherent to most wound beds. The common impregnated dressings are with silver, honey, iodine and methylene blue. Antibacterial dressings play an increasingly important role in bio-burden control and wound healing.

- *Silver impregnated dressings*: These are some of the popular forms of dressing agents, as silver is known to reduce the invasion and spread of bacteria and other pathogens. It can be combined with alginate or foam dressings, which adds to bacteria-fighting capabilities. Silver dressing can be used on almost any lower extremity wound, including heel abrasions and various ulcers.
- *Honey impregnated dressings*: Honey has been used as home remedy for wound healing since ages. Honey has an anti-bacterial activity because of its high sugar and low moisture content, gluconic acid which creates an acidic environment and hydrogen peroxide. When honey comes into contact with body moisture, the glucose oxidase enzyme introduced to the honey by the bee, slowly releases the antiseptic hydrogen peroxide.[11] Studies have shown that honey dressings decrease the pain levels, and odor in infected wounds.[12] Researchers have also reported that applying honey can be used to reduce amputation rates among diabetes patients.[13]
- *Iodine impregnated dressings*: Iodine is a chemical used extensively as a powerful disinfectant. It is available in two forms: povidone iodine and Cadexomer iodine. Both are available in impregnated tulle and dressings. Iodine is known to have a wide range of activity against gram-negative and gram-positive bacteria, fungi, viruses and protozoa. Iodine in different concentrations can affect fibroblasts, which are involved in wound healing. However, iodine can cause irritant and allergic contact dermatitis in sensitive individuals. It should be carefully used in patients with thyroid disorders.
- *Methylene blue dressings*: Methylene blue is normally paired with gentian violet. A foam dressing with added gentian violet and methylene blue (GV/MB) antibacterial agents has been shown to be effective against a wide spectrum of microorganisms found in wounds, including methicillin-resistant staphylococcus aureus (MRSA), vancomycin-resistant enterococcus (VRE) and Candida.[14] In a recently reported case series, authors found that GV/MB antibacterial foam dressings are safe and useful in managing chronic lower extremity and diabetic foot ulcers.[15]
- *Charcoal dressings*: Charcoal gets activated to adsorb by steaming or heating in a vacuum to approximately 1000°C in the absence of oxygen. As a consequence, activated carbon has a large pore volume and a large surface area, giving it a unique adsorption capacity.[16,17] Activated charcoal odor adsorbent dressing utilizes well-proven benefits of an activated charcoal layer. They are used in the treatment of malodorous and infected wounds. When applied onto a wound, they adsorb bacteria, locally released toxins and wound degradation products, thereby promoting wound healing.[18]

- *Unna boot*: Unna boot is a special dressing used for patients with venous leg ulcers and lymphedema who are mobile. It is composed of inelastic gauze which is impregnated with zinc, glycerin, or calamine. The dressing becomes rigid when it dries and when the patient walks, it restricts outward movement of the calf muscle, which directs the contraction force inward. This improves the calf-muscle pumping action and increases venous return.

Selection of Right Dressings

The three important factors that guide selection of suitable dressing are:
1. Wound related factors
2. Clinical effectiveness
3. Economic factors

Wound-related Factors

Wound related factors is an important factor in choosing the type of dressing (Table 9). For example:
- *Necrotic ulcers*: Normally, in any wound, the dead tissues are automatically debrided by the healthy tissue underneath. However, if dead tissue gets exposed to dry weather conditions it desiccates to form a hard-black eschar which delays autolytic removal of dead tissues making the ulcers painful. Management of such ulcers include rehydrating the wound with removal of eschar.[19] In such ulcers, hydrogel dressings which maintain hydration of the wound are preferred. Also hydrocolloid dressings can be used which are occlusive and prevent evaporation thus promoting moisture.
- *Sloughy wounds*: An open wound may rapidly get covered with slough which is nothing but a mixture of fibrin, proteins, leucocytes, serous exudates and bacteria. Sometimes it may be too thick to be removed by simple irrigation. It may require surgical debridement which is rapid but may not be practical in all situations. These require an adjuvant to naturally remove the slough and absorb excess exudates. In such situations, alginate dressing covered with a semipermeable film dressing or a hydrocolloid dressing is the choice as they maintain hydration and at the same time absorb exudates. If wounds have heavy exudates, hydrofibre dressings are useful.
- *Infected wounds*: Apart from systemic antibiotics, infected wounds require anti-microbial dressings with iodine, silver or honey impregnated in them. Charcoal dressings can be used if infected wounds are associated with bad odor.
- *Granulating wounds*: Granulating wounds requires a dressing that keeps the wound warm and moist. Depending on the size, depth and amount of exudates, dressings must be chosen. For superficial or low depth wounds, a non-adherent dressing or occlusive hydrocolloid dressings are effective. Occlusive hydrocolloid dressing improves granulating tissues by creating a hypoxic environment. If heavy exudates are present, alginate dressing is used for deep cavity granulating ulcers, polyurethane foam dressing can be used for packing the wounds.
- *Epithelializing wounds*: Aim of dressing at this stage is only to keep the wound moist as there is hardly any exudate. Hydrocolloid or any semi-permeable dressings are suitable at this stage. Care should be taken to avoid trauma as the epithelializing tissue is very delicate. Other dressings that can be used at the final stage are soft silicon dressings, knotted viscose and nylon sheet dressings. However, allergies to dressing material should be ruled out before using these dressings.

CONCLUSION

To conclude, a wide variety of dressings are available in market with various composition and mechanism of action each claiming superiority over each other. However, none of the studies have shown their advantages in managing ulcers. This needs further well-structured randomized controlled studies to prove their efficacy and cost effectiveness.

REFERENCES

1. Lim CS, Davies AH. Graduated compression stockings. CMAJ. 2014;186:E391-E398.

Table 9: Choice of dressings in different types of wounds.

Type of ulcer	Choice of dressing
Necrotic ulcers	- Hydrogel dressings - Hydrocolloid dressings
Sloughy wounds	- Alginate dressing covered with a semipermeable film dressing - Hydrocolloid dressing
Infected wounds	- Impregnated dressings
Granulating wounds	- Hydrocolloid dressings
Epithelializing wounds	- Hydrocolloid dressings

2. Motykie GD, Caprini JA, Arcelus JI, et al. Evaluation of therapeutic compression stockings in the treatment of chronic venous insufficiency. Dermatol Surg. 1999;25:116-20.
3. Moffatt C. Variability of pressure provided by sustained compression. Int Wound J. 2008;5:259-65.
4. Agu O, Baker D, Seifalian AM. Effect of graduated compression stockings on limb oxygenation and venous function during exercise in patients with venous insufficiency. Vascular. 2004;12:69-76.
5. Beidler SK, Douillet CD, Berndt DF, et al. Inflammatory cytokine levels in chronic venous insufficiency ulcer tissue before and after compression therapy. J Vasc Surg. 2009;49:1013-20.
6. Archer HG, Barnett S, Irving S, et al. A controlled model of moist wound healing: comparison between semipermeable film, antiseptics and sugar paste. J Exp Pathol. 1990;71:155-170.
7. Sussman 2010. Technology update: understanding foam dressings. Wounds International. Product Reviews. 2010;1(2):1-6.
8. O'Meara S, St. James MM. Foam dressings for venous leg ulcers. Cochrane Database of Systematic Reviews.2013. [online] Available from https://www.cochranelibrary.com/cdsr/doi/10.1002/14651858.CD009907.pub2/epdf/full [Accessed December 2018]
9. O'Meara S, St. James MM, Adderley UJ. Alginate dressings for venous leg ulcers. Cochrane Database of Systematic Reviews.2015. [online] Available from https://www.cochrane.org/CD010182/WOUNDS_alginate-dressings-venous-leg-ulcers [Accessed December 2018].
10. Ribeiro CTD, Dias FAL. Hydrogel dressing for venous ulcers. Cochrane Database of Systematic Reviews. 2013. [online] Available from https://www.cochranelibrary.com/cdsr/doi/10.1002/14651858.CD010738/full [Accessed December 2018].
11. Chirife J, Scarmato GA, Herszage L. Scientific basis for use of granulated sugar in treatment of infected Wounds. Lancet. 1982;1:560-561.
12. Dunford C, Hanano R. Acceptability to patients of a honey dressing for non-healing venous leg ulcers. J Wound Care. 2004;13:193-7.
13. Molan PC. Clinical Usage of Honey as wound Dressing. J Wound Care. 2004;13:353-356.
14. Karen Edwards. New Twist on an Old Favorite: Gentian violet and methylene blue antibacterial foams. Adv Wound Care (New Rochelle). 2016;5:11-18.
15. Coutts PM, Ryan J, Sibbald RG. Case series of lower-extremity chronic wounds managed with an antibacterial foam dressing bound with gentian violet and methylene blue. Adv Skin Wound Care. 2014;27:9-13.
16. Marsh H, Reinoso FR. Activated Carbon, 1st edition. New York: Elsevier; 2006.
17. Baker FS, et al. Activated carbon. Kirk-Othmer Encyclopedia of Chemical Technology. 1992;4:1015-37.
18. Kerihuel JC. Charcoal combined with silver for the treatment of chronic wounds. Wounds UK. 2009;5:87-93.
19. Bishop SM, Walker M, Rogers AA, et al. Importance of moisture balance at the wound—dressing interface. J wound care. 2003;12:125-8.

CHAPTER 16

Role of Skin Grafting in Managing Leg Ulcers

Smitha Segu, Suhas S

INTRODUCTION

Skin grafting is one of the most common surgical procedures in the area of non-healing wounds by which skin or a skin substitute is placed over a wound to replace and regenerate the damaged skin. Chronic leg ulcers are an important problem and a major source of expense.

Split thickness skin grafts offer stable, efficient and quick coverage of ulcers. Skin grafting is one of the most important procedures to obtain a stable, efficient and quick coverage of leg ulcers. The early reconstruction of leg ulcers cannot be overemphasized as they significantly reduce the morbidity, reduce pain, prevent further infection, and threat to the limb. Skin grafts in their various types have different indications and usage based on the etiology of ulcers and status of the wound. Due consideration to all these factors ensures uncomplicated healing and minimizes chances of skin graft failures.

Skin grafting was rediscovered during the First and Second world wars as the main treatment for wound closure.

Skin grafts (also called autograft) may be taken from the patient's own uninjured skin (e.g. thigh), may be grown by bioengineering patient's own skin cells (Kerationcyte epidermal culture), may be harvested from cadavers (allograft) or a dermal substitute such as Integra may be used.

Preserved skin from other animals, e.g. pigs, have also been used and these are known as xenografts.

Early optimization of the wound and auto skin grafting reduces the cost, the duration of hospital stay, pain during repeated dressings, use of antibiotics, constant mental trauma to the patients and relatives and helps in early rehabilitation.

APPLIED ANATOMY OF SKIN

The skin represents about 8% of our total body weight, with a surface area of 1.2–2.2 m^2. The skin is 0.5–4.0 mm thick and covers the entire external surface of the body. The main function of skin is to protect body contents from the environment, including pathogens, temperature, and excessive water loss. Insulation, temperature regulation, sensation, immune function, and the synthesis of Vitamin D are all important functions of the skin.

Skin has a complex three-dimensional structure characterized by two overlapping layers, the epidermis and the dermis.

Epidermis

Epidermis, as shown in Figure 1, is the outer or upper layer of skin, which is a thin, semitransparent, water-impermeable tissue, consisting primarily of keratinocytes. The basement membrane separates the epidermis from the dermis. Basal keratinocytes are partially differentiated stem cells of the epidermis that provide the proliferative and regenerative capacity of the skin epithelium. The epithelium is metabolically active and continuously self-renews to maintain an efficient barrier function. Homeostasis is maintained by the basal epidermal cells, which periodically cycle, executing their program of terminal differentiation, a process that takes approximately 28 days. Figure 2 shows the layers of epidermis—basal keratinocytes produce tonofilaments (precursor of keratin) and then transform into the stratum spinosum as the desmosomes stretch the cells into spikes visible with a microscope. Cells then start to produce keratohyalin, which aggregates in dense and

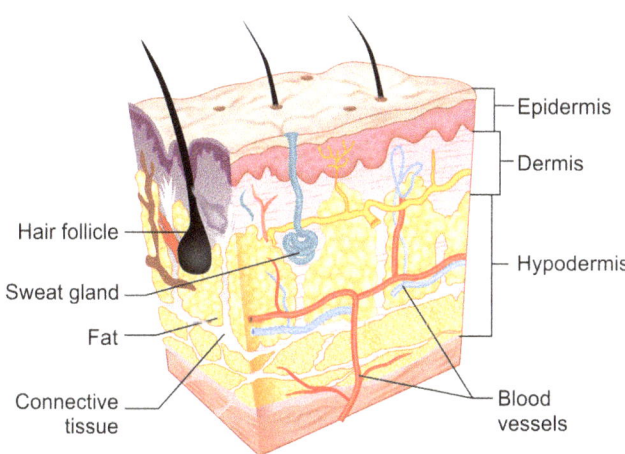

Fig. 1: Layers of the skin.

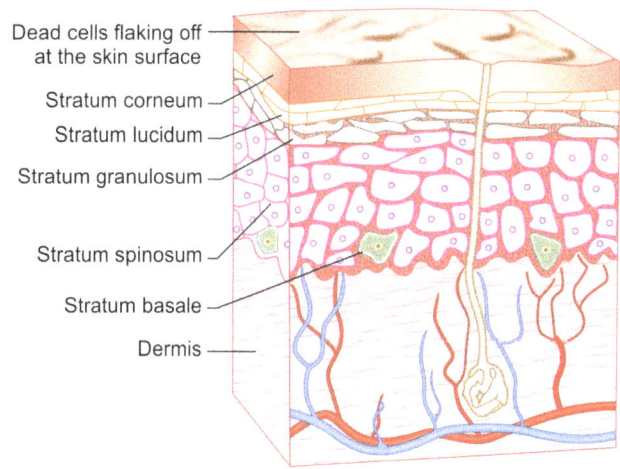

Fig. 2: Layers of epidermis.

basophilic granules, thus the name, stratum granulosum. As the cells divide and move up through the epidermis they transform into the stratum corneum, a layer of dead cells, which ultimately is highly mechanically and chemically resistant. The stratum corneum provides an extremely effective barrier layer to keep water in and microorganisms out. Other structures within the epidermis are melanocytes, Langerhans cells, Merkel cells, and sensitive nerves.

Dermis

The dermis is a tough fibrous layer that provides the mechanical strength of the skin. It is composed primarily of collagens, glycosaminoglycans, and elastins. Skin grafts without dermis result in a closed but often unstable skin. Grafting a part of the dermis is therefore very important to consider in terms of functionality of the future skin.

The upper part of the dermis has a particular architectural organization that is called papillary and contains blood vessels and nerve fibers. The papillary layer of dermis consists of fine collagenous fibers that form an undulating interface with the overlying basement membrane and epidermis. This increases the contact area between dermis and epidermis, allowing for maximal mechanical stability of the two layers and an exchange surface for diffusion. Deeper is the reticular dermis, with increasingly thicker collagenous fibers (mainly of type I). The reticular dermis has larger collagenous fibers with substantial strength. The mechanical properties of the dermis allow movement while providing stability and protection from mechanical trauma. The dermis has self-healing property, mainly due to the presence and activation of myofibroblasts following injury.[1]

STEM CELLS IN SKIN AND SKIN REGENERATION

Basal epithelial keratinocytes are the committed stem cells of the epidermis. Constant self-renewal provides a new protective layer at the skin surface. Hair follicles, as shown in Figure 3, contain multipotent stem cells that are activated upon the start of a new hair cycle and upon wounding to provide cells for hair follicle and epidermal regeneration. In the hair follicle, stem cells reside in the bulge area. Bulge cells are relatively quiescent compared with other cells within the follicle. However, during the hair cycle, bulge cells are stimulated to exit the stem cell niche, proliferate, and differentiate to form the various cell types of the hair follicle. In addition, bulge cells can be recruited during wound healing to support re-epithelialization.[2,3]

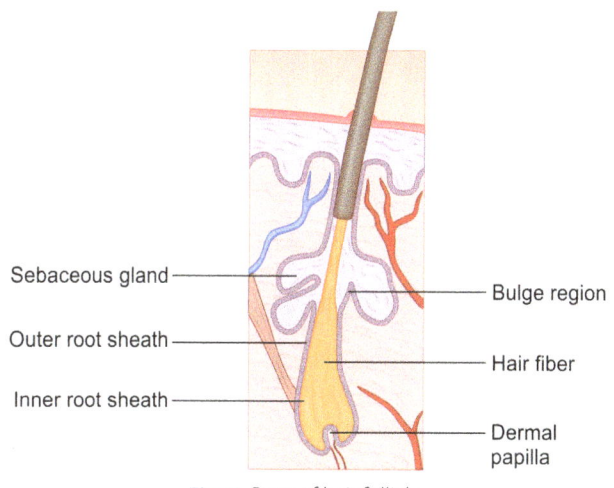

Fig. 3: Parts of hair follicle.

COMMON ULCERS AND ROLE OF SKIN GRAFTS

- *Arterial ulcers*: Usually seen secondary to peripheral vascular disease secondary to atherosclerosis or Buerger's disease.

  If leg is well perfused with at least a single parent artery or good collateral circulation—ulcers in such limbs are amenable to skin grafting.

  In critical limb ischemia—it is advisable to defer skin grafting until circulation is restored to the limb by vascular surgical procedures like stenting, thrombectomies or bypass grafts, thus optimizing the take in a well vascularized wound bed.

- *Venous ulcers*: In presence of saphenofemoral junction or saphenopopliteal junction insufficiency or perforator insufficiency, skin grafting is deferred until the venous incompetence is surgically corrected. Skin graft for venous ulcer can be done at the same time of the venous surgery or after the venous surgery.

- *Diabetic/neuropathic ulcers*: In trophic ulcers secondary to diabetic or any other neuropathy, first wound bed optimization is essential. This is achieved by a thorough surgical debridement under tourniquet control until all the slough and necrotic tissue is removed. This usually suffices to prepare wound bed for skin grafting, provided the infection is also well-controlled. Further optimization of the wound bed may be needed by way of negative pressure wound therapy or vacuum-assisted closure (VAC) therapy to hasten granulation tissue formation, improve vascularity of the wound bed and clear up further micro-slough. The red healthy wound is then skin grafted provided it is not a weight-bearing area of the foot and no critical structures are exposed in the wound bed. If wounds overlie weight bearing regions or regions of constant friction, they require flap cover for definitive treatment, with split thickness skin grafts reserved for immediate wound cover and to reduce exudate. This is very important so that the skin graft is not subjected to shearing forces or pressure strains while ambulating, which will hamper its take up.

- *Vasculitic/pyoderma ulcers*: These ulcers are associated with autoimmune conditions and routine management will not suffice. The first step is to make sure the active disease is controlled by medication like corticosteroids or disease modifying anti-rheumatic drugs (DMARDS). This can be confirmed by a fall in erythrocyte sedimentation rate (ESR) and C-reactive protein (CRP) levels. Till then, local wound care is best done by Dakin's solution (0.5% sodium hypochlorite), which prevents spread of the ulcer. Once active disease is controlled, then the debridement and skin grafting may be planned, under the medication cover. A preliminary VAC therapy (vide infra) may be beneficial in chronic ulcers.

OPTIMIZATION OF THE WOUND BED

The wound bed has to be optimized before application of a skin graft for the full "take" of graft. The important factors to be considered are:

a. Removal of non-viable tissue otherwise known as debridement, as in Figures 4A and B, which can be

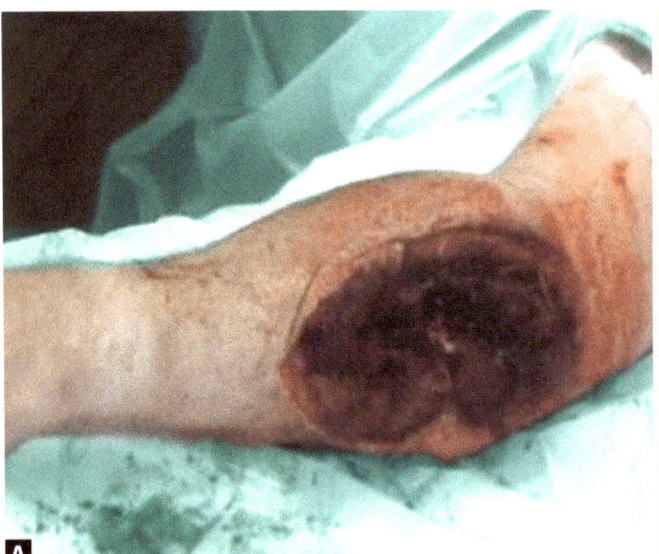 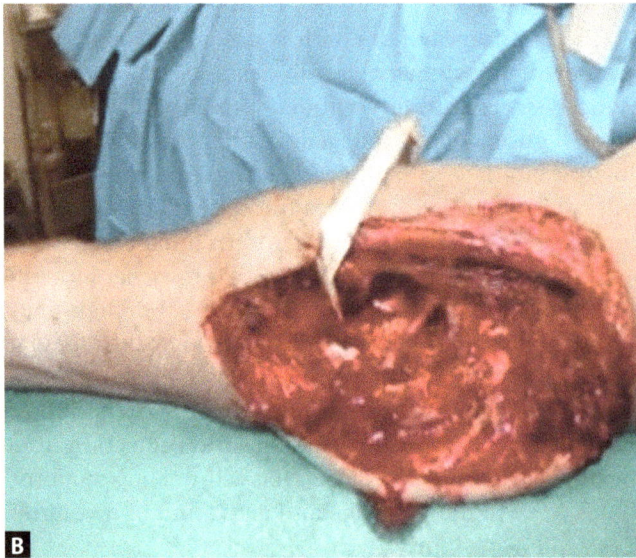

Figs. 4A and B: Wound debridement; (A) before and (B) after.

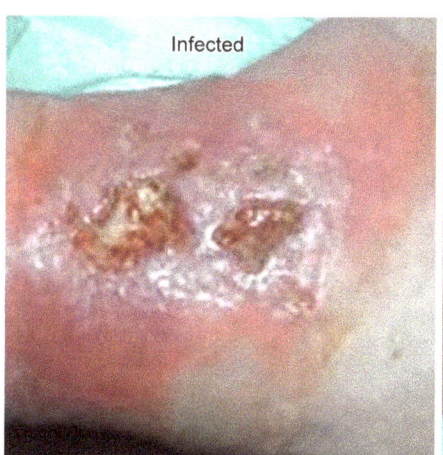 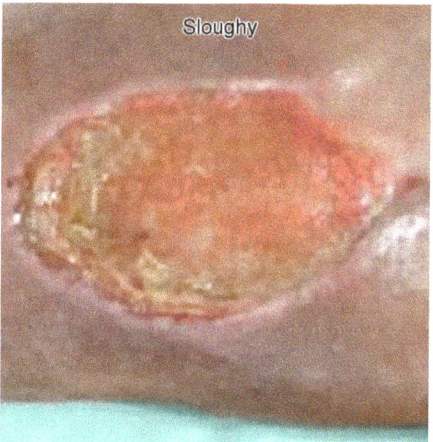 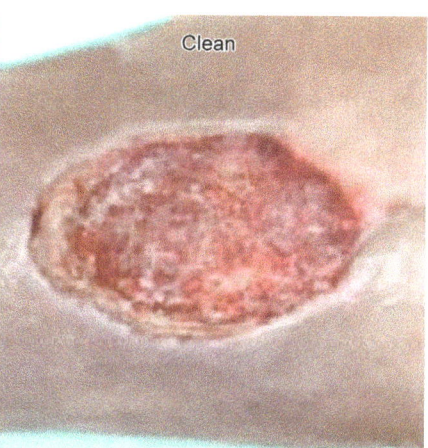

Fig. 5: Different stages of ulcer.

surgical, autolytic, mechanical, chemical or enzymatic, biological with maggots or larvae, ultrasonic or hydrosurgical.
b. Control of bacterial load with antimicrobials and antibiotics according to culture and sensitivity
c. Management of exudates with different kinds of dressing materials available like film dressings, foam dressings, hydrogel dressings, hydrocolloid dressings, alginate dressings, hydroactive dressings.

Capillary growth is the key for both vascularization of graft and granulation.

Wound granulation time co-relates directly with graft "take" time i.e. quickly granulated wounds accept and support grafts better. The different ulcers which are seen in practice are shown in Figure 5.

NEGATIVE PRESSURE WOUND THERAPY (VACUUM-ASSISTED CLOSURE THERAPY)

Negative pressure wound therapy (NPWT device), shown in Figures 6A and B, is a device which applies continuous or intermittent sub-atmospheric pressure, or suction, to the wound bed via a computerized vacuum pump attached to an open-cell foam sponge that is placed in the wound and secured with an adhesive semi-occlusive dressing. Wound fluids are evacuated via a tubing system placed on the foam at one end and connected to a disposable canister housed in the therapy unit on the opposite end.

Advantages of NPWT are:
- It maintains moist, protected environment
- It removes excess interstitial fluid from the wound periphery
- It increases local vascularity

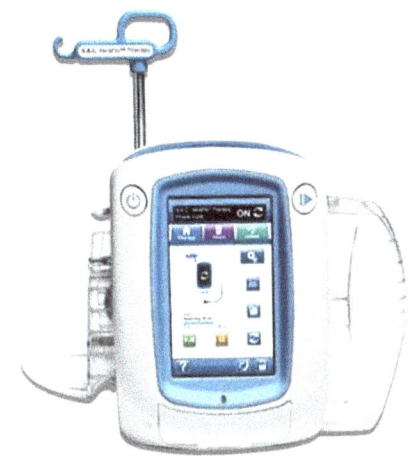

Fig. 6A: Negative pressure wound therapy.
Courtesy: KCI Medical, USA; V.A.C. Veraflo Therapy, 2018

- It decreases bacterial colonization
- It quantifies/qualifies wound drainage
- It increases rate of granulation tissue formation
- It increases rate of contraction of wound bed
- It increases rate of epithelialization.[4]

HYPERBARIC OXYGEN THERAPY

The use of 100% oxygen breathed at increased atmospheric pressure requires that:
- The patient be enclosed in a pressure vessel
- Subjected to an atmospheric pressure at least 1.5x sea level or ambient pressure and be breathing 100% oxygen
- Basis: Biochemical oxygen acts as a signal messenger for cell function

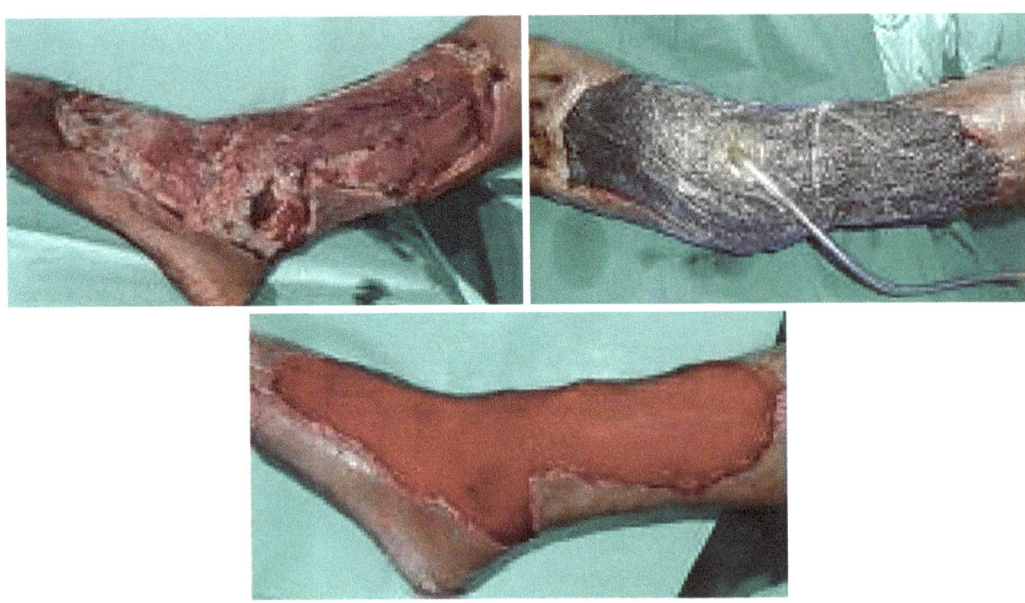

Fig. 6B: Negative pressure wound therapy (before and after).
Courtesy: Dr. Smitha Segu, Department of Plastic Surgery, Bangalore Medical College

- It improves fibroblast proliferation and collagen formation
- It helps endothelial budding and angiogenesis
- It stimulates functional receptor changes on neutrophils.[5]

PRE-REQUISITES OF WOUND BED FOR SPLIT THICKNESS SKIN GRAFT

- Wounds free of slough and active infection, as in Figure 7
- Post–debridement wounds with good vascularity
- Wounds exposing tendon with intact paratenon
- Wounds exposing bone with intact periosteum
- Wounds without exposed neurovascular structures
- Wounds without exposed orthopedic implants
- Wounds without too much dead space.

Note: Leg wounds exposing bare bone and tendon, neurovascular structures or orthopedic implants will require flap cover.

CONTRAINDICATIONS FOR SKIN GRAFTING

Absolute: Infection of wound bed with beta hemolytic Streptococcus- Cause of failure of graft is unknown although fibrinolysin may be a cause. Classically, these infected wounds are glazed and gelatinous in appearance with a tendency to bleed on touch.

Relative:
- MRSA Infection
- Anemia

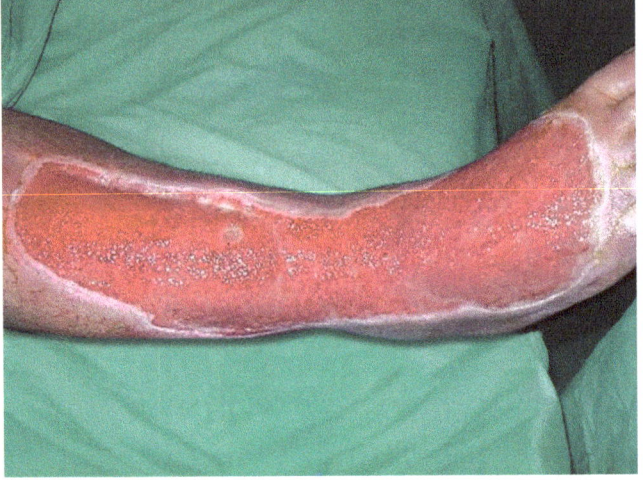

Fig. 7: Wound ready for skin grafting.

- Jaundice
- *Poorly vascularized limb*: Wound cover only after vascularity is established.

SKIN GRAFT

Skin grafts are a standard option for closing defects that cannot be closed primarily. A skin graft consists of epidermis and some or all of the dermis. By definition, a graft is something that is removed from the body, completely devascularized, and is replaced in another location. Grafts of any kind require vascularization from the bed into which they are placed for survival. Any tissue which is not completely removed prior to placement is not a graft.

Skin Graft Types

Skin grafts are classified as either split-thickness or full-thickness, depending on the amount of dermis included. Split-thickness skin grafts contain varying amounts of dermis, whereas a full-thickness skin graft contains the entire dermis.

All skin grafts contract immediately after removal from the donor site and again after revascularization in their final location.

Primary contraction is the immediate recoil of freshly harvested grafts as a result of the elastin in the dermis. The more dermis the graft has, the more primary the contraction that will be experienced.

Secondary contraction, the real nemesis, involves contraction of a healed graft and is probably a result of myofibroblast activity.

A full-thickness skin graft contracts more on initial harvest (primary contraction) but less on healing (secondary contracture) than a split-thickness skin graft. The thinner the split-thickness skin graft, the greater is the secondary contracture. Granulating wounds left to heal secondarily, without any skin grafting, demonstrate the greatest degree of contracture and are most prone to hypertrophic scarring.[6]

Instruments Used to Harvest a Skin Graft

- Dermatome, Humby's skin grafting handle for a split thickness graft
- Scalpel blade to harvest a full thickness graft

How Does a Skin Graft Take?

Graft take has 5 stages (Fig. 8):
1. Adhesion
2. Serum imbibition
3. Inosculation
4. Revascularization
5. Re-modelling.

Serum Imbibition

In the first days, before the graft revascularizes, oxygen and nutrients diffusing through the plasma between the graft and the wound bed will nourish the skin graft. This is "serum imbibition", as fibrinogen changes into fibrin that fixes the skin graft on to the wound bed. In the first hours, passive absorption of serum from the wound bed causes edema, which resolves when the revascularization is functional.[7]

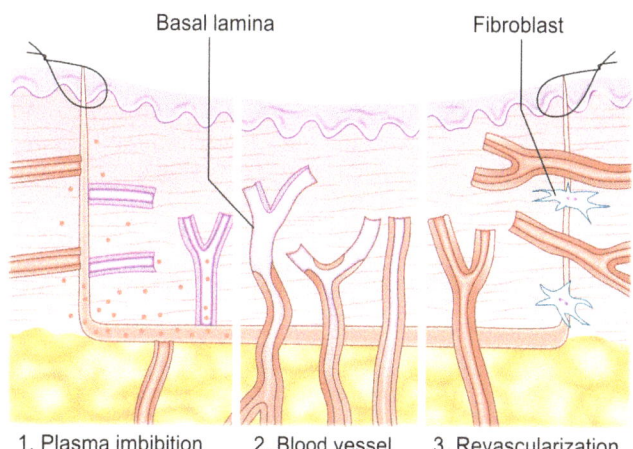

Fig. 8: Stages of skin graft take.
Source: Neligan PC. Plastic Surgery, 4th edition. Atlanta: Elsevier; 2012.

Revascularization

There are 3 stages of revascularization:
1. Anastomosis
2. Neovascularization
3. Endothelial cell in growth

Anastomosis is the process of reconnection between the blood vessels in the recipient site wound bed and the graft.

Neovascularization is characterized by new vessel ingrowth from the recipient site into the skin graft.

Endothelial cell proliferation, utilizing pre-existing vascular basal lamina as a structure, while in the graft endothelial cells gradually degenerate. The process of revascularization begins as early as 24–48 hours after grafting.[8]

Maturation

Once the skin graft is completely integrated, the same graft and surrounding tissues remodel and contract, similar to the last phase of wound healing after re-epithelialization is complete. Skin grafts take at least 1 year to complete maturation, with the extension of this process continuing for several years in chronic wounds, burn victims and children. Scars from skin grafts can continue to improve for a number of years, often making prolonged conservative therapy worth considering.[7]

Advantages and Disadvantages of Different Types of Skin Graft

Different advantages and disadvantages of several types of skin graft are described in Table 1.

Table 1: Advantages and disadvantages of different skin graft types.

Type of graft	Indication in leg ulcers	Advantage	Disadvantages
Thin split skin graft (0.15–0.3 mm) Thiersch Grafts	Debrided burn wounds; chronic wounds with less vascularized wound beds; exposed flap areas; acute well-vascularized wounds; non optimal wound bed	Fast donor site re-epithelialization; multiple possibilities to reharvest the same area; good graft take	Secondary contraction of the skin graft; graft quality limited because of minimal dermal thickness
Thick split skin graft (0.3–0.45 mm) Blair-Brown Grafts	Same as above	Less secondary graft contraction compared to thin split skin graft; more stable because of thicker dermal layer; good graft take	Slower donor site re-epithelialization
Full thickness graft (0.45–0.6 mm) Padgett Grafts	Reconstruction of functional areas such as in the feet; non-infected, well-vascularized wound beds, toe-tip injuries not exposing bone/tendon	Minimal to no secondary graft contraction; excellent skin quality; stability; hair re-growth and skin appendage function possible	Limited availability; nontake risk is higher in a less vascularized wound bed

Techniques of Split Skin Graft (Fig. 9)

- Prepare the wound bed for grafting (debridement and hemostasis)
- Estimate the needed skin graft size
- Clean the donor site from any residual disinfection (i.e. Betadine)
- Apply sterile paraffin or sterile lignocaine jelly to lubricate the donor site
- Set the dermatome at 0.2 mm thickness or skin graft handle only enough to pass a surgical blade
- Stretch the donor site skin by hands of assistant
- Apply the dermatome/skin graft handle at a 45° angle and apply light pressure and make the blade almost parallel to skin surface once the initial cut is made
- Slide the dermatome/handle along the skin while an assistant is lifting the skin graft with two forceps
- Lift the dermatome/handle upwards when the desired size of graft is obtained
- Dress the donor site with Vaseline gauze, dry gauze and bandages
- Spread evenly the graft (dermal site of the graft upwards) on a dermal carrier (rough surface of the carrier upwards) of the desired size (1:1.5, 1:3, etc.).
- Pass the graft through the graft mesher paying attention that it does not detach from the dermal carrier, as shown in Figure 10.

However, excessive meshing should be avoided, unless the wound is large and graft is inadequate, as it leads to a

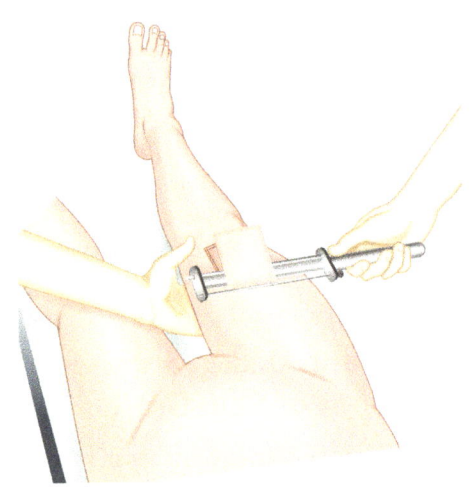

Fig. 9: Harvesting a split skin graft.
Source: Neligan PC. Plastic Surgery, 4th edition. Atlanta: Elsevier; 2012.

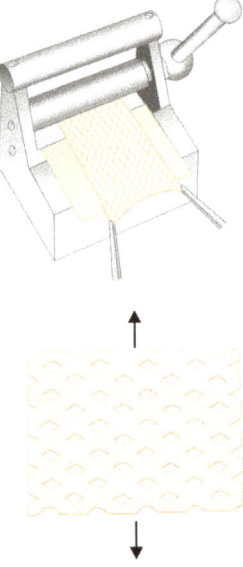

Fig. 10: Mesher for meshing the skin graft.
Source: Neligan PC. Plastic Surgery, 4th edition. Atlanta: Elsevier; 2012.

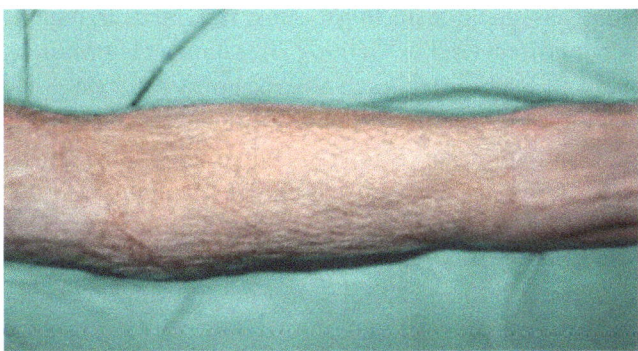

Fig. 11: Cobblestone appearance following meshing.

cobblestone appearance which is not aesthetically pleasing, as shown in Figure 11.
- Alternatively, meshing can be made manually with a surgical blade on the skin graft placed dermal side up stretched out on a smooth, stable surface
- Apply the graft on the recipient site by sutures, surgical staples or fibrin glue
- When indicated apply a bolster dressing by placing vaseline gauze on the skin graft, followed by a cotton sponge impregnated with Betadine or saline solution and tight sutures (4/0 nylon or polypropylene) from the opposite wound margins together at the center of the defect.
- First dressing change should be around 5-7 days postoperative.[9]

Full-thickness Skin Grafts

Full-thickness skin and composite grafts are limited in availability but show excellent function and sensitivity after engraftment. Full-thickness grafts (FTGs) should be considered in the reconstruction of aesthetically dominant (face) or functionally important (foot) areas.

Full-thickness skin grafts are taken in an area where loose surrounding skin is available to achieve primary closure. Skin grafts can be designed elliptical and excised with a knife. Most of the FTGs needs defatting and this can be easily performed by spreading the graft over the index finger and trimming the fat tissue tangentially to the skin. Defatting of the graft will encourage graft take.

Over time, the appearance of skin grafts tends to improve in both color and texture. Nevertheless, skin grafts rarely have the aesthetic appearance of normal skin and patients should be advised about the likely final appearance of the graft.

In leg, full thickness grafts are used less frequently, as optimal conditions necessary for FTG are rarely present in leg ulcers.[10]

Methods of Fixing the Skin Graft

One of the most important factors to achieve stable taking is the immobility of the graft during the revascularization process. Skin grafts are fixed through a series of sutures and overlying compressive dressing materials. Scattered sutures through the graft on to the wound bed can additionally immobilize larger skin grafts, like bolsters and tie-overs, as shown in Figure 12.

Fixation can be performed with staplers to shorten operation time. Vacuum-assisted pressure devices can be used with a protective interface of petroleum gauze or a silicone sheet to permit continuous compression on to the graft and fluid removal. This is useful if fast mobilization is desired in patients with wounds in joint regions or the lower extremities.

Compression to stabilize the graft on to the wound bed should be performed until 5-10 days after grafting, when the graft is usually stable and wound areas are completely closed.

Splints should be used as adjuncts if the risk of wound contraction is high, such as in wounds over popliteal fossa, ankle, or in joint and web space release of the foot. These splints or casts should be worn up to several months after grafting, in the beginning 24 hours per day, later during the night, to avoid the loss of mobility.

Physiotherapy and scar massage are also important elements for obtaining better results with skin grafts.

Sealants

Fibrin glue can be used to secure wounds to the graft bed, especially since the increase efficacy of natural fibrin found in a debrided and "scooped" wound bed.[11]

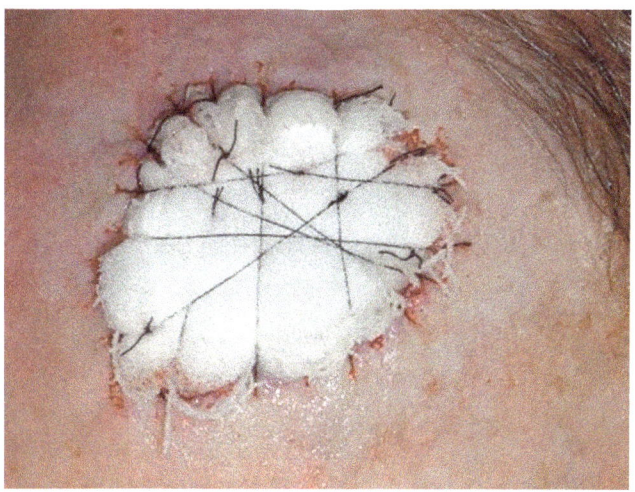

Fig. 12: Bolster and tie-over to immobilize the skin graft.

First Dressing Change

The first dressing change should occur once the skin graft is revascularized and has a stable physical connection to the wound bed. Early dressing change around the third day after grafting may allow for predicting the "take rate" of the graft but risks secondary graft loss through shear forces that disturb nascent vessel connections. More commonly the dressings are taken off for the first time 5–7 days after grafting. A good skin graft take is shown in Figures 13A and B.

Donor Site Considerations

The scarring or discoloration associated with donor sites must be considered when taking a skin graft. Common donor sites include the thigh, trunk, and buttocks, regions frequently covered by clothing. In traumatic leg wounds, avulsed (degloved) skin can often be prepared by extensive defatting and regrafted primarily or stored and used later.

Other common regions include the inguinal crease, which is often used to cover large defects. In this case it is important to harvest laterally and away from potentially hair-bearing regions of the pubis. This area generally heals well and is hidden. Donor sites from full-thickness skin grafts are generally closed primarily. Particular attention should be taken when supraclavicular donor sites are used, as this region is prone to develop hypertrophic scars. Sometimes large donor sites that cannot heal primarily are used for covering extensive defects, for example, in joints—

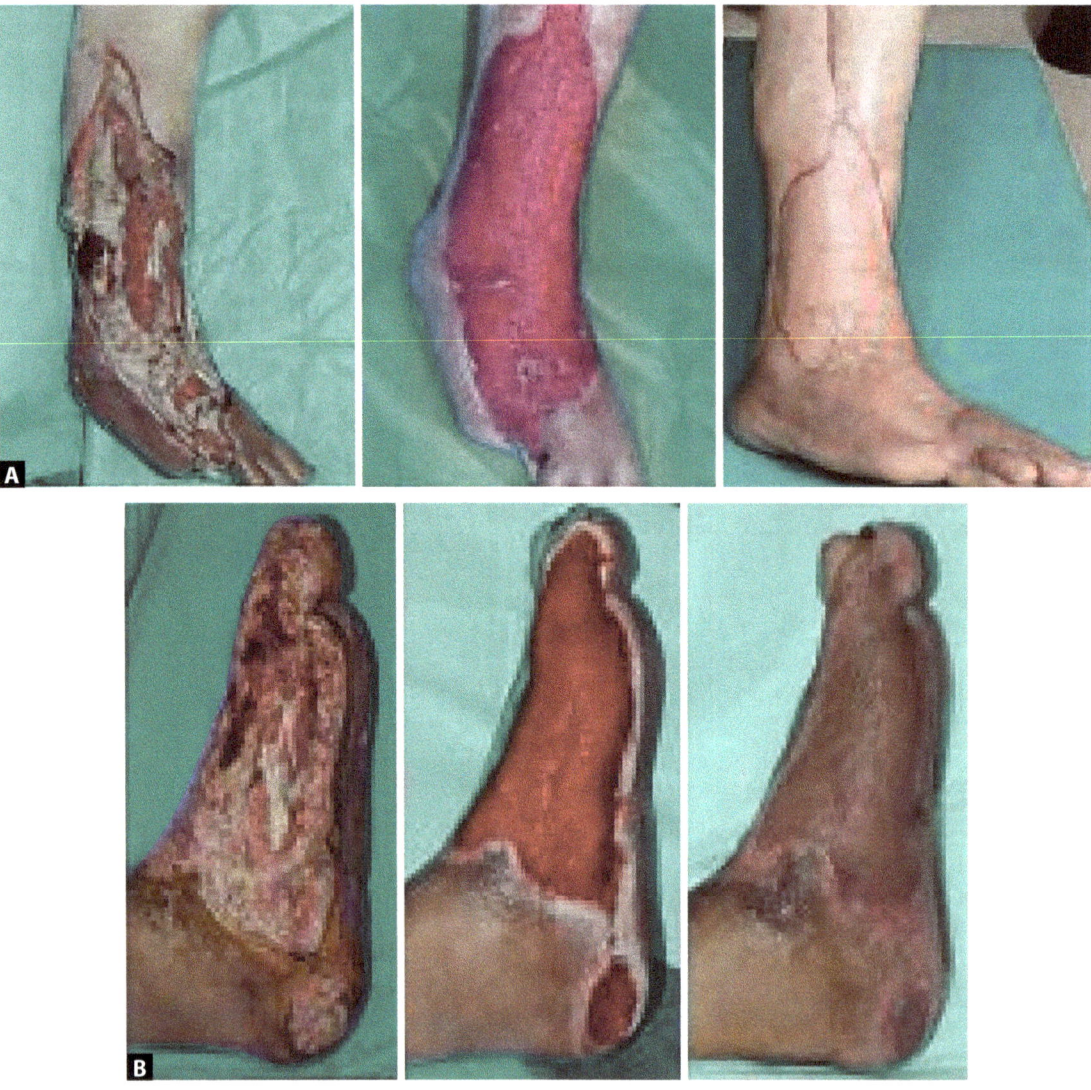

Figs. 13A and B: (A) Skin graft—full take; (B) Well settled skin graft.

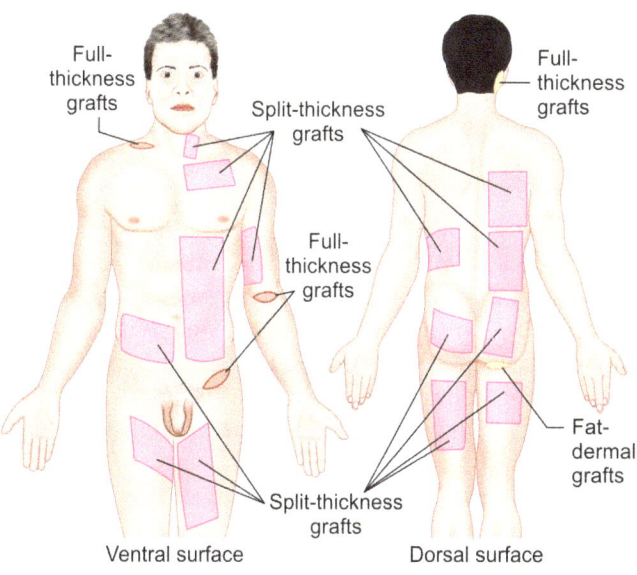

Fig. 14: Various donor sites for skin grafts.

knee and ankle. In this case, a split skin graft can be used to cover the donor site. All donor sites in body are represented in Figure 14.

Donor Site Dressing

The donor site of a split skin graft generally heals (re-epithelializes) in 7–21 days depending on the size and depth of the graft taken and the age of the patient. A myriad of donor site dressings are available with multiple studies on a variety of products. Traditionally, fine-meshed gauze, often impregnated with a petroleum-based product, is placed over the wound and fixed in place. Cotton gauze is placed over this and removed a day or two after the operation. The wound heals under this dressing and the dressing spontaneously comes off when healed. The advantages of this type of dressing system are its simplicity, low cost, and minimal wound care requirement. Generally, a moist wound heals faster. A large number of other dressings, including silver-based, absorptive, and biological, have been studied. When some complications occur, the harvest site can deepen and become a full-thickness defect, mainly due to infections in the elderly, infants, or critically ill patients. As a consequence, excision and grafting of the donor site may be required.[5,6]

SKIN GRAFT STORAGE

Skin grafts can be stored on moist gauze at 4°C for up to 2 weeks, although the viability decreases over time. Experimentally, storage can be extended using cell culture media. For degloving injuries, the skin can be defatted acutely and reapplied as a full-thickness graft.

COMPLICATIONS

Hematoma

Any liquid between the wound and skin graft can impair skin graft take. Bleeding represents one of the most important complications after excision and grafting. The surgeon must be certain that bleeding has stopped prior to dressing the wound. Suture ligation or cautery can be used to control larger bleeding vessels; oozing can be controlled with pressure and/or pharmacological methods such as topical thrombin, epinephrine, or fibrin glue. To reduce bleeding during excision the area can be primarily injected with epinephrine diluted in saline (tumescent technique).

Seroma

Serum imbibition is essential for early skin graft survival. Excessive serum, such as a seroma, will prevent or delay skin graft take. Seromas are better tolerated than hematomas, and adequate fenestrations (pie crusting) can prevent this problem.

Infection

When skin graft infections occur, pus often accumulates beneath the skin graft and can rapidly spread. If an infection is found early, prompt incision and drainage of the fluid beneath the graft can often salvage some or all of the skin graft. A large number of dressings have been developed that carries a variety of topical antimicrobial agents. Silver nitrate, mafenide acetate, and silver ion dressings are commonly used. Bacteria seem not to develop resistance easily to silver products, making these products desirable.

A contaminated wound will not heal and will reject a graft. Some microorganisms, such as *Pseudomonas* spp., can contaminate the wound and cause nonpurulent infections. Even systemic or non skin-localized infections have been proven to delay or prevent skin graft taking.

Non-take

Unfavorable conditions such as malnutrition, vasculitis, malignant diseases, steroids, and chemotherapeutic medications have all been shown to cause or accelerate non-take of the graft.

Wound Contraction

Wounds covered with skin grafts can still undergo wound contraction leading to a scar contracture. After the acute inflammation phase the contraction starts. Fibroblasts from surrounding tissues and from blood circulation start to be activated and repopulate the wound between the graft and the wound bed. Cells at the interface need to build new collagen-rich tissue to replace fibrin and anchor the graft to the wound bed.

Instability

Shear forces are a major cause of skin graft failure that can disrupt the nascent fragile blood vessel connections. Later, thin skin grafts have less collagen content and are prone to frequent ulcerations due to shear forces.

Cosmetic Issues

Unpleasant cobblestone-like patterns of meshed Split skin grafts are much more prominent than non meshed or full-thickness grafts. Color differences are a common problem if donor sites could not be optimally chosen. If excess skin surrounds the grafted area, the skin graft can be excised in multiple steps until primary closure can be reached.

Donor Site

Infection at donor sites can occur from bacterial contamination during the operation or in the postoperative period. These infections are treated with topical antimicrobial agents, including silver dressings. The delay in healing of donor sites due to infection can lead to hypertrophic scar formation. Hypertrophic scar or keloid formation can also result from deep donor sites or in patients with a propensity for scarring. Itching is a common reaction to donor sites as well as hypersensitivity to changes in temperature.

RECENT ADVANCES IN SKIN REPLACEMENT

Dermal Substitutes

Integra®, is a bovine-derived collagen type I cross-linked matrix with glycosaminoglycans that is similar to the dermal structure and covered by a silicone sheet to recreate temporarily the function of the epidermis. Integra® can be applied to a vascularized wound bed which is followed by blood vessels and cell growth into the collagen matrix to create a vascularized neodermis after 2–3 weeks. During the avascular period, the dermal graft is very sensitive to infection, one of the main disadvantages of the two-step strategy. Once revascularization is accomplished, the silicone layer can be removed and the epidermal replacement can be granted by either keratinocyte cultures or a thin STSG.[12]

After the invention of Integra®, a number of other human-and animal-derived dermal substitutes are now commercially available. Another synthetically engineered dermal substitute is **MatriDerm**®(MedSkin Solutions Dr. Suwelack), a bovine-derived collagen matrix with non cross-linked collagen fibers of types I, III, and V matrix coated with elastin fibers. Synthetic dermal substitutes such as Integra® and MatriDerm® are permanent dermal regenerative templates that will be ultimately covered by an epidermal autologous graft.[13]

Cell Cultures

Cultured epithelial autografts (CEA) are keratinocytes harvested from a small biopsy of the same patient that are then expanded manifold in the laboratory, as represented in Figure 15.

The time needed to expand keratinocyte cultures *in vitro* for clinical use is dependent upon the delivery method. In order to obtain sheets of confluent keratinocytes as in normal epidermis, it may take up to 5 weeks. This time can be shortened to less than 2 weeks 57 by expanding the cultures on bioscaffolds that allow cell attachment and proliferation prior to transplantation.

Hyaluronan or collagen scaffolds have been demonstrated to be very useful in delivering cell-seeded sheets with approximately 80% confluence up to even multi layered epithelial tissue constructs. Cell suspensions have the advantage of being delivered faster, reducing the *in vitro* time to only 5–7 days.[14]

Bioengineered Cultured Allogeneic Bilayered Constructs

Neonatal skin cells are very efficient in accelerating wound healing. Neonatal foreskin keratinocytes and fibroblasts were then used in combination with biological or synthetically engineered scaffolds to stimulate wound healing in topically applied allogeneic skin constructs. Other than autologous cells, which seem to integrate into wound tissues, allogeneic constructs rather stimulate healing by growth factor release and initial production of extracellular matrix proteins, but are rejected eventually. **Apligraf**® (Organogenesis, Canton, MA and Novartis Pharmaceuticals, East Hanover, New

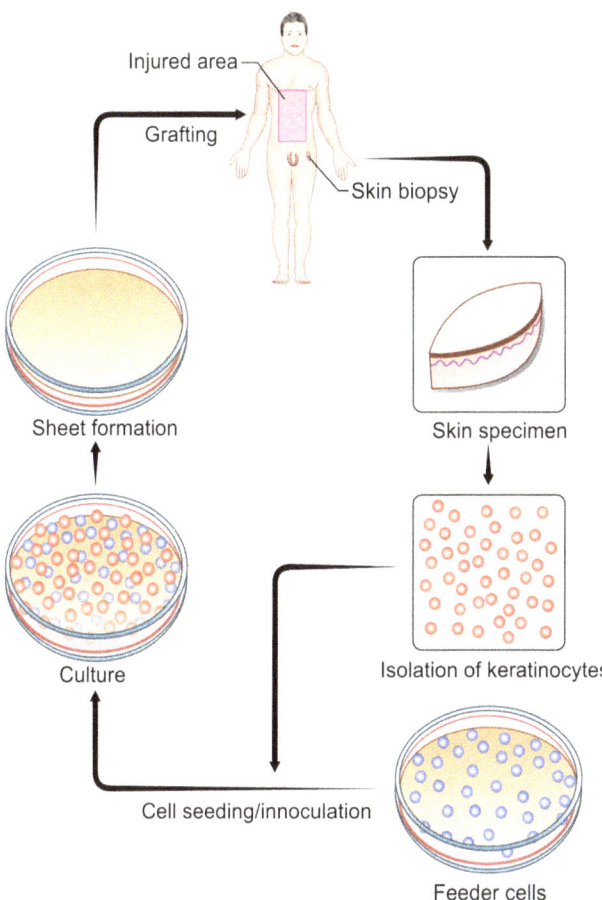

Fig. 15: Keratinocyte cell cultures.

Jersey) is a bilayered living skin equivalent composed of type I bovine collagen and allogeneic keratinocytes and fibroblasts obtained from neonatal foreskin. Fibroblasts are cultured in the collagen matrix where they proliferate and augment the extracellular matrix with all types of proteins. Keratinocytes are then added and build up the epidermal layer. The living skin construct supports skin graft take in difficult wounds, such as burn wounds in leg, or accelerates healing in chronic wounds. With a shelf-life of 5 days at room temperature, Apligraf® has to be applied fresh either as a temporary dressing or over meshed STSGs. If used as temporary dressing, it will subsequently require STSG coverage, thus buying time for donor sites to heal.[15]

Cadaveric Allografts from Skin Bank

Skin harvested, processed and stored from cadavers within 6 hrs of death can be used over large areas of ulcers when conditions are not viable for an auto graft. This helps in covering of the wound, preventing infection acts as a biologic cover until autograft is a possibility.

CONCLUSION

The full epithelization of an ulcer may take several months or even years if left to heal primarily. Sometimes an ulcer does not fully heal for several years with conservative treatment. Auto Skin grafting is a method of treatment that decreases the area of chronic leg ulcers or heals them completely, and it improves quality of life for the patient.

Early optimization of the wound and autografts reduces the cost, the duration of hospital stay, pain during repeated dressings, use of antibiotics, constant mental trauma to the patients, and relatives and helps in early rehabilitation.

REFERENCES

1. Fuchs E. Scratching the surface of skin development. Nature. 2007;445:834-842.
2. Myung P, Andl T, Ito M. Defining the hair follicle stem cell (Part I). J Cutan Pathol. 2009;36:1031-4.
3. Myung P, Andl T, Ito M. Defining the hair follicle stem cell (Part II). J Cutan Pathol. 2009;36:1134-7.
4. Korber A, Franckson T, Grabbe S, et al. Vacuum assisted closure device improves the take of mesh grafts in chronic leg ulcer patients. Dermatology. 2008;216:250-6.
5. Neligan PC. Plastic Surgery, 4th edition. Philadelphia: Elsevier; 2017. Pp. 214-30.
6. Thorne CH, Barlett SP, Beasley RW. Grabb and Smith's Plastic Surgery, 6th edition. Philadelphia: Lippincott Williams Wilkins; 2006. Pp. 07-10.
7. Haller JJBR. Studies of the origin of the vasculature in free skin grafts. Ann Surg. 1967;166:896-901.
8. Capla JM, Ceradini DJ, Tepper OM, et al. Skin graft vascularization involves precisely regulated regression and replacement of endothelial cells through both angiogenesis and vasculogenesis. Plast Reconstr Surg. 2006;117:836-44.
9. Tanner JC Jr, Vandeput J, Olley JF. The mesh skin graft. Plast Reconstr Surg. 1964;34:287-92.
10. Birch J, Branemark PI. The vascularization of a free full thickness skin graft: I. A vital microscopic study. Scand J Plast Reconstr Surg.1969;3:1-10.
11. Foster K, Greenhalgh D, Gamelli RL, et al. Efficacy and safety of a fibrin sealant for adherence of autologous skin grafts to burn wounds: results of a phase 3 clinical study. J Burn Care Res. 2008;29:293-303.
12. Wood FM, Stoner ML, Fowler BV, et al. The use of a non-cultured autologous cell suspension and Integra dermal regeneration template to repair full-thickness skin wounds in a porcine model: a one-step process. Burns. 2007;33:693-700.
13. Orgill DP, Butler CE, Barlow M, et al. (1998). Method of skin regeneration using a collagen-glycosaminoglycan matrix and cultured epithelial autograft. [online] Available from https://patents.google.com/patent/US5489304 [Accessed December 2018].
14. Rheinwald JG, Green H. Serial cultivation of strains of human epidermal keratinocytes: the formation of keratinizing colonies from single cells. Cell.1975;6:331-43.
15. Boyce ST, Goretsky MJ, Greenhalgh DG, et al. Comparative assessment of cultured skin substitutes and native skin autograft for treatment of full-thickness burns. Ann Surg. 1995;222:743-52.

CHAPTER 17

Role of Platelet Rich Plasma and Platelet Rich Fibrin in Managing Leg Ulcers

Reena Rai, Yuvasri Gunasekaran

INTRODUCTION

Regenerative medicine in dermatology is a newer branch that emphasizes on the repair and regeneration of cells and tissue of the skin.[1] A major revolution in treatment of leg ulcer is cellular therapy where the blood from the patient is used that contains growth factors and cytokines. Platelet derived products have shown promising results in wound healing.

ROLE OF PLATELET-DERIVED PRODUCTS

Platelets play an important role in hemostasis and wound healing. The alpha granules of platelets contain various growth factors and cytokines. These potent wound healing factors helps in inflammation and tissue repair.

The Table 1[2,3] lists the various growth factors and their role in wound healing. Mechanism of action of growth factors at cellular level has been shown in Flowchart 1.

Table 1: Various growth factors and their role in wound healing.

S. No	Growth factors	Role
1.	Platelet derived growth factor (PDGF)	Helps in angiogenesis, macrophage activation Stimulates neutrophil chemotaxis Enhances collagen synthesis, bone cell proliferation
2.	Transforming growth factor-beta	Regulates collagen synthesis, fibroblast proliferation Induces deposition of bone matrix
3.	Insulin like growth factor–1	Activates protein synthesis Enhance proliferation and differentiation of osteoblast Stimulates fibroblast chemotaxis
4.	Vascular endothelial growth factor	Angiogenesis Increases vascular permeability
5.	Epidermal growth factor	Angiogenesis Exerts collagen secretion, endothelial chemotaxis, epithelial mitogenesis
6.	Fibroblast growth factor	Promotes growth and differentiation of chondrocytes and osteoblasts
7.	Connective tissue growth factor	Angiogenesis Cartilage regeneration Helps in fibrosis and platelet adhesion
8.	Platelet factor-4	Exerts neutrophil and fibroblast chemotaxis
9.	Leucocytes	Prevents infection

Flowchart 1: Mechanism of action of growth factors at cellular level.[4]

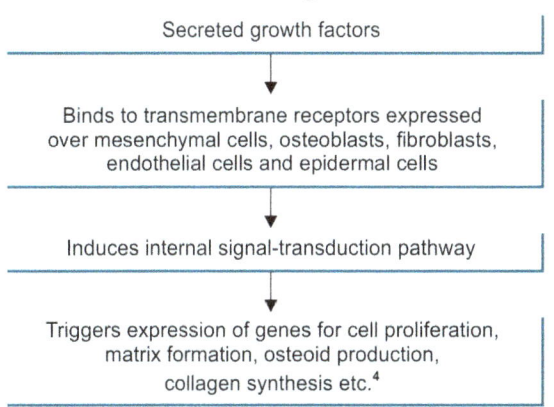

```
Secreted growth factors
        ↓
Binds to transmembrane receptors expressed
over mesenchymal cells, osteoblasts, fibroblasts,
endothelial cells and epidermal cells
        ↓
Induces internal signal-transduction pathway
        ↓
Triggers expression of genes for cell proliferation,
matrix formation, osteoid production,
collagen synthesis etc.[4]
```

The growth factors bind to the transmembrane receptors present over the mesenchymal cells and various other cells involved in wound healing. It induces the signal transduction pathway and thereby causing expression of genes for proliferation of cells and collagen synthesis.

PLATELET RICH PLASMA (FIGS. 1 TO 9)

Marx defined platelet rich plasma as autologous plasma with platelet concentration above blood baseline.[5] Platelet rich plasma means abundant platelets that are concentrated into a small volume of plasma.

Preparation[6] (Flowchart 2)

Platelet rich plasma (PRP) is found to be used to augment wound healing without any adverse effects. The growth factors in PRP helps in regulating the mesenchymal cell and extracellular matrix proliferation and synthesis. There have been various studies in which leg ulcers have been managed successfully with platelet rich plasma.

Flowchart 2: Preparation of platelet rich plasma.[6]

```
20 mL venous blood collected in a test tube containing
acid citrate dextrose in ratio of 9:1 (blood:ACD)
        ↓
Centrifuge at 5000 rpm for 15 min
        ↓
A buffy coat with RBCs below and supernatant
plasma above is obtained
        ↓
Supernatant and buffy coat transferred into a
separate plain test tube
        ↓
Centrifuge at 2000 rpm for 5 min
```

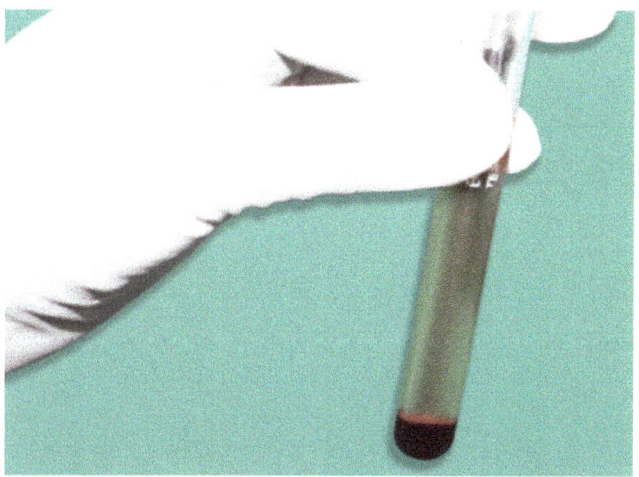

Fig. 1: Test tube with platelet rich plasma after double centrifugation method.

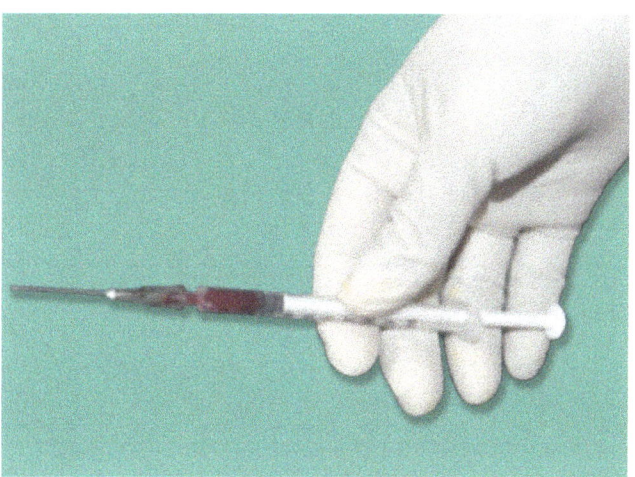

Fig. 2: Syringe with PRP.

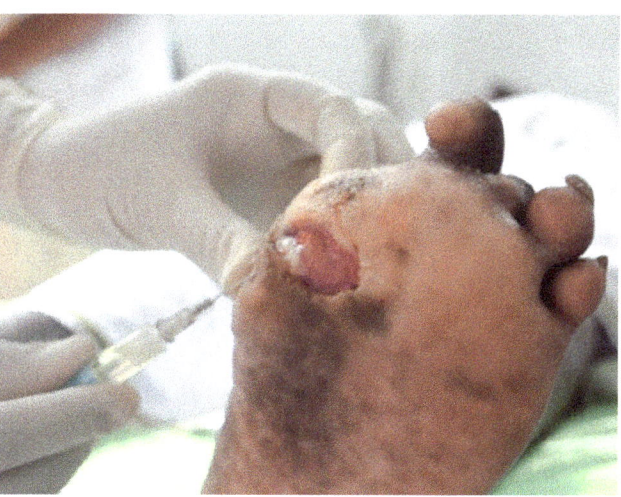

Fig. 3: Injecting PRP around the ulcer.

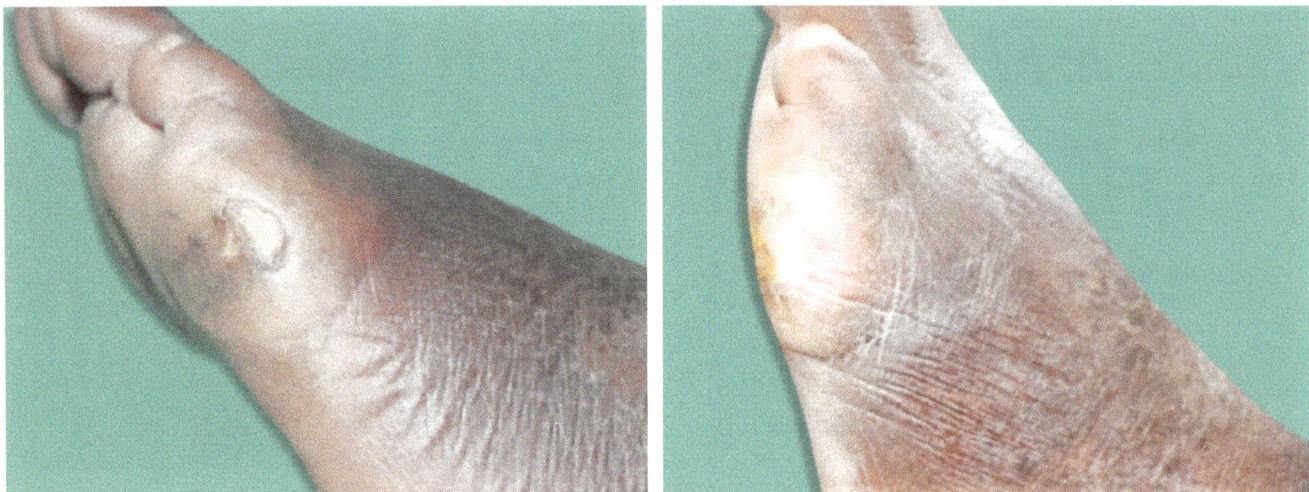

Fig. 4: Ulcer before and after 2 weeks of PRP dressing.

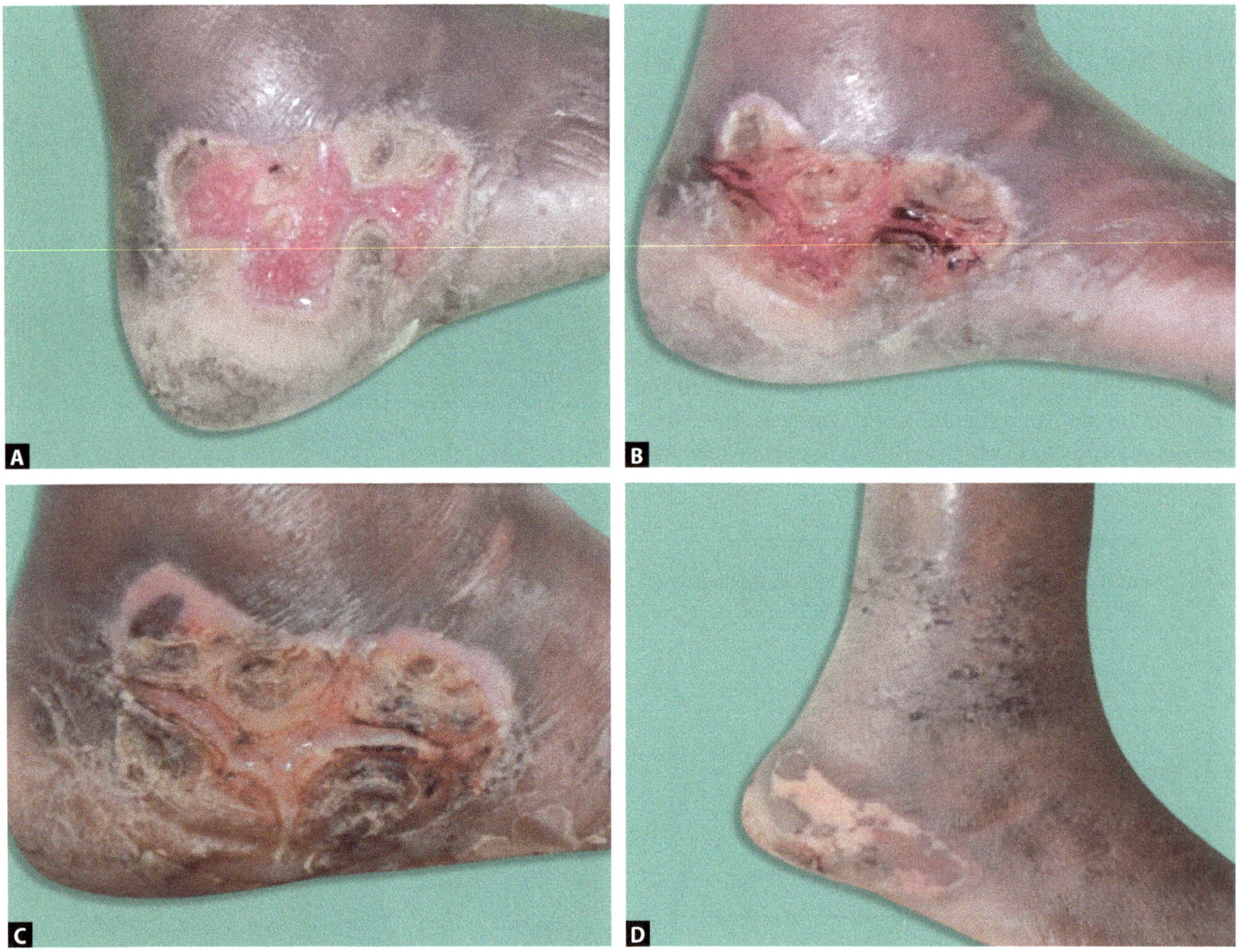

Figs. 5A to D: (A) Ulcer before PRP; (B) Day 6; (C) Day 13; (D) Day 32 (after PRP dressing).

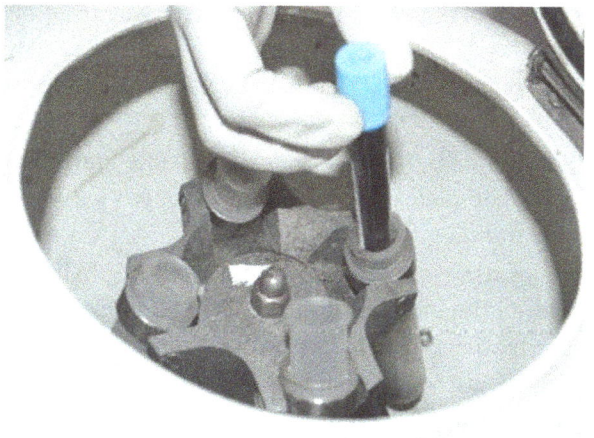
Fig. 6: Placing the test tube in a centrifuge.

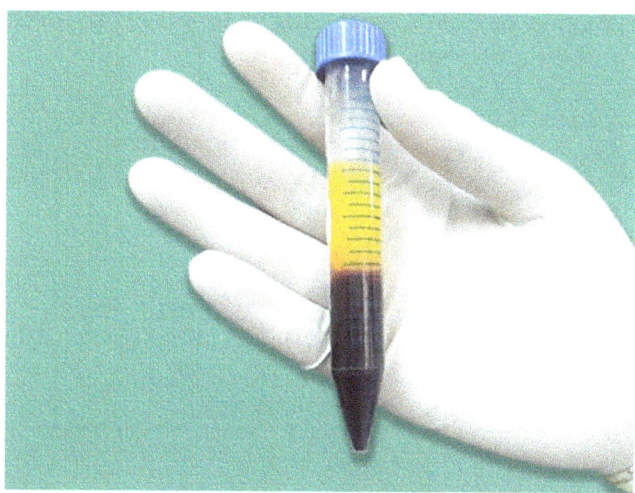
Fig. 7: Test tube with PRF.

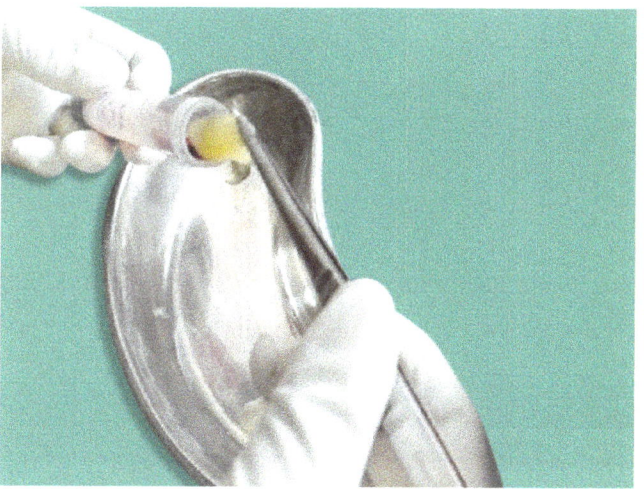
Fig. 8: Using blunt forceps PRF gel.

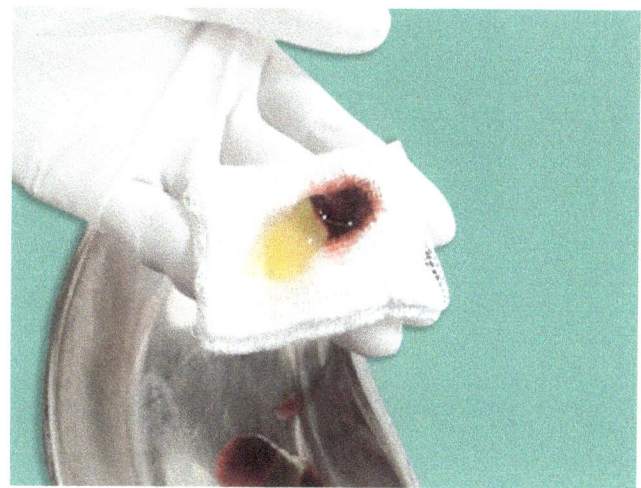
Fig. 9: PRF gel with RBCs being removed.

A randomized uncontrolled study done by Sacchidanand Sarvajnamurthy et al. reported 94.7% and 95.6% improvement in ulcers treated with PRP in area and volume respectively.[6]

Deepak et al. reported a case with complete closure of a nonhealing ulcer with PRP in 7 weeks.[7]

In another study by Shwetha Suryanarayan et al. showed 91.7% and 95 % reduction in area and volume of the ulcer with platelet rich plasma.[8]

PLATELET RICH FIBRIN (FIGS. 10 TO 13)

- Platelet rich fibrin (PRF) is a second-generation platelet concentrate.
- PRF is obtained by separation of blood after centrifugation into various components like RBCs, plasma, WBCs and platelets.[9]
- The finally derived PRF acts as a biodegradable scaffold for cell migration, proliferation and differentiation and delivers growth factors.[10]
- Platelets trapped within the 3-D mesh ensures slow and continuous release of growth factors over time which lasts until day 28.[11]
- PRF also acts as a pool of growth factors and living autologous cells, a delivery system.[9]

Preparation[12] (Flowchart 3)

On an average, 10 mL of blood yields 2.5 mL of clot.

Studies have shown excellent results with platelet rich fibrin for leg ulcers. A randomized controlled trial conducted by Reena Rai et al. in chronic venous leg ulcers comparing efficacy of autologous PRF versus saline dressing concluded the mean reduction in the area of ulcer size in

PRF group was 85.51% and in saline group was 42.74% which was statistically significant.[12]

Flowchart 3: Preparation of platelet rich fibrin.[12]

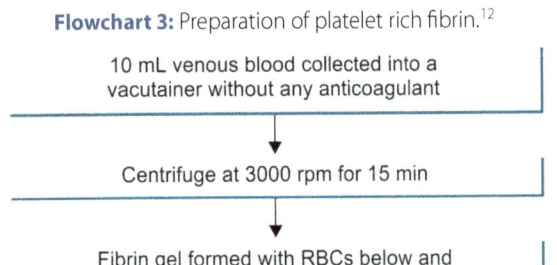

A study conducted by Umashankar Nagaraju et al. showed 93.52% and 97.74% improvement in area and volume respectively at the end of 2 weeks/second sitting treated with PRF.[13]

Study done by Seam O'Connell et al. PRF for leg ulcers achieved complete closure of 66.7% in venous leg ulcers in 7 weeks duration.[14]

In another study conducted by Pravin AJS et al. compared the efficacy of PRP and PRF in chronic non-healing leg ulcers concluded that mean duration of healing of ulcers were 5.7 weeks and 6.5 weeks in PRF and PRP group respectively.[15]

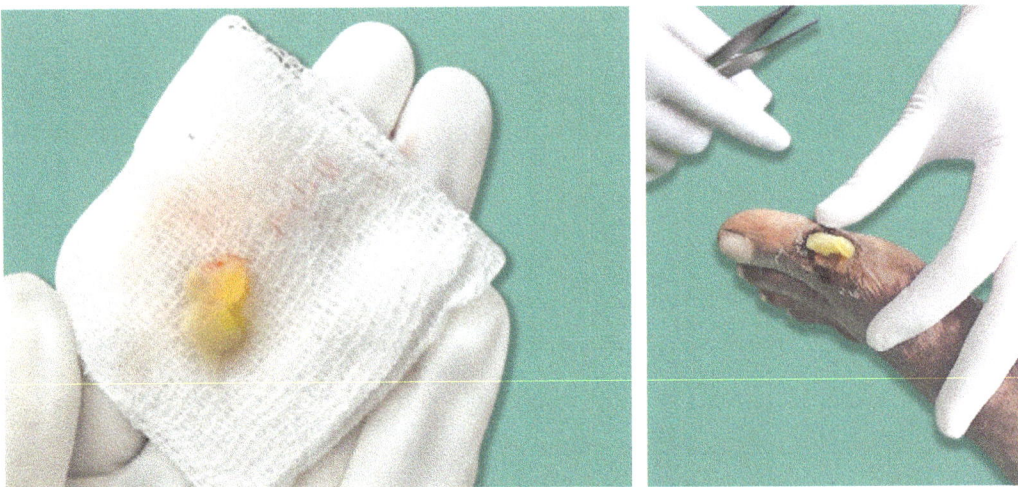

Fig. 10: PRF gel after removing the RBC layer and placed over the ulcer.

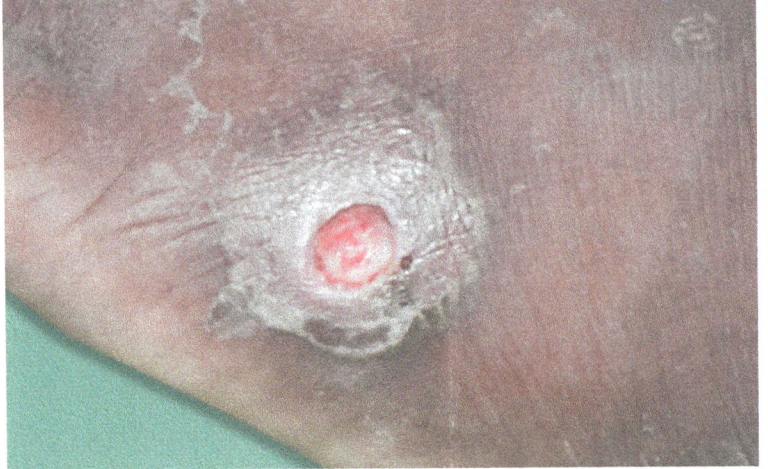
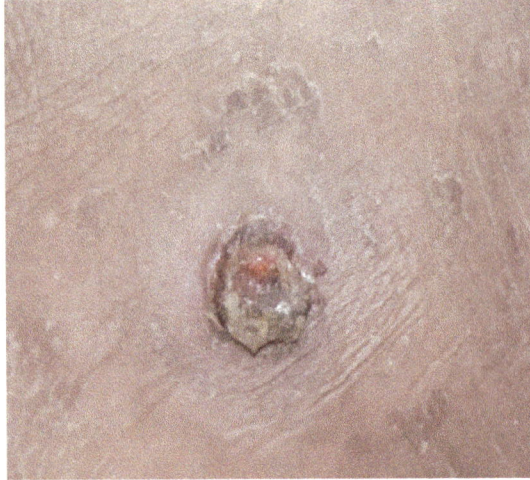

Fig. 11: Ulcer before and after 4 weeks of treatment with platelet rich fibrin.

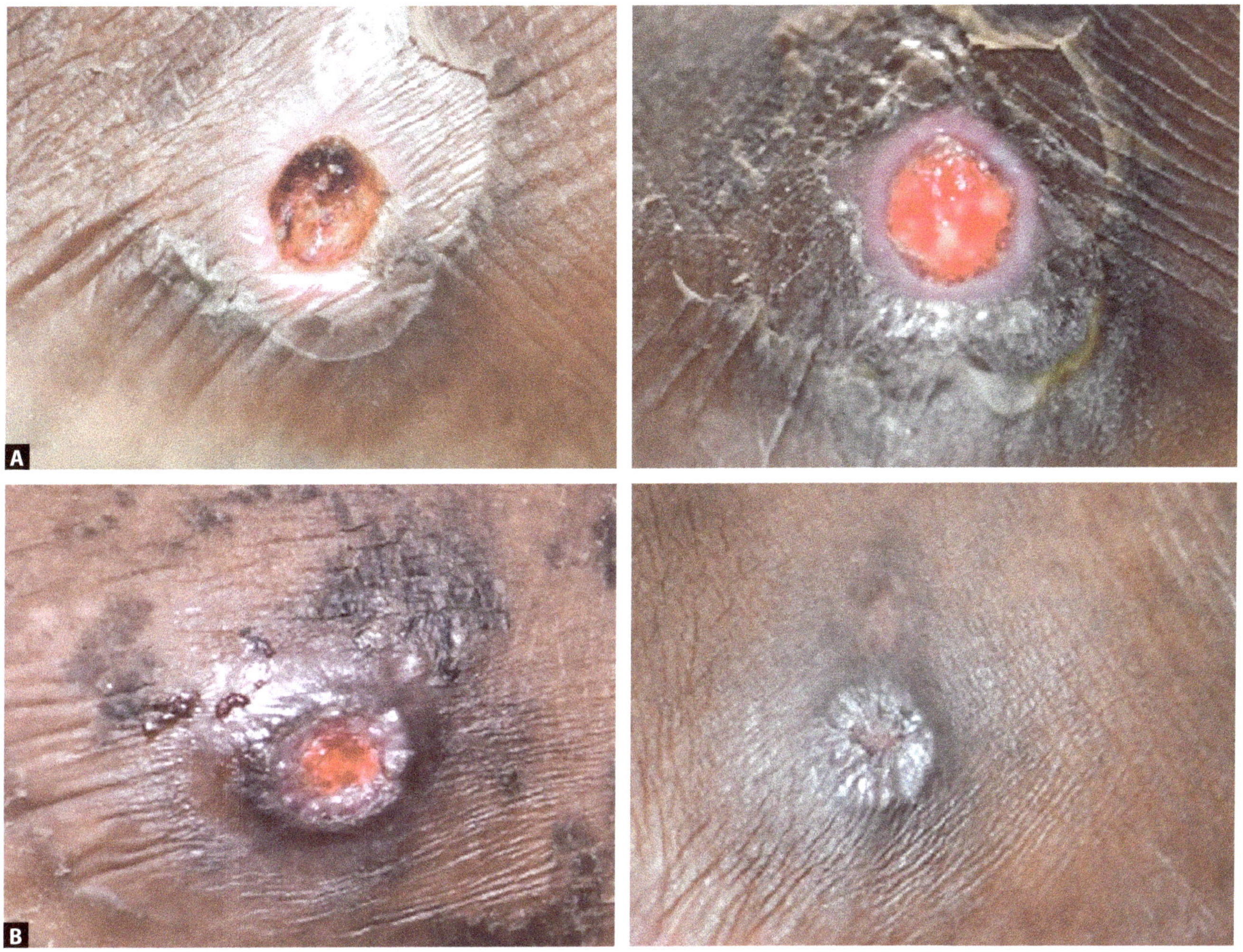

Fig. 12A and B: (A) Ulcer before and after 1st week of treatment with platelet rich fibrin; (B) At 3rd week and complete closure at 4th week of treatment with PRF.

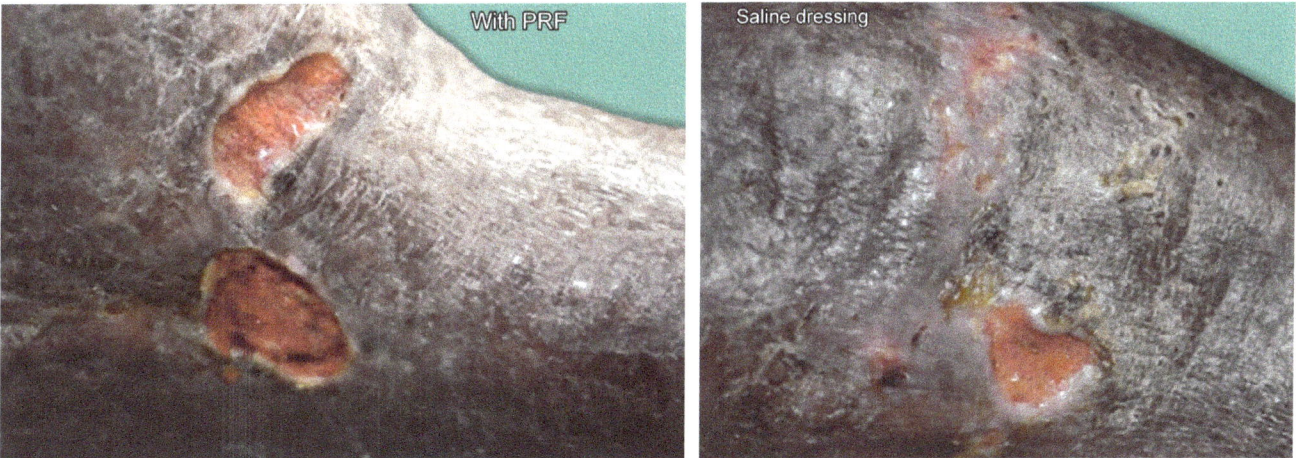

Fig. 13: Ulcers before and after 4 weeks of dressing with PRF (complete closure) and saline.

CONCLUSION

Though there are multiple therapies available for chronic leg ulcers platelet derived products have shown promising results in wound healing. We conclude that these procedures are simple, feasible, safe, cost-effective and above all can be done as an out-patient procedure.

REFERENCES

1. Khunger N. Accelerated wound healing: Harnessing the power of platelets, biomaterials, stem cells and gene therapy. J Cutan Aesthet Surg. 2017;10:1-2.
2. Sunitha RV, Naidu EM. Platelet-rich fibrin: evolution of a second-generation platelet concentrate. Indian J Dent Res. 2008;19: 42-6.
3. Hotwani K, Sharma K. Platelet rich fibrin-a novel acumen into regenerative endodontic therapy. Restor Dent Endod. 2014;39:1-6.
4. Arshdeep, Kumaran MS. Platelet-rich plasma in dermatology: Boon or a bane?. Indian J Dermatol Venereol Leprol. 2014;80: 5-14.
5. Babo PS, Reis RL, Gomes ME. Periodontal tissue engineering: current strategies and the role of platelet rich hemoderivatives. Journal of Materials Chemistry B. 2017;5:3617-28.
6. Sarvajnamurthy S, Suryanarayan S, Budamakuntala L, et al. Autologous platelet rich plasma in chronic venous ulcers: study of 17 cases. J Cutan Aesthet Surg. 2013;6:97-9.
7. Suresh DH, Suryanarayan S, Sarvajnamurthy S, et al. Treatment of a non-healing diabetic foot ulcer with platelet-rich plasma. J Cutan Aesthet Surg. 2014;7:229-31.
8. Suryanarayan S, Budamakuntla L, Khadri SI, et al. Efficacy of autologous platelet-rich plasma in the treatment of chronic nonhealing leg ulcers. Plast Aesthet Res. 2014;1:65-9.[online] Available from https://parjournal.net/article/view/37 [Accessed December 2018].
9. Khiste SV and Tari RN.Platelet-Rich Fibrin as a Biofuel for Tissue Regeneration. International Scholarly Research Notices 2013:2013:6 Available at http://dx.doi.org/10.5402/2013/627367.
10. Borie E, Oliví DG, Orsi IA, et al. Platelet-rich fibrin application in dentistry: a literature review. Int J Clin Exp Med. 2015;8:7922-9.
11. Chignon-Sicard B, Georgiou CA, Fontas E, et al. Efficacy of leukocyte-and platelet-rich fibrin in wound healing: a randomized controlled clinical trial. Plast Reconstr Surg. 2012;130:819e-829e.
12. Somani A, Rai R. Comparison of efficacy of autologous platelet-rich fibrin versus saline dressing in chronic venous leg ulcers: A randomised controlled trial. J Cutan Aesthet Surg. 2017;10: 8-12.
13. Nagaraju U, Sundar PK, Agarwal P, et al. Autologous platelet-rich fibrin matrix in non-healing trophic ulcers in patients with Hansen's disease. J Cutan Aesthet Surg. 2017;10:3-7.
14. O'connell SM, Impeduglia T, Hessler K, et al. Autologous platelet-rich fibrin matrix as cell therapy in the healing of chronic lower-extremity ulcers. Wound Repair and Regen. 2008;16:749-56.
15. Pravin AJS, Sridhar V, Srinivasan BN. Autologous platelet rich plasma (PRP) versus leucocyte-platelet rich fibrin (l-PRF) in chronic non-healing leg ulcers—a randomised, open labelled, comparative study. J. Evolution Med. Dent. Sci. 2016;5:7460-7462.[online] Available from https://jemds.com/latest-articles.php?at_id=12468 [Accessed December 2018].

CHAPTER 18

Novel Research and Recent Advances in Managing Leg Ulcers

Eswari L, S Sacchidanand

INTRODUCTION

Recent advances in diagnosing and managing leg ulcers with evidence-based update has been attempted to cover in this chapter. Leg ulcers will continue to be a major burden on the health care system. They have an immense impact on the cost of therapy, quality of life and psychosocial status. In spite of various advances in the therapy, nonhealing ulcers continue to exist and is challenging.

The various recent advances discussed in this chapter are:
- *Role of stem cell therapy*: Mesenchymal stem cell therapy
- Biopharmaceuticals
- Endothelial progenitor cell EPC therapy
- Novel drug delivery systems
- Tissue engineered skin equivalents
- Human amniotic cellular/tissue-based products
- Recent advances in topical therapy
- Advances in dressings
- Oral nutritional supplements
- Balneotherapy
- Photodynamic therapy and other light-based therapy
- Negative pressure wound therapy (NPWT)
- Hyperbaric oxygen therapy (HBOT)
- Electric stimulation (ES)
- Pulsed Radiofrequency Electromagnetic field therapy PEMF
- Surgical advances

THE ROLE OF STEM CELLS

Research is still in the early phases with a very few clinical trials, but stem cells could prove to be an important method for advancing wound healing in difficult leg ulcer cases. Overall, stem cells are known to produce high quantities of chemokines and growth factors and have the ability to generate into different cell types, giving potential benefit to wound healing. Stems cells can be categorized as allogenic or autologous. Allogenic stem cells include placental, umbilical cord, and embryonic stem cells. Placental mesenchymal stem cells (MSC) have been shown to be useful for improving blood flow and ischemic complications of chronic wounds. MSCs derived from umbilical cord blood are noted to increase cutaneous healing. Embryonic stem cells can be induced to differentiate into any cell type and have shown increased wound healing in a diabetic rat model with topical application.[1] Autologous stem cells include bone marrow–derived MSCs, endothelial progenitor cells, hematopoietic stem cells, and adipose-derived stromal cells.[2]

Mesenchymal Stem Cell (MSc) Therapy

Mesenchymal stem cells are the promising source of adult progenitor cells which are capable of developing into various cell lineages[3] which can have therapeutic applications in wound healing. Under hypoxic conditions as in chronic nonhealing wounds, the MSC show improved growth factor such as basic fibroblast growth factor (b-FGF), keratinocyte growth factor (KGF), transforming growth factor beta (TGF-b), hepatocyte growth factor (HGF), and vascular endothelial growth factor (VEGF), cytokine release and regulates hypoxia-inducible factor (HIF-1) which enhances regenerative ability.[4] This enhances fibroblast activation, keratinocyte proliferation and migration, angiogenesis and increase in collagen synthesis. All these play a key role in wound healing strategies. MSC can be injected or administered through a scaffold. Recent studies have shown that MSCs migrated towards the wound site and control regeneration processes via the paracrine mechanism, fusion and differentiation into keratinocytes or dermal fibroblasts.[5] Fernado et al. showed that MSC-containing scaffold for dermal regeneration (SDR) pre-incubated in hypoxia show higher infiltration of endothelial cells. Cell-assisted lipotransfer (CAL) is another promising technique to improve stem-cell based treatments.

BIOPHARMACEUTICAL AGENTS (TABLE 1)

The positive effect of rh-GM-CSF was shown in a randomized controlled study where patients treated with 400 mcg dose of rh-GM-CSF (Leucomax) showed better healing compared to placebo controls.[15]

Beclapermin a topical recombinant human rhPDGF, is the only growth factor approved by the US Food and Drug Administration for the treatment of diabetic foot ulcers.[16] Patel et al.[17] studied the efficacy of topical PDGF and platelet rich plasma in the Chronic Non-Healing Ulcer where complete healing was seen in 73.33% ulcers.

Efficacy of topical Rh-KGF-2 (Repifemin) in the treatment of venous ulcer was studied in a randomized, double-blind study where 75% wound closure was achieved.[18]

Penn et al. showed that TGF-β is involved in a number of processes in wound healing.[19] To establish MSC therapy, we need to study the tissue engineering process involving collection of a cell source, scaffold biomaterial, and native microenvironment to contribute for cell growth. There are no adverse effects of MSC therapy.

Connexin43-based Peptide Gel

The gap junction protein, connexin43 (Cx43), has critical roles in the inflammatory, edematous, and fibrotic processes following dermal injury and during wound healing, and is abnormally upregulated at the epidermal wound margins of venous leg ulcers (VLUs). Targeting Cx43 with ACT1, a peptide mimetic of the carboxyl-terminus of Cx43, accelerates fibroblast migration and proliferation, and wound re-epithelialization. In a prospective, multicenter clinical trial conducted in India, adults with chronic VLUs were randomized to treatment with an ACT1 gel formulation plus conventional standard-of-care (SOC) protocols and was found that the group treated with ACT1 gel showed greater reduction in the ulcer area.[20]

ENDOTHELIAL PROGENITOR CELL THERAPY (EPC)

Endothelial progenitor cell (EPC) transplantation therapy is a promising method in the field of regenerative therapy. EPCs, which were identified in adult peripheral blood, have the ability to differentiate into endothelial cells (ECs). Because of the potential for EPCs to promote tissue regeneration, transplantation of autologous EPCs is now recognized as a novel therapeutic option for revascularization and blood vessel repair in ischemic diseases, diabetic refractory limb ulcers, and other conditions. However, aging and various conditions and disease states, such as diabetes and arteriosclerosis, are associated with reduced numbers and dysfunction of EPCs, which may result in decreased efficacy of autologous therapies.[21]

Current EPC-based therapies[22] (Fig. 1):
- *Nonselective EPC therapies* are performed by transplanting bone marrow-derived mononuclear MNCs, including both the EPC fraction and the non-EPC fraction.
- *Selective EPC therapies* are performed by transplanting purified EPCs from peripheral blood or bone marrow-derived MNCs.

NOVEL DRUG DELIVERY SYSTEMS

Current advances in novel drug delivery systems (DDSs) to release growth factors (GFs) play an important role in wound healing and skin repair. To this end, biocompatible biomaterials have been extensively studied to improve in vivo integration of DDSs, to enhance the bioactivity of the released drugs and to deliver bioactive molecules in a localized and controlled manner. The following are the various DDs (Fig. 2) and Table 2:

i. Polymeric micro and nanospheres
ii. Lipid nanoparticles
iii. Nanofibrous structures
iv. Hydrogels
v. Scaffolds

An ideal drug delivery system should[23]:
- Maintain its bioactivity through protection from proteolysis in the wound bed.
- Localize its bioavailability by preventing rapid dilution in wound fluid and systemic uptake and distribution.
- Facilitate its release or presentation within the wound at a physiologically relevant rate and duration.

Table. 1: The various growth factors, their functions and clinical applications in managing nonhealing wounds.

Growth factors	Functions	Clinical applications
Transforming growth factor TGF beta	cell proliferation, differentiation, apoptosis, migration, epithelial-to-mesenchymal transition (EMT), extracellular matrix (ECM) remodeling, immune function, and roles in cancer.	clinical form of recombinant human TGF-β3, avotermin (Juvista, Shire), had the potential to reduce scarring.[6]
Epidermal growth factor (EGF)	promotes re-epithelialization by stimulating keratinocyte proliferation and migration.	Topical application of EGF in clinical studies has been shown to increase re-epithelialization and shorten healing time in venous leg ulcers and diabetic foot ulcers.[7]
Fibroblast growth factor (FGF)	important roles in re-epithelialization through promotion of keratinocyte proliferation and migration, granulation tissue formation, angiogenesis, and tissue remodelling.	the use of bFGF in the treatment of pressure ulcers has been reported in two studies to result in improved healing.[8]
Platelet-derived growth factors (PDGF)	mediates cellular infiltration during the inflammatory stage of wound healing through chemotaxis. It also stimulates the release of TGF-β from macrophages and mediates tissue debridement. It is further implicated in the processes of granulation tissue formation, angiogenesis, and reepithelialisation.	Becaplermin (Regranex, Smith and Nephew Inc.) is a recombinant PDGF approved by the FDA for the treatment of diabetic ulcers that extend into the subcutaneous tissue and have adequate blood supply [35]. It has been shown to improve wound closure in diabetic ulcers.
Granulocyte macrophage-colony stimulating factor (GM-CSF)	It is a potent mitogen for keratinocytes and upregulates proliferation and migration in keratinocytes, fibroblasts, endothelial cells, monocytes, macrophages, and dendritic cells, which is thought to be mediated by stimulating release of other cytokines and growth factors.	Sagramostin and its analogue molgramostim (Leucomax, Schering-Plough) are commercially available, injectable recombinant human GM-CSF formulations that are used in patients with venous leg ulcers, pressure ulcers, diabetic foot ulcers, and diabetic foot infections.[9]
Connective tissue growth factor (CTGF)	involved in granulation tissue formation and re-epithelialization, as well as matrix formation and remodelling.	Reduction in CTGF levels with antisense oligonucleotide technology showed reduced hypertrophic scarring in a preclinical rabbit model.[10] A self-delivering RNAi (ds-rxRNA) compound is in development by RXi Pharmaceuticals to reduce CTGF in patients.[11]
Interleukin 10 (IL-10)	a powerful, broad-spectrum, anti-inflammatory cytokine helping to initiate the post-inflammatory phases of wound healing. IL-10 is one of the family of anti-inflammatory cytokines expressed in the skin.	Treatment with viral IL-10 showed improved healing in full-thickness murine wound models.[12]
Connexins	These junctional proteins are expressed in both the epidermis and the dermis, and they are acutely regulated following injury to the skin.	A significantly greater reduction in mean percent ulcer area from baseline to 12 weeks was associated with the incorporation of ACT1 (a peptide mimetic of the carboxyl-terminus of Cx43) therapy when compared to compression bandage therapy alone.[13]
Matrix Metalloproteinase 9 (MMP9)	delaying wound healing by degrading extracellular matrices associated with normal tissue remodelling processes.	In Diabetic Foot Ulcer (DFU), this protein is highly expressed especially at the stage where wound healing is poor. Therefore, by inhibiting the MMP activity, the Extra Cellular Matrix ECM is less degraded leading to a rapid wound healing.[14]

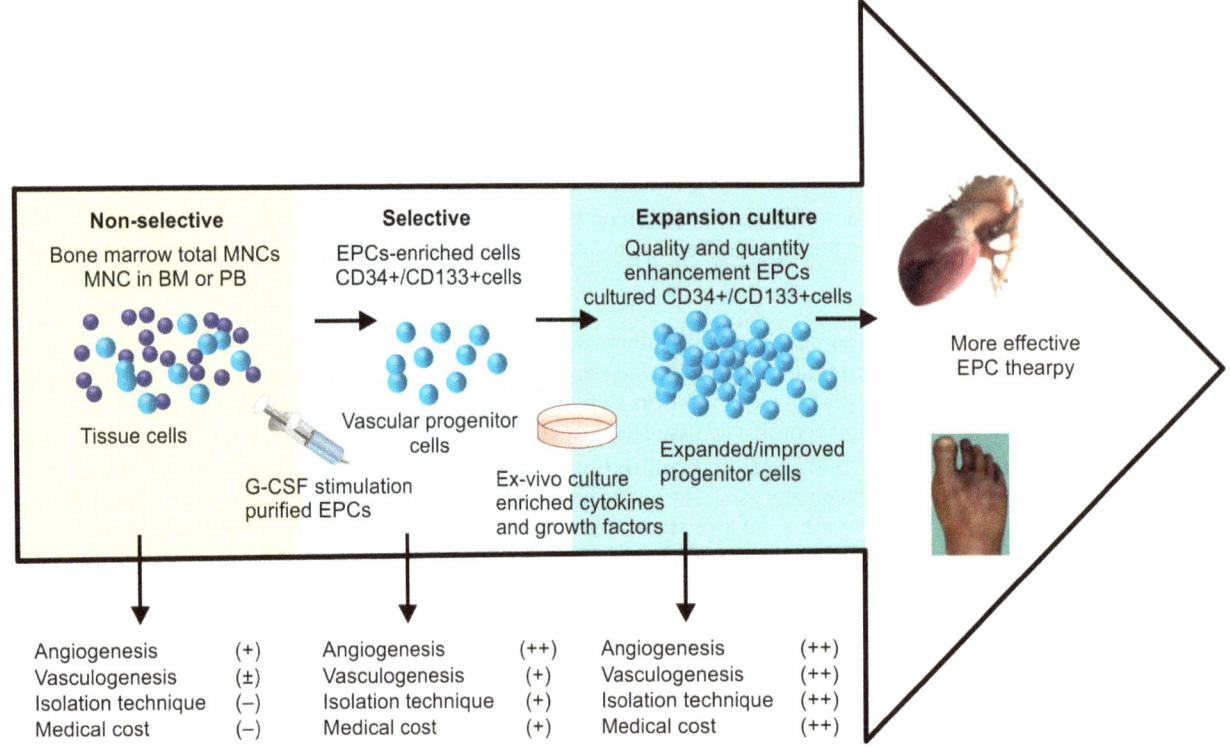

Fig. 1: Evolution of autologous endothelial progenitor cell therapy.
(BM: bone marrow; EPC: endothelial progenitor cells; G-CSF: granulocyte colony stimulating factor; PB: peripheral blood)

Table 2: Drug delivery systems DDs.		
Types	*Examples*	*Functions*
Polymeric micro and nanospheres	poly lactic-co-glycolic acid (PLGA), alginate, gelatine, chitosan.	they allow controlled drug release over time, reduce drug degradation by wound proteases, avoid frequent administration and prolong treatment effectiveness.[24] Moreover, occasionally, dose can be lessened and thus, side effects related to high doses may be reduced, significantly improving treatment safety.
Lipid nanocarriers	solid lipid nanoparticles (SLN), and nano-structured lipid carriers (NLC).	remain on the skin and release drugs in a sustained manner, also improving skin hydration
Nanofibrous structures (NFs)	silk protein NFs poly (ethylene glycol)-poly (DL-lactide) (PELA) polymer.	higher healing rates, re-epithelization, dermis proliferation and collagen synthesis.
Hydrogels	chitosan, fibrin, hyaluronic acid, collagen, gelatine or synthetic polymers e.g. cellulose derivatives or poly(ethylene oxide)-poly (propylene oxide) copolymers.	hold moisture at the wound surface, providing an ideal environment for healing, maintaining skin hydration and allow the body to rid itself of necrotic tissue.
Scaffolds	Topical hyaluronic acid HA sponges Chitosan Collagen	They are 3 dimensional structures that mimic the natural ECM and provide an adequate environment for cell growth and differentiation

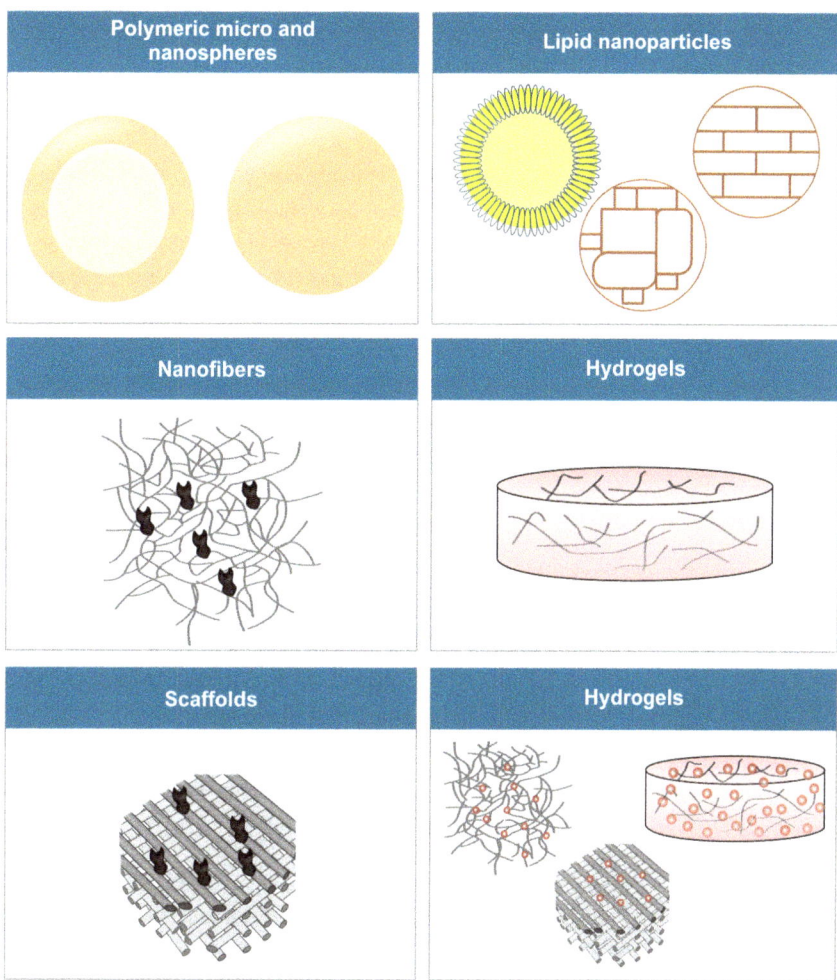

Fig. 2: The various drug delivery systems.

BIOLOGICALLY ACTIVE SKIN GRAFT SUBSTITUTES/ TISSUE ENGINEERED SKIN EQUIVALENTS

Tissue engineering and regenerative medicine aim at generation of implantable or *in situ* forming tissues and organs. They can be dermoinductive, where cells or other protein factors are imbedded into the material or dermoconductive, where products serve as scaffolds with no active agents integrated. In the tissue engineering approach, cells are seeded in a biodegradable matrix or scaffold which provides adequate three-dimensional structure of the target tissue. While the cells proliferate and differentiate, producing extracellular matrices (ECM), the matrix/scaffold degrades; these processes can eventually result in the formation of functional tissues.[25] Regenerative medicine approaches share the same principles as tissue engineering but emphasize more the utilization of patients' only cells, e.g. stem cells.

Some of the commercially available skin equivalents[26] are mentioned in Table 3 and the simple algorithm to use bioengineered skin substitutes is shown in Fig. 3.

US FDA has approved biologically active skin graft substitutes which contain viable human skin cells in treating chronic nonhealing venous leg ulcers.

Apligraf is a living, bilayered skin substitute consisting of an outer layer of keratinocytes derived from neonatal foreskin and a deeper layer of type I bovine collagen impregnated with cultured, foreskin-derived neonatal fibroblasts. Apligraf does not contain melanocytes, Langerhans cells, macrophages, lymphocytes, blood vessels, hair follicles, or sweat glands. It is a circular disc of 75 mm in diameter and 0.75 mm thick.

TheraSkin (procured and processed by Life Net Health, Virginia Beach, VA, USA, and distributed by Soluble Systems, Inc., Newport News, VA, USA) is a cryopreserved human split-thickness skin allograft harvested within 24 hours postmortem from an organ donor who clears standard

Table 3: Tissue engineered skin equivalents.

	Trade name	Graft composition
Epidermal	Epicel	Keratinocyte from skin biopsy.
	Epidex	
	Bioseed	Keratinocyte in fibrin sealant
	Epiderm	Neonatal human-derived epidermal keratinocytes (NHEK) cultured to form a multi-layered, model of the human epidermis.
Dermoinductive (cellular)	Dermagraft	Allogenic—neonatal foreskin fibroblast in polyglactin suture.
Dermoconductive (acellular)	Alloderm	Cadaveric decellularized dermis.
	Theraskin	
	Integra	Bovine tendon collagen and shark chondroitin.
	OASIS	Porcine intestine collagen type I and extracellular matrix.
Full thickness/ Bilayered	Apligraf	Allogenic—engineered neonatal foreskin keratinocytes and fibroblasts plus bovine collagen type I.
	PermaDerm	Keratinocytes and fibroblasts seeded into a collagen sponge.

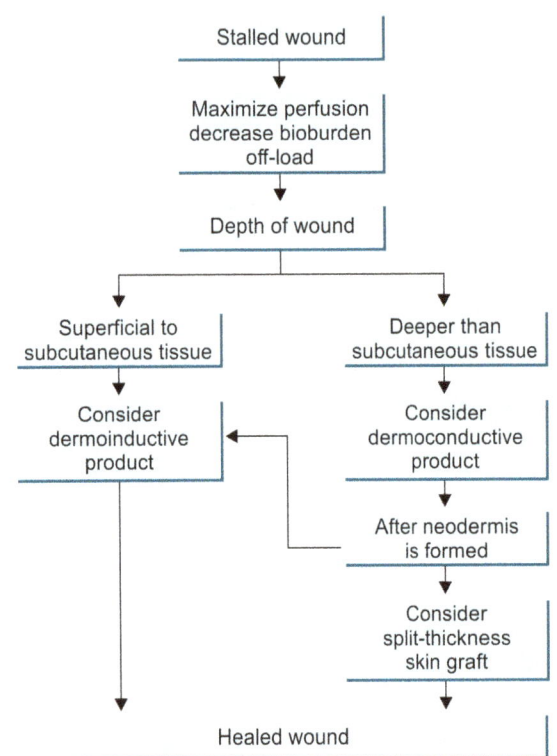

Fig. 3: A simplified algorithm to use the bioengineered skin substitutes.

safety screenings for organ procurement. When harvested, TheraSkin is washed with antibiotics in accordance with FDA specifications and cryopreserved up to 5 years, until it is delivered on dry ice. It is thawed to room temperature just before application.[27]

Both of them when used with compression, form an effective therapy in managing refractory venous leg ulcers.

Kirsner et al. conceptualized a cell-based biotherapy for leg ulcers, where human growth-arrested neonatal allogeneic fibroblasts and keratinocytes are applied in a modified fibrin spray.[28]

ACELLULAR REGENERATIVE TISSUE SCAFFOLD

Regenerative scaffolds provide a matrix to facilitate cell migration, chemoattraction, angiogenesis, wound bed granulation, and expedite wound closure. Acellular tissue scaffolds are classified as allogeneic, derived from adult human cadaveric tissue; xenogenic, derived from animals; or synthetic, derived from synthetic materials.[29] The cellular components are removed from the tissues while the native collagen matrix and the biochemical components are retained. This avoids the inflammatory and immune response, but appropriate signals are provided to guide revascularization and cellular repopulation throughout the 3-dimensional structure, after transplantation (Fig. 4).

Biomechanically, suture retention is supported, and the surrounding soft tissues are reinforced.[30] Thus, acellular matrices with the mesenchymal stem cells lead to intrinsic regeneration of normal, physiologic tissue and wound closure.

Factors to be considered while selecting grafts for individual patients are:
- Difference source of matrices (allograft, xenograft, synthetic material) (Table 4)
- Tissue processing
- Sterilization procedures
- Application duration (temporary vs permanent)
- Cost

Table 4: Advantages and disadvantages of acellular dermal regenerative matrix.		
Source	*Advantages*	*Disadvantages*
Allogeneic sources	resemble the native matrix	carry a risk of disease transmission (i.e. hepatitis, human immunodeficiency virus).
Xenogenic sources	less expensive and easier to produce, given the availability of the materials.	the derivation from an animal introduces the potential for an inflammatory response as well as the presence of giant cells.[31] Porcine dermis can become infected, acellular, and encapsulated, requiring explanation.[32]
Synthetic materials	Sterile	undergo rapid absorption.

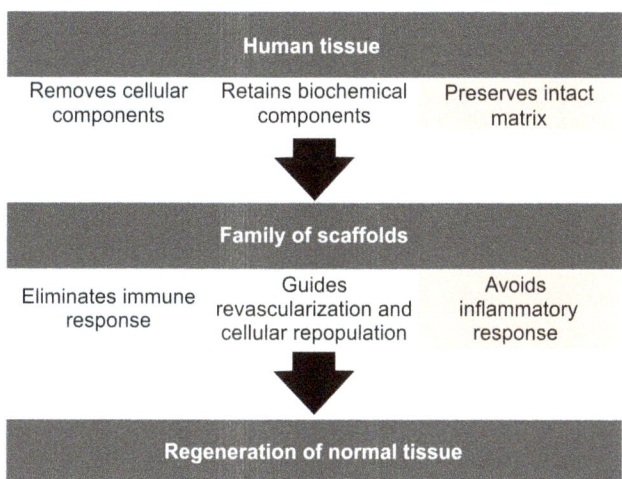

Fig. 4: Acellular dermal regenerative matrix.

Patient age, comorbidities, activity level, and ability to comply with protocol as well as wound etiology, duration, depth, surface area, exudate, bacterial burden, location, vascular status, ischemic status, and presentation are all critical components that have to be considered.

After full thickness debridement, removal of necrotic tissue, and creating a bleeding wound bed, the acellular dermal graft is cut to fit the defect and stapled if required ensuring that the entire scaffold is in contact with the wound bed. A moist wound environment must be maintained postoperatively to facilitate graft uptake.

Acellular flowable dermal scaffold is also available which can be injected onto the wound bed.

The acellular dermal scaffolds have found clinical applications in patients with diabetic ulcers, full-thickness wounds penetrating to bone, traumatic wounds, sinus tract wounds, and wounds with substantial tissue loss. Seroma formation and drying of the grafts are the few complications that can be encountered which can be avoided by using mineral oil based moist dressings.

HUMAN AMNIOTIC CELLULAR/TISSUE BASED PRODUCTS (CTP)

Human amniotic CTPs are non-immunogenic and have anti-inflammatory effects, facilitate the release of growth factors and cytokines that stimulate ulcer healing in the wound bed.[33] Dehydrated amniotic membrane allograft (DAMA)[34] is a CTP with an intact extracellular matrix to support skin repair, reconstruction, and replacement. It is procured from consenting women during live births via planned cesarean section and undergoes sterilization and proprietary processing to maintain inherent extracellular matrix components, growth factors such as fibroblast growth factor, insulin-like growth factor and vascular endothelial growth factor, and cytokines. Barr et al.[35] conducted a study where 3 to 8 applications of dehydrated amniotic membrane allograft (DAMA) was used in 7 patients and complete wound healing was observed in 6 of 7 patients, with an average time to closure of 7.9 weeks.

TOPICAL THERAPY

0.5% Timolol Maleate

A study conducted by Thomas et al.[36] suggested adding topical timolol to local antibiotics and dressings to accelerate healing of chronic venous and diabetic leg ulcers. Beta-adrenergic receptor antagonists enhance the ability of keratinocytes to migrate by increasing ERK (Extra cellular signal related Kinases) phosphorylation and ultimately accelerate wound re-epithelialization. Topical Timolol improves wound healing in chronic ulcer irrespective of gender, smoking, and alcohol habits of the patient.

Topical Simvastatin

Recent research suggests that statins might be useful in the process of wound healing, playing a positive immune-modulatory role, improving microvascular function and reducing oxidative stress. Anyhow, topical Simvastatin is not available in market by prescription and it is just experimental at present time.[37]

Topical Sevoflurane

Irrigating leg ulcers with 1 mL of liquid sevoflurane for every square centimeter of wound size has an intense analgesic effect in painful leg ulcers.[38]

DRESSINGS

An adequate supply of oxygen has long been recognized as key to successful wound healing. Active hydrogel dressings incorporate an enzyme system intended to optimize the conditions within the wound bed. There is a programmed production of iodine and pH is optimized by the generation of gluconate. Dissolved oxygen is the byproduct at the interface between the wound and dressing. This leads to enhanced autolytic debridement, healthy granulation and orderly epithelization.

The Oxyzyme[39] (Archimed, Knutsford, UK) dressing contains glucose oxidase to make hydrogen peroxide and a halide, iodide, to make hypoiodite (similar to hypochlorite) which leads to iodine. When the dressing is removed from its airtight package and the two layers are brought into contact with each other, the oxidase enzyme within the top layer is ready to start its reaction with oxygen. Just as leukocytes activate their oxidase enzyme to generate hydrogen peroxide, so the assembled 2-layer dressing uses oxygen from the air to produce a steady flow of hydrogen peroxide in the dressing. While the dressing is in contact with the wound surface, the hydrogen peroxide is converted to water and dissolved oxygen by serum catalase in the wound. The wound bed becomes rich in locally available oxygen, which enhances the antimicrobial effects of iodine.

Iodozyme (Archimed, Knutsford, UK) is preferred in ulcers with chronic infection or bacterial burden. It is based on the same dressing characteristics and differs only in the amount of iodine produced and the absorptive capacity of the wound contact gel. The assembled dressing ready for use comprises two layers, composite hydrogel. As with Oxyzyme, it absorbs wound fluid while the gel conforms to the wound bed, maintaining an optimized moist environment. The level of iodine produced in the dressing is substantially higher than produced by the Oxyzyme product. However, both dressings have lower levels of iodine compared with other iodine-based dressings but have similar antimicrobial properties.

BALNEOTHERAPY

Balneotherapy (spa hydromassage with thermal waters) is suggested (grade 2B) to reduce trophic skin changes and improve quality of life in patients with advanced venous disease.[40]

ORAL NUTRITIONAL SUPPLEMENTS (ONS)

More recently, research has focused more on wound-specific ONS, namely arginine-enriched ONS. Arginine holds a key position in the cellular functions and interactions that occur during inflammation and immune responses Arginine enhances wound strength and collagen deposition in artificial wounds in rodents and humans.[41] Arginine improves protein anabolism and cellular growth and donates nitric oxide which increases blood flow to the wound area and acts as an immune response mediator and increases the release from the bone marrow of endothelial progenitor cells which are directly involved in new blood vessels and tissue regeneration.

PHOTODYNAMIC THERAPY

It is used as an alternative to antimicrobial therapy in infected leg ulcers. It involves the use of photosensitizer, light of a particular wavelength and molecular oxygen which generates reactive oxygen species ROS. Patients with chronic leg ulcers usually have infections with antibiotic resistance.

Photodynamic inactivation (PDI)/antimicrobial photodynamic therapy (aPDT)/photodynamic antimicrobial chemotherapy (PACT) is the most promising treatment of infectious diseases because photogenerated ROS leads to complete eradication of a variety of resistant bacteria strains.[42] The presence of a positive charge in the Photosensitizer structure is important to target Gram-negative bacteria and negatively charged molecules may be more effective for Gram-positive bacteria and also should be more selective against bacteria than the host cells.[43] Phenothiazinium dyes, psoralens, chlorophyll derivatives, fullerenes and synthetic macrocycles (porphyrins, chlorins, bacteriochlorins, phthalocyanines, porphycenes) are the novel photosensitizers with enhanced antimicrobial activity (Table 5).[44]

Table 5: Various photosensitizers and antimicrobial activity.		
5- aminolevulinic acid (5-ALA)	Red light irradiation	*Pseudomonas aeruginosa* MRSA *Staphylococcus epidermidis*
5-aminolevulinic acid methyl ester (MAL)	Red light (630 nm)	*S. aureus* and *E. faecalis*[45]
Methylene blue (MB)[46]	Red light	*P. aeruginosa* and *Fusarium* spp. *S. aureus, S. epidermidis,* and *E. coli*
Zinc phthalocyanine derivative - RLP068/Cl	Red Light	MRSA
Phenothiazine derivative, toluidine blue and Chlorine[47]	Red light	*Staph. epidermidis* MDR-SA
Nanoparticles like hypericin loaded poly (lactic-co-glycolic acid)[48]	Red light	*E. coli* *N. gonorrheae*

Recent studies have shown that the PDI procedure increases fibroblastic activity with the production of neocollagen, modulation of matrix metallopeptidases (MMP1, MMP3) as well as the production of vascular endothelial growth factor (VEGF) and keratinocyte growth factor (FGF-7).[49]

The mechanisms of PDT of ulcers can be summarized as:
i. Marginal keratinocyte photoactivation
ii. Anti-inflammatory action
iii. Immunomodulatory activity
iv. Antimicrobial activity

This is the only therapeutic method that leads to complete cure of the disease and improves the quality of life.

Other Light-based Therapies

Low-level laser therapy (LLLT) and light emitted diode (LED) are both light therapy which act on the skin at several depths; they can shorten the time period needed to achieve complete healing of venous leg ulcers. Low-level laser therapy (LLLT) is a medical procedure that uses red and near-infrared monochromatic light (600–1000 nm) to enhance the body's natural healing processes. When the light source is placed in contact with the skin, the light energy (photons) penetrates into the tissue, where it alters the healing process at a cellular level.[50]

Photonic Technology

The combined effects of photodynamic therapy, LLLT and cellulose biomembrane were investigated on the healing of venous and arterial leg ulcers and the results showed a great reduction of area of ulcer in seven patients treated in a study conducted by Coelho et al.[51]

NEGATIVE PRESSURE WOUND THERAPY

Negative pressure wound therapy (NPWT) is the delivery of subatmospheric pressure to the wound bed. In this system, polyurethane or polyvinyl alcohol foam or gauze is cut and placed on the wound surface and secured airtight. A vacuum pump is connected to this space which provides a negative pressure environment. The suction effect causes deformation of the extracellular matrix and promotes cellular proliferation.[52] NPWT was found to be safe and effective for the postsurgical treatment of acute diabetic wounds, but it has not shown effectiveness in chronic nonhealing wounds.[53]

HYPERBARIC OXYGEN THERAPY

Hyperbaric oxygen therapy (HBOT) involves intermittent administration of 100% oxygen, usually in daily sessions of 90 minutes each, at pressures of 1.5–3.0 atmospheres absolute (ATA) in an airtight cabin. It increases the blood oxygen content and enhances the wound healing. It increases the expression of vascular endothelial growth factor (VEGF) and fibroblast growth factor (FGF), thus enhancing angiogenesis and fibroblast proliferation. Hyperoxia causes vasoconstriction, thereby decreasing tissue edema. It reduces the expression of pro-inflammatory cytokines and enhances bacterial killing activity of leukocytes.[54]

Low level of evidence, high costs of HBOT, the burdensome nature of a full HBOT regimen, add to insufficient evidence to support the routine use of HBOT as an adjunct to standard wound care in diabetic patients with foot ulcers. Although there is some indication of a beneficial effect on wound healing, it is currently unknown which patients are likely to benefit from HBOT and which patients are not.

ELECTRICAL STIMULATION

Electrical stimulation (ES) aids in wound healing by imitating the natural electrical current that occurs in injured skin. The body naturally creates and uses electrical energy that aids in the recruitment of cells necessary for healing through a process called galvanotaxis or electrotaxis. The undamaged skin contains an electropotential of 30–100 mV between the *Stratum corneum* and the dermis; however, when the epithelial cells break down because of injury, this difference in potential is lost. This initiates cell migration, and re-epithelization and many epithelial cells including human keratinocytes have the ability to detect electric fields and respond with directed migration. It also has antibacterial effects. Usually, the ES is applied using an external device by placing the electrodes on the skin and often directly onto the wound.[55] Many different modalities of ES have been described for each wound type with varying voltages, currents, electrical waveforms, modes, and duration of time of application, and no device-related complications or adverse effects have been reported.

Bioelectric dressings (BED) are emerging as a useful method of delivering ES to the wound site. This device combines the beneficial wound repair characteristics of both an occlusive dressing and an electrical gradient. A new bioelectric bandage based on the PROSIT™ technology was approved by the FDA to treat partial and full-thickness wounds. The application of an electric field generated by Ag/Zn BED increases keratinocyte migration, a critical event in wound re-epithelization, via redox-dependent processes, resulting in faster wound epithelization and improved scar appearance.[56] They can be cut to the size of the wound and conforms to irregular surfaces and to wound edges. The main advantage of these devices is that they are wireless with no need for an external power source.

PULSED RADIOFREQUENCY ELECTROMAGNETIC FIELD

The use of pulsed radio frequency electromagnetic field (PEMF) therapy has shown notable success in healing of chronic wounds. PEMF is a nonionizing energy at the shortwave radio frequency band of the electromagnetic spectrum, commonly at a frequency of 27.12 MHz. There is no sufficient clinically relevant evidence in the treatment of leg ulcers.[57]

Extremely Low Frequency Magnetic Field

Cellular and animal models investigating extremely low frequency magnetic fields (ELF-MF) have reported promotion of leukocyte-endothelial interactions, angiogenesis, myofibroblast and keratinocyte proliferation, improvement of peripheral neuropathy and diabetic wound healing. In humans, it has also been reported that systemic exposure to ELF-MF stimulates peripheral blood mononuclear cells, promoting angiogenesis and healing of chronic leg ulcers.[58]

SURGICAL THERAPY

Early Venous Reflux Ablation Trial

UK National Institute for Health Research, Health Technology Assessment funded Early Venous Reflux Ablation (EVRA) trial[59] which randomized 450 venous leg ulcers to either early (within 2 weeks) or delayed (after 6 months) endovenous ablation of superficial truncal reflux in addition to standard compression management. Early endovenous ablation was associated with a reduction in healing time from a median of 82 to 56 days.

Lateral Fasciectomy

The technique of lateral fasciectomy (LF) sparing the superficial peroneal nerve with mesh graft coverage is a novel treatment of non-healing lateral leg ulcers of various vascular origin affecting the fascia. LF locally interrupts any superficial circulation and in particular all kinds of superficial venous reflux. It is thought that pain in lateral leg ulcers is often the result of "inflammatory nervous compression syndrome" of the superficial peroneal nerve, which is located in a small and narrow fibrous channel of the anterior crural intermuscular septum underneath lateral leg ulcerations. Covering the liberated nerve with nearby muscles during the procedure is thought essential to prevent postoperative pain.[60]

Hair Follicle Punch Grafts and Follicular Unit Grafting

Bishop[61] pioneer experiments demonstrated that re-epithelialization started around the remaining hair

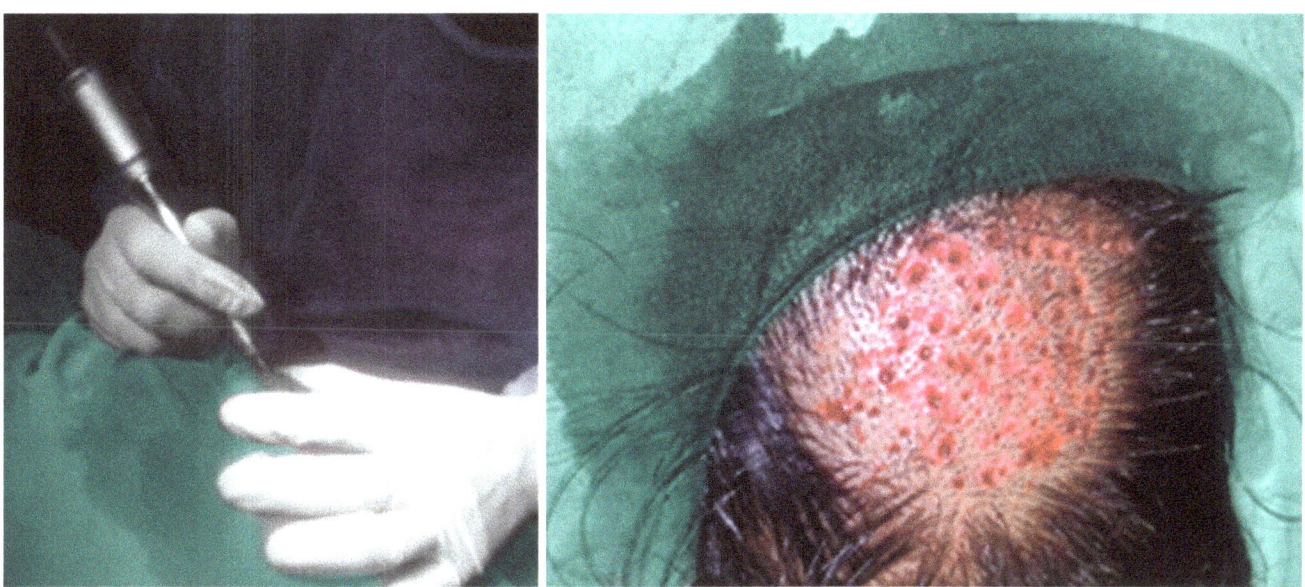

Follicular unit extraction using micromotor punch and implantation in ulcer bed

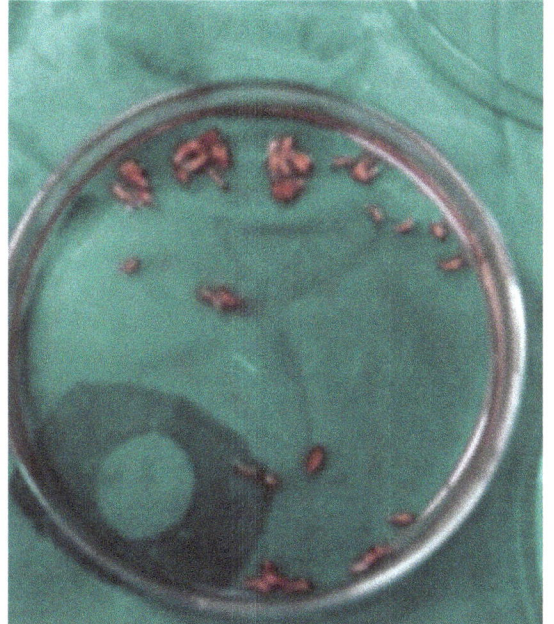
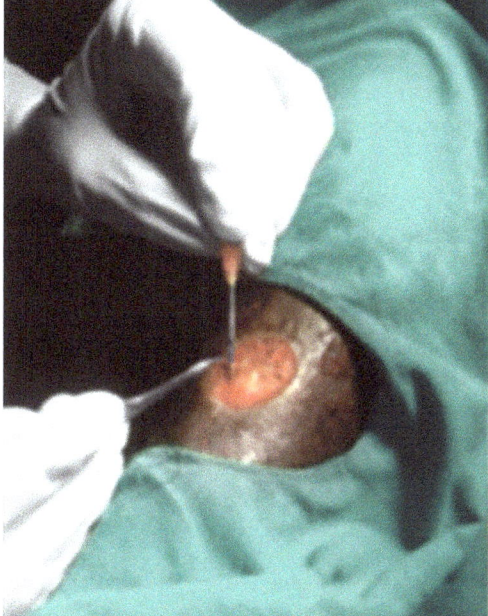

Fig. 5: Follicular unit extraction.

follicles, and that when the skin was destroyed down to the reticular dermis, the granulation tissue originated from the connective tissue surrounding the follicles. A pilot study showed that hair scalp punch grafts transplanted into the wound bed of chronic leg ulcers stimulated healing in majority of patients.[62] Similar study was conducted where excellent results were found following Follicular hair units extracted by micromotor device was implanted into the ulcer bed[63] (Fig. 5). Wound healing is faster when anagen hair follicles are grafted compared to telogen. Volume repletion is faster than the closure of area of wounds (Figs. 6A and B).

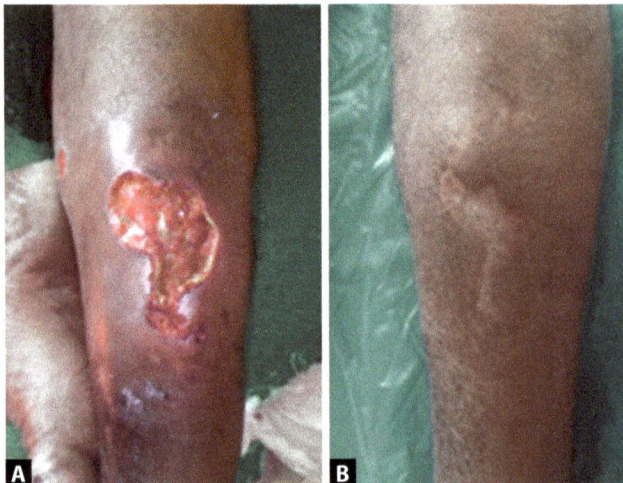

Figs. 6A and B: Pyoderma gangrenosum ulcer healed completely 12 weeks after FUE and implantation. (A) before FUE; (B) after FUE.

CONCLUSION

Managing leg ulcers is an ever-challenging task involving quality of life of patients and treatment costs. So there is an unbaiting advances and research in terms of newer therapies ranging from regenerative medicine to novel surgical techniques.

REFERENCES

1. Lee KB, Choi J, Cho SB, et al. Topical embryonic stem cells enhance wound healing in diabetic rats. J Orthop Res. 2011;9:1554-62.
2. Gu C, Huang S, Gao D, et al. Angiogenic effect of mesenchymal stem cells as a therapeutic target for enhancing diabetic wound healing. Int J Low Extrem Wounds. 2014;13:88-93.
3. Chen JS, Wong VW, Gurtner GC. Therapeutic potential of bone marrow-derived mesenchymal stem cells for cutaneous wound healing. Front Immunol. 2012;3:192.
4. Kaufman DS. HIF hits Wnt in the stem cell niche. Nat Cell Biol. 2010;12:926-7.
5. Ebrahimian TG, Pouzoulet F, Squiban C, et al. Cell therapy based on adipose tissue-derived stromal cells promotes physiological and pathological wound healing. Arterioscler Thromb Vasc Biol. 2009;29:503-10.
6. Occleston NL, O'Kane S, Laverty HG, et al. Discovery and development of avotermin (recombinant human transforming growth factor beta 3): a new class of prophylactic therapeutic for the improvement of scarring. Wound Repair Regen. 2011;19:s38-48.
7. Berlanga-Acosta J, Gavilondo-Cowley J, Lopez-Saura P, et al. Epidermal growth factor in clinical practice—a review of its biological actions, clinical indications and safety implications. Int Wound J. 2009;6:331-46.
8. Ohura T, Nakajo T, Moriguchi T, et al. Clinical efficacy of basic fibroblast growth factor on pressure ulcers: case-control pairing study using a new evaluation method. Wound Repair Regen. 2011;19:542-51.
9. Cianfarani F, Tommasi R, Failla CM, et al. Granulocyte/macrophage colony-stimulating factor treatment of human chronic ulcers promotes angiogenesis associated with de novo vascular endothelial growth factor transcription in the ulcer bed. Br J Dermatol. 2006;154:34-41.
10. Sisco M, Kryger ZB, O'Shaughnessy KD, et al. Antisense inhibition of connective tissue growth factor (CTGF/CCN2) mRNA limits hypertrophic scarring without affecting wound healing in vivo. Wound Repair Regen. 2008;16:661-73.
11. Rxipharma.com. (2019). RXI-109 | RXi Pharmaceuticals. [online] Available at: http://www.rxipharma.com/technology/rxi-109/ [Accessed 4 Jan. 2019].
12. Wise LM, Stuart GS, Real NC, et al. Orf virus IL-10 accelerates wound healing while limiting inflammation and scarring. Wound Repair Regen. 2014;22:356-67.
13. Qiu C, Coutinho P, Frank S, et al. Targeting connexin43 expression accelerates the rate of wound repair. Curr Biol. 2003;13(19):1697-703.
14. Krishnan JSS. Study on matrix metalloproteinases in diabetic foot ulcer disease. Journal of Biomedical and Pharmaceutical Research [Internet]. 30 Oct. 2017 [cited 4 Jan. 2019];4(3).
15. Da Costa RM, Ribeiro Jesus FM, Aniceto C, et al. Randomized, double-blind, placebo controlled, dose-ranging study of granulocyte-macrophage colony stimulating factor in patients with chronic venous leg ulcers. Wound Repair Regen. 1999;7:17-25.
16. Bennett SP, Griffiths GD, Schor AM, et al. Growth factors in the treatment of diabetic foot ulcers. Br J Surg. 2003;90:133-46.
17. Barrientos S, Brem H, Stojadinovic O, et al. Clinical application of growth factors and cytokines in wound healing. Wound Repair Regen. 2014;22:569-78.
18. Robson MC, Phillips TJ, Falanga V, et al. Randomized trial of topically applied repifermin (recombinant human keratinocyte growth factor-2) to accelerate wound healing in venous ulcers. Wound Repair Regen. 2001;9:347-52.
19. Penn JW, Grobbelaar AO, Rolfe KJ. The role of the TGF-β family in wound healing, burns and scarring: a review. Int J Burns Trauma. 2012;2:18-28.
20. Ghatnekar GS, Grek CL, Armstrong DG, et al. The effect of a connexin43-based Peptide on the healing of chronic venous leg ulcers: a multicenter, randomized trial. J Invest Dermatol. 2015;135:289-98.
21. Hagiwara H, Tanaka R. Evolution of autologous endothelial progenitor cell therapy for tissue regeneration and vasculogenesis. Personalized Medicine Universe. 2016;5:8-15.
22. Tateishi-Yuyama E, Matsubara H, Murohara T, et al. Therapeutic angiogenesis for patients with limb ischemia by autologous transplantation of bone-marrow cells: a pilot study and a randomised controlled trial. Lancet. 2002;360:427-35.
23. Noah RJ, Wang Y. Drug Delivery Systems for Wound Healing. Current Pharmaceutical Biotechnology. 2015;16:621-9

[online] Available from http://www.eurekaselect.com/128240 [Accessed December 2018].
24. Gainza G, Aguirre JJ, Pedraz JL, et al. rhEGF loaded PLGA-Alginate microspheres enhance the healing of full thickness excisional wounds in diabetised Wistar rats. Eur J Pharm Sci. 2013;50:243-52.
25. Langer R, Vacanti JP. Tissue engineering. Science. 1993;260: 920-6.
26. Zhang Z, Michniak-Kohn BB. Tissue engineered human skin equivalents. Pharmaceutics. 2012;4:26-41.
27. Towler MA, Rush EW, Richardson MK, et al. Randomized, prospective, blinded-enrollment, head-to-head venous leg ulcer healing trial comparing living, bioengineered skin graft substitute (Apligraf) with living, cryopreserved, human skin allograft (TheraSkin). Clin Podiatr Med Surg. 2018;35:357-365.
28. Kirsner RS, Marston WA, Snyder RJ, et al. Spray-applied cell therapy with human allogeneic fibroblasts and keratinocytes for the treatment of chronic venous leg ulcers: a phase 2,multicentre, double-blind, randomised, placebo-controlled trial. Lancet. 2012;380:977-85.
29. Shevchenko RV, James SL, James SE. A review of tissue-engineered skin bioconstructs available for skin reconstruction. J R Soc Interface. 2010;7:229-58.
30. Brigido SA, Boc SF, Lopez RC. Effective management of major lower extremity wounds using an acellular regenerative tissue matrix: a pilot study. Orthopedics. 2004;27:s145-9.
31. Mulder G, Wallin K, Tenenhaus M. Regenerative materials that facilitate wound healing. Clin Plast Surg. 2012;39:249-67.
32. Chavarriaga LF, Lin E, Losken A, et al. Management of complex abdominal wall defects using acellular porcine dermal collagen. Am Surg. 2010;76:96-100.
33. Ueta M, Kweon MN, Sano Y, et al. Immunosuppressive properties of human amniotic membrane for mixed lymphocyte reaction. Clin Exp Immunol. 2002;129:464-470.
34. Dermasciences.com. (2019). AMNIOEXCEL | Derma Sciences. [online] Available at: http://www.dermasciences.com/amnioexcel [Accessed 4 Jan. 2019].
35. Barr SM. Dehydrated amniotic membrane allograft for treatment of chronic leg ulcers in patients with multiple comorbidities: A case series. J Am Coll Clin Wound Spec. 2014;6:38-45.
36. Thomas B, Kurien JS, Jose T, et al. Topical timolol promotes healing of chronic leg ulcer. J Vasc Surg Venous Lymphat Disord. 2017;5:844-50.
37. Raposio E, Libondi G, Bertozzi N, et al. Effects of topic simvastatin for the treatment of chronic vascular cutaneous ulcers: a pilot study. J Am Coll Clin Wound Spec. 2015;7:13-8.
38. Imbernon-Moya A, Ortiz-de Frutos FJ, Sanjuan-Alvarez M, et al. Pain and analgesic drugs in chronic venous ulcers with topical sevoflurane use. J Vasc Surg. 2018;68:830-835.
39. Moffatt CJ, Stanton J, Murray S, et al. A randomised trial to compare the performance of Oxyzyme® and Iodozyme® with standard care in the treatment of patients with venous and mixed venous/arterial ulceration. Wound Medicine. 2014;6:1-0.
40. O'Donnel TF Jr, Passman MA, Marston WA, et al. Management of venous leg ulcers: clinical practice guidelines of the Society for Vascular Surgery—and the American Venous Forum. J Vasc Surg. 2014;60:3S-59S.
41. Singer P. Nutritional care to prevent and heal pressure ulcers. Isr Med Assoc J. 2002;4:713-6.
42. Goslinski T, Konopka K, Piskorz J, et al. Prospects for photodynamic antimicrobial chemotherapy-PACT. Postepy Mikrobiologii. 2008;47:447-56.
43. Pucelik B, Paczyński R, Dubin G, et al. Properties of halogenated and sulfonated porphyrins relevant for the selection of photosensitizers in anticancer and antimicrobial therapies. PloS One. 2017;12:e0185984.
44. Pucelik B, Gürol I, Ahsen V, et al. Fluorination of phthalocyanine substituents: Improved photoproperties and enhanced photodynamic efficacy after optimal micellar formulations. Eur J Medicinal Chem. 2016;124:284-98.
45. Devirgiliis V, Panasiti V, Fioriti D, et al. Antibacterial activity of methyl aminolevulinate photodynamic therapy in the treatment of a cutaneous ulcer. Int J Immunopathol Pharmacol. 2011;24:793-5.
46. Aspiroz C, Sevil M, Toyas C, et al. Photodynamic therapy with methylene blue for skin ulcers infected with pseudomonas aeruginosa and fusarium spp. Actas Dermosifiliogr (English Edition). 2017;108:e45-e48.
47. Winkler K, Simon C, Finke M, et al. Photodynamic inactivation of multidrug-resistant *Staphylococcus aureus* by chlorin e6 and red light (λ = 670 nm). J Photochem Photobiol B. 2016;162: 340-347.
48. M. Parani, G. Lokhande, A. Singh, et al. Engineered nanomaterials for infection control and healing acute and chronic wounds. ACS Appl Mater Interfaces. 2016;8:10049-10069. [online] Available from https://pubs.acs.org/doi/pdf/10.1021/acsami.6b00291 [Accessed December 2018].
49. Devirgiliis V, Panasiti V, Fioriti D, et al. Antibacterial activity of methyl aminolevulinate photodynamic therapy in the treatment of a cutaneous ulcer. Int J Immunopathol Pharmacol. 2011;24:793-5.
50. Farivar S, Malekshahabi T, Shiari R. Biological effects of low-level laser therapy. J Lasers Med Sci. 2014;5:58-62.
51. Coelho VHM, Alvares LD, Carbinatto FM, et al. Photodynamic therapy, laser therapy and cellulose membrane for the healing of venous ulcers: Results of a pilot study. J Nurs Care. 2017;6:1-4. [online] Available from https://www.omicsonline.org/open-access/photodynamic-therapy-laser-therapy-and-cellulose-membrane-for-the-healing-of-venous-ulcers-results-of-a-pilot-study-2167-1168-1000387.php?aid=88196 [Accessed December 2018].
52. Woo K, Ayello EA, Sibbald RG. The edge effect: current therapeutic options to advance the wound edge. Adv Skin Wound Care. 2007;20:99-117.
53. Armstrong DG, Marston WA, Reyzelman AM, et al. Comparative effectiveness of mechanically and electrically powered negative pressure wound therapy devices: a multicenter randomized controlled trial. Wound Repair Regen. 2012;20:332-41.

54. Stoekenbroek RM, Santema TB, Legemate DA, et al. Hyperbaric oxygen for the treatment of diabetic foot ulcers: a systematic review. Eur J Vasc Endovasc Surg. 2014;47:647-55.
55. Ud-Din S, Bayat A. Electrical stimulation and cutaneous wound healing: a review of clinical evidence. Healthcare (Basel). 2014;2: 445-467.
56. Banerjee J, Ghatak PD, Roy S, et al. Improvement of human keratinocyte migration by a redox active bioelectric dressing. PLoS One. 2014;9:e89239.
57. Aziz Z, Cullum N, Flemming K. Electromagnetic therapy for treating venous leg ulcers. Cochrane Database Syst Rev. 2013;2:CD002933.
58. Canedo-Dorantes L, Soenksen LR, García-Sánchez C, et al. Efficacy and safety evaluation of systemic extremely low frequency magnetic fields used in the healing of diabetic foot ulcers–Phase II Data. Archives of medical research. 2015;46: 470-8.
59. Gohel MS, Heatley F, Liu X, et al. A randomized trial of early endovenous ablation in venous ulceration. N Engl J Med. 2018;378:2105-2114.
60. Obermayer A, Maier A, Zacherl J, et al. Lateral fasciectomy sparing the superficial peroneal nerve with simultaneous mesh graft in non-healing lateral leg ulcers of diverse vascular origins: surgical technique, short-and long-term results from 44 legs. Eur J Vasc Endovasc Surg. 2016;52:225-32.
61. Bishop B. Regeneration after experimental removal of skin in man. Am J Anat. 1945;76:153-81.
62. Jimenez F, Garde C, Poblet E, et al. A pilot clinical study of hair grafting in chronic leg ulcers. Wound Repair Regen. 2012;20:806-14.
63. Budamakuntla L, EswariLoganathan SA, Nataraj HV. Follicular unit grafting in chronic nonhealing leg ulcers: A clinical study. J Cutan Aesthet Surg. 2017;10:200.

Index

Page numbers followed by *b* refer to box, *f* refer to figure, *fc* refer to flow chart, and *t* refer to table.

A

Abdomen 71
   and pelvis, ultrasonography 103
Acellular dermal regenerative matrix 161*f*
   advantages of 161*t*
   disadvantages of 161*t*
Acellular regenerative tissue scaffold 160
Aching 40
Acid glycerol lysis test 110
Acid-fast bacilli, multiple 106*f*
Acne 80
Activated partial thromboplastin time 108
Adalimumab 83
Alcohol 29
Alginate 158
   dressing 53, 130
      covered 134
Allergic contact dermatitis 91
Allergic diathesis 43
Allergy
   to sclerosant 42
   to stocking material 128
Allograft 160
Alpha-benzopyrones 42, 120
Ambulatory venous pressure 96, 98
Aminolevulinic acid 163
   methyl ester 163
Amorphous hydrogel 132
Amputation 79
   prevention 56
Anakinra 83
Anaphylactic shock 44
Anemia 66, 74
Angiogenesis 23, 24, 148
   stage of 25*f*
Angiogram 104
Angiography 100, 102
Angiotensin-converting enzyme 110

Ankle 30
   edema 38
   flare 39, 39*f*
   perforator 10, 11
   pressure 99
   systolic pressure, ratio of 71
Ankle brachial
   index 51, 99
   pressure
      clinical category 100*t*
      index 39, 71, 72*f*
Antibacterial agents 53
Antibiotic 41, 42, 76, 120, 121
   therapy, guidelines on 53*t*
   use of 52
Anticardiolipin 108
   antibody 89
Antiembolism stockings 127
Antiglomerular basement membrane 103
Anti-infectives, use of 52
Anti-inflammatory action 163
Antimicrobial activity 163, 163*t*
Antimicrobial photodynamic therapy 162
Antineutrophilic cytoplasmic autoantibody 104
Antinuclear antibody 89, 103, 110
Antioxidant agent 26
Antiphospholipid antibodies
   presence of 37
   workup, complete 103
Antiphospholipid syndrome 68
Anti-rheumatic drugs, disease modifying 84, 138
Antiseptic 41
Antistreptolysin O titers 103
Antithrombin 108
   deficiency of 37
Aortic coarctation 68
Aorto-bifemoral bypass 78

Arch vein 6
   posterior 6
Arm-foot venous pressure 96
Arterial brachial pressure index 128
Arterial disease 39, 48, 68
   management of peripheral 77, 77*t*
   peripheral 45, 47, 68, 73*t*, 99, 114
Arterial insufficiency 30, 32, 32*f*
   evaluation for 33
Arterial leg ulcers 68
   pathophysiology of 15*fc*
Arterial occlusive disease, peripheral 28, 42, 128
Arterial reconstruction surgery 76, 91
Arterial ulcer 40*t*, 72, 72*t*, 73, 74*t*, 91, 138
   management of 76, 76*t*
   pathophysiology of 14
   treatment 68
Arteriography 74, 100
Arteriosclerosis obliterans 68
Arteriovenous
   fistulae 37
   malformation 34, 68
Artery 34
Aspirin 41, 42, 90, 121
Asthma 43
Atherectomy 79
Atheromatous embolism, investigations for 102, 103*b*
Atherosclerosis 14, 68, 69, 73, 138
   development of 68
   pathophysiology of 69*f*
Atmospheres absolute 163
Atrophic blanche 30, 32, 39, 89
Atrophic papulosis, malignant 16, 110
Auscultation 34
Autoamputation 29
Autoimmune disease 84, 114

Autolytic debridement 89
Autonomic nerve 62
    fibers 16
Autonomic neuropathy 48
Azathioprine 83

B

Bacterial index 105
Bacterial infection, levels of 21f
Balneotherapy 155, 162
Basal cell carcinoma 2, 13, 17
B-cell lymphoma 17
Becaplermin 76
Bedside tests 31
Bedsores 1
Behcet's disease 16, 110
Bicuspid valves 8
Bilayer cellular construct 54
Biochemical profile 74
Bioelectric dressings 164
Bioengineered skin substitutes 116
Biopharmaceutical agents 156
Biopsy 103
Blood
    culture 103
    pressure 71
    tests, routine 103, 110
    vessels 23
Blood sugar
    and hypertension, control of 91
    estimation 96
    random 65
Blood urea 96
    nitrogen 99
Body mass index
    high 40
    increased 37
Bone marrow
    biopsy 110
    sampling 110
Bony prominences 50
Bowel bypass syndrome 29
Boyd's perforators 10
Brodie-Trendelenburg test 33, 33f, 33t, 38
Buerger's angle 34
Buerger's disease 138
Buerger's test 34, 71
Bullous diseases 16
Bullous pemphigoid 110

Bullous pyoderma gangrenosum 81f
Bullous vasculitis 15f
Burns 2, 62

C

Cadaveric allografts from skin bank 147
Cadexomer iodine 115
Calciphylaxis 29, 109, 114
Calcium
    channel blockers 90
    dobesilate 42, 90, 120, 122
Calf muscle functioning, insufficient 37
Canakinumab 83
Capillary refill
    normal 40
    time 71
Carbon dioxide angiography 102
Cardiovascular system 71
Catheter-based intravascular ultrasound 102
Causative organism 80
Cell cultures 146
Cell mediated immunity, defective 80
Center for disease control and prevention 2
Central nervous system 108
Cerebrospinal fluid 107, 108
Cerebrovascular accident 71
Charcoal dressings 133, 134
Charcot arthropathy 56, 57
Charcot foot 49f, 50, 56
    basic treatment algorithm 57fc
Charcot fracture 57
Charcot joint 107
Charcot neuroarthropathy 49
Charcot neuropathic osteoarthropathy 50
Charcot's deformity 32
Charcot-Marie-Tooth disease 107
Chilblains 16
Chlamydia 14
Chlorambucil 83
Chlorhexidine 90
    impregnated dressings 90
Chlorine 163
Cholesterol 104
    emboli 68
Chromate glycerine 42
Churg-Strauss syndrome 85
Cilostazol 123
Clammy extremities 29

Claudication 100
    pain 29, 88
Claw toes 63
Clofazimine 83
Clotting disorders 17, 108
Colchicine 83
Cold 29
    leg 32
Collagen
    dressings 132
    vascular disorders 29
Common femoral artery, color Doppler of right 100f
Common iliac artery, right 100f, 101f
Compartment syndrome, chronic 73
Complement deficiency 81
Complete blood count 65, 99, 103, 108, 109
Compression stockings 128
    types of 126, 127t
Compression therapy 41, 91, 126
    and dressings 126
Computed tomography
    angiography 74, 101
    venography 94
Concealed ulcer, stage of 62
Connective tissue
    disease-associated ulcers, mixed 85t
    growth factor 148, 157
    remodeling of 23, 25
        stage of 26f
Connexins 157
Coombs test 110
Corona phlebectatica 39
Coronary artery disease 29
Cosmetic issues 146
Cosmetically unacceptable linear swellings 28
Cosmetic-spider webs 42
Cough impulse test 31
C-reactive protein 65, 68, 103, 138
Creatine phosphokinase 103
Creatinine 99
Critical limb ischemia
    clinical signs of 71t
    symptoms of 70t
Cryofibrinogenemia 68
Cryofibrinogens 89
Cryoglobulinemia 13, 17, 17f
Cryoglobulins 89, 104
Cryoproteins 15

Cutaneous discoid 16
Cutaneous T-cell 17
Cyclophosphamide 83
Cyclosporine 83
Cysteine proteinase 25
Cytokine 117
    dysregulation 37
    inflammation and release of 14
Cytomegalovirus 14

D

Da Vinci vein 6
Dakin's solution 138
Dapsone 83, 121
D-dimer assays 95
Deep fascial plexus group 9
Deep fungal infections 82
Deep mycotic infections 17
Deep venous
    competence of 97
    plexus 5
        of lower limb 9f
    system 9
    thrombosis 10, 13, 37, 40, 42, 43, 73, 126
        diagnosis of 94
Deep wound biopsy 75, 76
Defibrotide 42, 123
Deformities 65
Dehydrated amniotic membrane allograft 161
Deoxyribonucleic acid 106
Dermal neutrophilia, epidermal necrosis with 16f
Dermal regeneration, scaffold for 156
Dermal substitutes 117, 146
Dermal tissue 118
Dermatitis 40
    chronic 91
    contact 16
Dermatological manifestations 38
Dermis 137
DeWeese's test 34
Diabetes 2, 13, 29, 75
    long standing 42
    mellitus 29, 40, 45, 61, 68, 74, 88, 104
    related amputations 55
Diabetic foot 51
    disease 47
    infection 47
        system of 49t

    pathology, multifactorial etiology of 48f
    physical examination 50
    surgery classification 55f
    ulcer 2, 15, 30, 32, 47, 48, 51t, 56, 61, 63, 104
        classification systems 51
    ulceration, etiology of 47
Diabetic revascularization 57
Diabetic ulcer 2, 138
    classification 51
Digital subtraction angiography 75, 101
Diosmine 120
Donor site 146
    considerations 144
    dressing 145
Dorsiflexors, clinical test for 36f
Doxycycline 121
Dragging pain 28
Dressing 52, 129, 162
    advances in 155
    aim of 129
    change, first 144
    choice of 134
    types of 129, 130t, 131f
Drug 17
    delivery systems 156, 159f
        novel 155, 156
    eluting stents 79
Dry foam 44
Dry skin 62
Duplex Doppler ultrasonography 96
Duplex ultrasonography 94, 100
Duplex ultrasound 40
    scan 74
Dyslipidemia 68
Dysproteinemia 17

E

Ecthyma gangrenosum 21
Eczema 32
    gravitational 38
Eczematous pigmented skin 32f
Edema 32, 42, 44
    gross 128
    mild 128
Egyptian eye 8f
Electric stimulation 155, 164
Electrocardiogram 103
Electrocardiography 110
Electrolyte 99

Electromyography 103
Electroneuromyography 104, 107
Embolism, investigations for 102
Emission tomography scans, positive 51
Endocrine disorders 29
Endothelial cell 156
    proliferation 141
Endothelial progenitor cell 155, 156
    therapy 156
Endovascular laser therapy 92
Endovenous ablation 45
Enterobacter 19
Enterococcus 19
Enzymatic debridement 89
Enzyme linked immunosorbent assay 95
Enzyme, topical 54
Eosin-5'-maleimide binding test 110
Eosinophil count, absolute 103
Eosinophilia 103
Epidermal growth factor 24, 148, 157
    inhibitor 80
    receptor inhibitor 16
Epidermal stem cells 24
Epidermal substitutes 117
Epidermis 136
    layers of 137f
Epithelial autografts, cultured 117, 146
Epithelializing wounds 134
Epithelioid cell infiltrate 105f
Epithelioma 17
Ergotamine 17
Erysipelas 21
Erythema 44, 108
    elevatum diutinum 16, 110
    exudativum multiforme 16
    induratum 16
Erythermalgia 16
Erythrocyte sedimentation rate 103, 104, 109, 138
Erythromelalgia 16
Escherichia coli 19, 50
European Society of Vascular Surgeons 69
Exercise therapy 77
Extensor hallucis longus 34
Extracellular matrices 116, 159
Eye of horus 8f

F

Factitious panniculitis 82
Familial neuropathies 29
Fasciectomy, lateral 164

Fat necrosis 16
Fegan's technique 43
Femoral artery, superficial 79
Femoral vein
   common 95f
   left deep 95f
   superficial 9
Fever 20, 108
Fibrin cuff
   around capillaries 14f
   theory 14, 37
Fibrinogen 103
Fibrinoid necrosis of vessel wall 15f
Fibrinolytic enhancers 123
Fibroblast growth factor 24, 148, 157, 163
Fibroplasia 23
Flattened plantar arch 63
Flavonoids 122
   address deficiencie 122
Foam
   dressings 130
   types of 44
Foam preparation 45f
   injection of 45f
Foam sclerotherapy 44
   advantages of 44
   disadvantages of 44
Follicular unit
   extraction 165f
   grafting 164
Fontaines classification of critical ischemia 70t
Foot 10, 16
   and ankle, perforating veins of 6f
   architectural changes in 32
   infection 51
   perforators 11
   pressures 50
   reducing pressure on 65
   ulcers, surgical management of complicated 66
Footwear 66
   type of 63
Fossa ovalis 32f
Frequency-rhythmic electrical modulation system 118
Frostbite 62
Frozen autologous plasma 123

G

Gamma-benzopyrones 42, 120
Gangrene 100
   dry 71
   gas 21
   wet 71
Gastrointestinal diseases 29
Gastrointestinal disorders 122
Gelatinases 25
Gelatine 158
General health and nutrition 87
Glucose deficiency 26
Glucose-6-phosphate dehydrogenase 110
   deficiency 17
Glycation, advanced 26
Gout 109
Graduated compression stockings 127f
Graft, type of 142
Gram's stain 21f
Granular casts 103
Granulating wounds 134
Granulation tissue, formation of 25, 25f
Granulocyte
   colony-stimulating factor 17, 65, 80
   macrophage colony 115
      stimulating factor 90, 157
   stimulating factor 16
Granulomatosis 85
Great saphenous vein 5, 31, 42, 45, 97, 98f
Growth factor 53, 54, 148, 156, 157, 157t
   at cellular level 149fc
   beta, transforming 37, 148, 155
   insulin like 148
   role of 90
   transforming 14

H

Hair follicle
   parts of 137f
   punch grafts 164
Hair loss 32
Hallux rigidus 63
Halogenoderma 82
Halogens 17
Hammer toes 63
Hansen's disease 29, 35, 35f
Healing 23
   by first intention 27
   by second intention 27
Healthcare, cost of 2
Heart failure, decompensated 128
Hemangioma 16
Hemangiosarcoma 17
Hematological disorders 17, 29
Hematoma 145
Hematoproliferative disorders 76
Hemoglobin 104
   electrophoresis 110
   estimation 96
   spray, topical 116
Hemogram, complete 103
Hemosiderin staining 40
Hemostasis 23
Heparin 83
Hepatitis 81
   B 103
   C 103
Hepatocyte growth factor 155
Hereditary sensory
   motor neuropathy 61
   neuropathy 107
Hereditary spherocytosis 17, 110
Herpes virus 14
Hidradenitis suppurativa 80
Hodgkin disease 17
Holiday ulcers 61
Homocysteine 14
   levels 74
Homocystinuria 109
Honey 65
   impregnated dressings 54, 133
Horse chestnut extract 42
Horus eye 7
Human amniotic cellular 155, 161
Human immunodeficiency virus 61, 80
   infection 17
   test 103
Human leukocyte antigen 16
Human skin equivalents 54
Hyaluronic acid, topical 158
Hydrated polymer dressings 132
Hydrocolloid dressing 53, 131, 134

Hydrogel 156, 158
　dressings 53, 132, 134
　impregnated 132
　wound dressings 132t
Hydrosurgical debridement 64
Hydroxyethylrutosides 122
Hydroxyureum 17
Hyperbaric oxygen 54
　therapy 83, 139, 155, 163
Hypercoagulability 43
Hypercoagulable disorders 17
Hypercoagulable state 68
Hypercoagulable status with embolization 29
Hyperglycemia 16, 26, 48
　role of 16
Hyperhomocysteinemia 37, 68
Hyperimmunoglobulin E syndrome 81
Hyperlipidemia 29
Hyperoxaluria 109
Hypertension 13, 29, 40, 68, 75
　control 77
Hyperthyroidism 42
Hypertonic saline 42, 43
　dextrose 42
Hyperviscous state 68
Hypogammaglobinemia 81
Hypostatic ulcer 37
Hypoxia 88
　inducible factor 155

I

Ibroblasts 23
Iliac artery
　endofibrosis of external 68
　proximal external 101f
　right external 101f
　syndrome 68
Iliac spine, anterior-superior 34
Iliac vein thrombus, common 95f
Immobility 42
Immunohistochemical reaction 104, 106
Immunomodulatory activity 163
Impregnated dressings 134
Infected ulcer, investigations in suspected 65b
Infection 13, 19, 48, 82, 88, 114, 145
　control 114
　local 42
　management of secondary 64
　signs of 20b

Infectious diseases 17
Infectious Diseases Society of America classification 49t
Inflammation 14, 23, 24
　laboratory markers of 103
Inflammatory bowel disease 76, 80
Infliximab 83
Infra-inguinal revascularization 78
Innate immunity, aberrant response of 80
Insect bites 16, 82
Interleukin 10 157
Interstitial collagenases 25
Intradermal reaction 104, 105
Intralesional injection 17
Intravascular ultrasound 102
Intravenous immunoglobulin 83
Iodine 90
　impregnated dressings 133
Iodozyme 162
Iron profile 104
Ischemia 51
　acute 100
Ischemic arterial ulcers 68
Ischemic leg ulcer, etiology of 68b
Ischemic subcutaneous arteriolosclerosis 75
Ischemic ulcer
　classification of 68t
　hypertensive 76
　pathogenesis of 69fc
　risk factors for 68b
Isotretinoin 16, 80
Itching 40

J

Jaundice 140
Joint contractures 50

K

Kaposi sarcoma 17
Keratinocyte 117
　cell cultures 147f
　growth factor 155
　photoactivation, marginal 163
　proliferation of 23
Keratosis actinica 16
Kidney transplant 75
Klebsiella 19
Klippel-Trenaunay syndrome 28

Knee
　compression stockings, below 127f
　perforators 11
Kyrle's disease 29

L

Laboratory screening tests 108
Lactic-co-glycolic acid 163
Laser therapy 44
　low-level 65, 163
Leg
　acute ischemia of 99
　edema, chronic 126
　elevation 41
　extreme deformity of 128
　fracture, history of 37
　heaviness of 28
　perforators 11
Leg ulcer 1, 3, 13, 18, 20, 84, 85, 85t, 87, 87t, 88, 89t, 94, 110, 115, 120, 128, 155
　arterial cause of 99
　case of 87
　causes of 2t, 13t, 108, 110t
　chronic 1, 13, 87, 92, 114, 136
　　nonhealing 1
　　venous 37
　complications of 19
　due to antineutrophil cytoplasmic antibody-associated vasculitis 85t
　etiology of 13
　examination in chronic 28
　formation, chronic 69f
　in rheumatoid arthritis 84t
　indication in 142
　infectious causes of 108
　investigating atypical 108
　investigation for 94
　management of 88, 114, 136, 148
　　principles of 87
　metabolic causes of 108, 109t
　microbiology of 19
　microbiota of 19
　pathology of 13
　radiological diagnosis of 94
　systemic therapy of 120
　topical therapy for 114
　treatment
　　of chronic 28
　　of nonhealing 28

Leishmaniasis 17
Lepromatous leprosy 106, 106f
    borderline 106
Leprosy 2, 61, 104
    mid borderline 106
    trophic ulcers 13, 63
Leukemia 17, 80, 110
Leukocyte 14, 148
    adhesion molecules 15
    counts, differential 104
    entrapment theory 37
Leukocytosis 103
Levamisole 121
Lichen planus 16
Light emitted diode 163
Light-based therapy 155
Limb edema 40
Limb ischemia
    acute 70t
    critical 69, 138
Limited joint mobility 50, 63
Lipedema 16
Lipid carriers, nanostructured 158
Lipid control 77
Lipid nanocarriers 158
Lipid nanoparticles 156
Lipodermatosclerosis 10, 30, 32, 38
Lipoprotein 68
    low-density 15
Liver
    biopsy 109
    failure, chronic 61
    function test 103, 104, 110
Local therapy 83
Lorenzo Tessari's tourbillon technique 44
Lower extremity
    pain, left 94f
    ulcer, management of 28
    venous anatomy of 5
Lower limb
    eponymous perforators of 10f
    lymphatic insufficiency of 126
    microcirculation of 5
    motor power of 35
    motor weakness of 36t
    nerve examination 36t
    swelling of 28
    vessels, anatomical landmark for 34t
Lupus anticoagulant 89, 108
Lymphangiosarcoma 17
Lymphangitis 20
Lymphatic obstruction 29
Lymphedema 16, 114, 126
Lymphocytes 24
Lymphoma 17
    leukemia 82
Lymphosarcoma 17

M

Macrophages 24
Maggot debridement therapy 64
Magnetic resonance imaging 65, 94, 107, 110
    of spine 107
    techniques 95
Magnetic resonance venography 95
Malleolar flare 39
Malnutrition 66
Mantoux test 103
Maritime pine tree extract 42, 120
Marjolin ulcer 17
Martorell's ulcer 72f
Mass spectroscopy 110
Matrix metalloproteinases 13, 25, 26, 64, 116, 132, 157, 163
Maturation 141
McConkey agar, culture on 20f
Mechanical blistering disorders 29
Mechanical debridement 89
Medication glucocorticoids 26
Melanoma, malignant 13, 17
Mesalazine 83
Mesenchymal stem cell 155
    therapy 155
Mesher for meshing skin graft 142f
Mesoglycans 123
Metabolic disorders 29
Metastasis 17
Methicillin-resistant *Staphylococcus aureus* 90, 133
Methotrexate 17, 83
Methylene blue 163
    dressings 133
Methylprednisone pulse 83
Metronidazole 53
Mezlocillin 83
Microangiopathy theory 37
Microbial culture 65
Microcellular rubber 66
Microhematuria 103

Micronized purified flavonoid fraction 42, 120, 122, 124
Microthrombotic disease 68
Migraine 43
Minocycline 83
Moisture 88
    balance 114
Monoclonal gammopathy 80
Morphological index 105
Motor nerves, involvement of 61
Motor neuropathy 16, 48
Multidisciplinary team, structure of 58b
Multiglycoside 83
Muscle cramps 28
Mycobacteria, atypical 17
Mycobacterium leprae 104
    bacillus 104, 106
Mycophenolate mofetil 83
Myelodyplasia 80
Myeloproliferative disease 80
Myocardial decompensation 43
Myocardial infarction 71
Myxedema 16

N

Nanofibrous structures 156, 158
Necrobiosis lipoidica 2, 13, 109
Necrosis 88
Necrotic ulcers 134
Necrotizing fasciitis 21
Neonatal human foreskin fibroblasts 118
Neovascularization 141
Nerve
    accompanying 10
    conduction studies 103
    examination of peripheral 35
Neuropathic ulcer 31, 34, 63, 64f, 138
    causes of 61, 61t, 108t
    infection in 64b
Neuropathy 48
    advanced peripheral 128
    minor peripheral 128
    peripheral 47, 61
Neutrophilic dermatoses 82
    of dorsal hand 81
Neutrophilic dysfunction 80
Neutrophilic infiltration 15f
Neutrophils 24, 80
    release nitric oxide 116

New endovascular techniques 79
New omental transfer surgery 76
Nicorandil 82
Nitric oxide 15
Nodules 89
Nonmedical support hosiery 127
Nutritional deficiencies 29

O

Obesity 26, 40, 68
Open ulcer, stage of 62
Open venous surgery 45
Oral corticosteroid cover 83
Oral nutritional supplements 155, 162
Osmotic fragility 110
Osteoarthritis 81
    diagnosis of 52
Oxygenation 88

P

Pain 42, 70, 73
    associated with heel raising 33
    increased 20
    onset of 73
    relief of 73
    type of 73
    uncontrolled 45
Palpable purpura 89
Pancreatic fat necrosis 16
Panniculitis 13, 16, 110
PAPA syndrome 16
Papillary dermal plexus 5
Paraplegia 61, 108
Paraproteins 15
Paratibial perforators 10
Paravasal injection 17
Patch testing 41
Peak systolic velocity 100
Pegfilgrastim 80
Pemphigoid 16
Pentoxifylline 41, 42, 120
Percussion test 33
Perforator incompetence, evaluation of 97
Perforator reflux 42
Perforator vein 11
Periarteritis nodosa 16
Periodic acid-Schiff stain 109
Peristomal pyoderma gangrensoum 83

Perniosis 16
Peroneal nerves, superficial 35*f*, 36
Persistent sciatic artery 68
Perthes test 33
    demonstration of 34*f*
    interpretation of 33*t*
    modified 33
Pes cavus 63
Phagedenisme geometrique 80
Phase-contrast techniques 95
Phenothiazine derivative 163
Phenytoin 115
    sodium 65
    topical 115
Phlebography 97
Phlebotonics 122
Phlegmasia cerulea dolens 128
Photodynamic antimicrobial
        chemotherapy 162
Photodynamic inactivation 162
Photodynamic therapy 155, 162
Photonic technology 163
Photoplethysmography 40
Placing test tube in centrifuge 151*f*
Plantar ulceration, mechanisms of 62*b*
Plasma spectrofluorimetry 109
Plasminogen activator inhibitor 123
Platelet derived
    growth factor 148
    products, role of 148
Platelet factor-4 148
Platelet rich
    fibrin 90, 148, 151, 153*f*
        preparation of 152*fc*
        treatment with 152*f*
    plasma 41, 90, 123, 149
        preparation of 149*fc*
        role of 148
        test tube with 149*f*
Platelet-derived
    fibrin 65
    growth factor 65, 116, 157
Plethysmographic techniques 96
Plethysmography 100
Polar tuberculoid leprosy 105
Polidocanol 42, 43
Poliomyelitis 61, 108
Polyangiitis 85
    microscopic 85
Polyarteritis nodosa 13

Polycythemia 17, 74
    vera 68, 80
Polyiodinated iodine 42
Polylactic-co-glycolic acid 158
Polymerase chain reaction 106, 108
Polyurethane
    films 53
    foam 53
Popliteal entrapment 68
Popliteal nerves, lateral 35*f*, 36
Popliteal vein 9
Porcine small intestine submucosa 54
Porphyria cutanea tarda 109
Post-sclerotherapy compression 44
Post-thrombotic
    syndrome 94, 126
    venous insufficiency 128
Potassium iodide 83
Prealbumin levels 104
Precursor of keratin 136
Prednisolone 83
Prednisone 122
Pregnancy 40, 126
    first trimester 42
Pressure measurement 99
Pressure off-loading 91
Pressure sites 30
Pressure wound therapy, negative 139, 139*f*, 140*f*, 155, 163
Pricking and burning sensation 29
Prolidase deficiency 109
Propylthyuracil 80
Prostacycline analoges 123
Prostaglandin 123
Protein
    C 108
        deficiency 37
        topical 90
    deficiency 26
    S 108
        deficiencies 37
Proteinuria
    mild 103
    urinalysis for 103
Proteus 19
Prothrombin mutation 37
Prothrombin time 108
Protozoa 13
Provocative tests 34
Pruritus 28
Pseudoclaudication 73

Pseudoepitheliomatous hyperplasia 17
Pseudo-Kaposi sarcoma 17
Pseudomonas aeruginosa 90, 163
Pseudoxanthoma elasticum 68
Psoriatic arthritis 80
Pulses, peripheral 40, 73
Pyoderma gangrenosum 2, 13, 16, 16f, 29, 30, 31f, 32, 68, 72, 73, 80, 82, 82b, 83b, 114, 122
    associations of 80b
    classical ulcer of 81f
    clinical course of 81t
    differential diagnosis of 82b
    treatment of 83b
    types of 81b
    ulcer 166
Pyoderma ulcers 138
Pyogenic arthritis 80
Pyostomatitis vegetans 81

Q

Quantiferon gold test 103

R

Radionuclide scintigraphy 96
Recurrent phlebitis 40
Red blood cells 15
    extravasation of 15f
Renal disease 29
Renal disorders 29
Renal failure 61
    dialysis in 66
Renal function test 65, 103, 104, 109, 110
Renal insufficiency, chronic 68
Rest pain 70, 100
Reticular vein 43, 44
Retiform purpura 32, 89
Rheumatoid
    arthritis 76, 80, 84
    factor 89
    polyarthritis 128
Ridley's logarithmic scale 105
Rifampicin 83
Right dressings, selection of 134
Rocker bottom foot 50

S

Saphenofemoral junction 6, 7, 33, 42, 97, 98f

Saphenopopliteal junction 7, 97
Saphenous fascia 6f
Saphenous femoral artery, right 101f, 102f
Saphenous nerve 10
Saphenous vein 6f
    accessory 7
    lesser 31
    long 5, 42
    short 45, 97
    small 6, 7
    tributaries of 7f
Saponins 42, 120
Sarcoidosis 16, 80, 110
Sarcoma 17
Scaffold 156, 158
Scar 30, 32
    formation 23
Scarless healing 26
Scleroderma 16, 85T, 110
Sclerosis, multiple 108
Sclerotherapy 41, 45
    complications of 44
    injection, technique of 44f
Sedentary lifestyle 68
Semipermeable film dressing 134
Semmes-Weinstein filaments 34
Sensorimotor neuropathy, peripheral 91
Sensory
    nerves, involvement of 61
    neuropathy 16
    test 34
Septic phlebitis 128
Serological testing 104, 106
Seroma 145
Serum
    creatinine 96
    electrophoresis 110
    glucose 104
    imbibition 141
Sevoflurane, topical 162
Sheet hydrogel 132
Sickle cell
    anemia 2, 17, 68, 110
    disease 13
Sickling test 110
Sigg's technique 43, 44
Silver compounds 90
Silver impregnated dressings 133
Simvastatin, topical 161
Single-photon emission computed tomography 51

Skin
    and peripheral nerve 104
    applied anatomy of 136
    around ulcers, examination of 29
    autoimmune blistering disorders of 29
    biopsy 109, 110
    changes 32t
    condition 71
    dryness of 29
    irritation 28
    layers of 137f
    pigmentation 28
    regeneration 137
    replacement, recent advances in 146
    smear microscopy 105
    wounds, healing of 27
Skin graft 45, 76, 136, 140, 141, 144f
    advantages of 141
    contraindications for 140
    disadvantages of 141
    donor sites for 145f
    full-thickness 143
    harvest 141
    harvesting split 142f
    methods of fixing 143
    role of 136, 138
    split thickness 136
    stages of 141f
    storage 145
    substitutes, biologically active 159
    types 141
        advantages of different 142t
        disadvantages of 142t
Slit skin smear 104
Sloughy wounds 134
Smoking 40
    avoidance of 65
    cessation 77
Sodium
    dodecyl sulfate 110
    hypochlorite 138
    morrhuate 42, 43
    tetradecyl sulfate 42, 43
Soleus muscle pump 9
Solid lipid nanoparticles 158
Spider veins 30
Spina bifida 61, 108
Split skin graft, techniques of 142
Spondylitis 80
Squamous cell carcinoma 2, 13, 17
Standard Doppler examination 96

Stanozolol 42, 90, 123
Staphylococcus aureus 19, 50, 52
Staphylococcus epidermidis 163
Stasis dermatitis 11, 38, 39f, 42
Stasis eczema 89
Stasis ulcer 37
Stellate scarring 32
Stem cell 159
   in skin 137
   role of 155
   therapy, role of 155
Sterilization procedures 160
Steroid 17
   topical 116
Stewart-Bluefarb syndrome 16
Stratum corneum 164
Streptococcus pyogenes 17
Streptococcus sanguis 17
Strokes 29
Stromeolysins 25
Subcutaneous plexus group 5
Subepidermal bulla 15f
Submuscular plexus 9
Sudomotor dysfunction 48
Suflamethyoxy pyridazine 83
Sulfapyridine 83
Sulfasalazine 83
Sulodexide 123
Supra-inguinal revascularization 78
Sural nerve 10, 36
   examination of 35f
Surgery, role of 91
Surgical methods 55
Surgical therapy 164
Swabbed material, culture of 20f
Sweet's syndrome, atypical 82
Synthetic phlebotonics 42, 120
Syphilis 61
Syringomyelia 2, 13, 61, 108
Systemic disease, severe 42
Systemic examination 71
Systemic involvement 87
Systemic lupus erythematosus 13, 16, 110
Systemic steroids 83, 122
Systemic therapy 83

T

Tabes dorsalis 2, 107
Tacrolimus 83
Takayasu's disease 80
Tap test 33
Telangiectasia 42, 44
Tetracyclines 83
Thalassemia 17, 110
Thalidomide 83
Thermal injuries 62
Threatened ulcer, stage of 62
Throbbing 40
Thromboangiitis 68
   obliterans 68, 73, 103
      diagnosis of 103
Thrombocythemia 74
   essential 17
Thrombocytopenia 103
Thrombophilia 43
   screen 74
Thrombophlebitis, superficial 10, 126
Thrombosis 10
   acute 68
Thrombotic thrombocytopenic purpura 17
Thrombus 95f
Thyroid
   disease 29
   disorders 29, 81
Tibia, anterior 30
Tibial nerve, posterior 35f, 36
Timolol maleate 161
Tissue
   based products 155, 161
   engineered skin equivalents 155, 159, 160t
   inhibitors 26
   injury, external 82
   ischemia 88
   processing 160
   removal 114
Tobacco 14
   use 29
Toe 30
   brachial index 71
   in Hansen's patient, second 31f
   typically unilateral 30
Topical regimen, choice of 52
Topical therapy 161
Total contact cast 55, 55f, 65
Transcutaneous pressure of oxygen 100
Transesophageal echocardiography 103
Trauma 40, 114
   acute 68
Trendelenburg test 33
   modified 33
Triglycerides 104
Tripterygium wilfordii 83
Tuberculoid leprosy, borderline 105
Tuberculosis 2, 103
Tulle dressings 53
Tumor 13
   necrosis factor-alpha 14
   pressing on arteries 29

U

Ulcer 29, 40, 45, 62, 63, 71, 75, 76, 78, 79, 150f
   atypical distribution of 45
   biopsy in diagnosis 75t
   cause of 30
   chronic 72f, 129
   chronicity of 37
   common 138
   developments 63
   examination 29
   formation
      sequence of chronic 63fc
      stages of 62
   gravitational 37
   irregular large and deep 31f
   ischemic 68
   liable 61
   local care of 76
   management of 63
   multiple 81f
   neuropathic 88t
   of various etiologies 30t
   prone 61
   size, increased 20
   stages of 62f, 139f
   trophic 61
   type of 134
   vaccination 17
   venous 88t
   with heavy discharge 83
   with purulent discharge 83
Ulcerating pyoderma 21
Ulcerating skin diseases 16, 110, 110t
Ulcerating tumors 17
Ulceration 28, 30, 100, 126
Ulcerative pyoderma gangrenosum 81
Ulcus rodens 17
Ulcus tropicum 17
Ultrasound machine 96f
University of Texas classification system 51

Unna boot 134
Urinary albuminuria levels 104
Urine 109
    dipstick 103
    for albumin 96
    for sugar 96
Ustekinumab 83

V

Vacuum compression therapy 76
Vacuum therapy 54
Vacuum-assisted closure 138
    therapy 64, 139
Valsalva, junction on 96*f*
Valves 8
Valvular incompetence 13
Valvular system of superficial veins 8*f*
Vancomycin 83
    resistant *Enterococcus* 133
Varicography 97
Varicose ulcer 37
Varicose veins 10, 32, 37, 40, 43, 126
    complication 42
    during pregnancy 128
    early 128
    emptying of 33
    gross 128
    interventional treatment of 126
    of medium severity 128
    sclerotherapy for 42, 44
    superficial 128
    uncomplicated 126
Varicosities 40
    of lateral venous system 42
Vascular disease 40
    management of peripheral 78, 79
    peripheral 16, 47, 61, 68
Vascular endothelial growth factor 115, 148, 155, 163
Vascular insufficiency 48
Vascular tumors, primary 68
Vasculitic ulcer 15, 30, 68, 83, 138
    management of 86*fc*

Vasculitis 2, 13, 15, 29, 31*f*, 32, 68, 82-84, 114
    disease 84
    exclude 104
    mimics, exclusion of 103
    screen 74
    type of 104
Vasculopathy 17*f*
Veins
    direct perforating 9*f*
    superficial 5
Venae comitantes 9
Venereal disease research laboratory test 107
Venography 96, 97
Venous disease 40, 82
    classification of chronic 97*t*
    primary chronic 126
    signs of 38
Venous eczema 38, 126
Venous hypertension 13, 37, 38
    and stasis 13
Venous insufficiency 28, 30, 32, 32*f*, 96*b*
    chronic 11, 37, 38*t*, 42, 87, 98, 126
    classification of chronic 38
    symptoms of 28*b*
Venous leg ulcer 13, 37, 45, 120, 156
    pathophysiology of 13, 14*f*, 13*fc*
Venous reflux 97
    ablation trial, early 164
Venous sinuses 9
Venous system, superficial 5
Venous thromboembolism, prevention of 126
Venous ulcer 2, 37, 39, 40*f*, 40*t*, 42, 72, 73, 73*f*, 96, 138
    chronic 39
    etiology of 37
    recurrence 45
    surgery for 45
Venous ulceration 11, 76
    risk factors for 37*t*
Venulectasia vein 44

Vitamin
    A deficiency 26
    C 26
        deficiency 26
    E 26
        deficiency 26
    K antagonists 76
von Kossa stain 109

W

Wagner and Texas classification systems 51*t*
Wagner classification 51
Wagner method 51
Waldenstrom disease 110
Wave Doppler ultrasonography 96
Wearing footwear 29
Wegener's granulomatosis 85, 104
White blood cells 14
Wound 51
    bed, optimization of 138
    chronic 26
    cleansing 88
    closure with healing 63
    contraction 146
    debridement 52, 89, 138*f*
    dressing 41, 89
        impregnated 133
        transparent 132
    edge of 114
    healing 23, 26, 27, 52, 148*t*
        mechanism of delayed 21*f*
    infected 134
    management 64
    of leg, chronic 13
    ready for skin grafting 140*f*
    strength 27
    types of 134*t*
Wound-related factors 134

X

Xenograft 136, 160

Z

Zinc 42, 90, 121
    phthalocyanine derivative 163

EU GSPR Authorised Reprsentative
Logos Europe, 9 rue Nicolas Poussin
1700, La Rochelle, France
Phone: +33 (0) 6 67 93 73 78
E-mail: contact@logoseurope.eu

www.ingramcontent.com/pod-product-compliance
Ingram Content Group UK Ltd.
Pitfield, Milton Keynes, MK11 3LW, UK
UKHW061409121225
465990UK00036B/148